Skin Manifestat

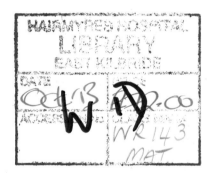

Marco Matucci-Cerinic • Daniel Furst
David Fiorentino
Editors

Skin Manifestations
in Rheumatic Disease

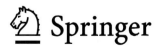 Springer

Editors
Marco Matucci-Cerinic
Department of Biomedicine
Division of Rheumatology
University of Florence
Florence, Italy

Daniel Furst
Department of Medicine
Division of Rheumatology
UCLA Medical Center
Los Angeles, CA, USA

David Fiorentino
Department of Dermatology
Stanford University School of Medicine
Redwood City, CA, USA

ISBN 978-1-4614-7848-5   ISBN 978-1-4614-7849-2 (eBook)
DOI 10.1007/978-1-4614-7849-2
Springer New York Heidelberg Dordrecht London

Library of Congress Control Number: 2013944232

Springer is part of Springer Science+Business Media (www.springer.com)

Foreword

Skin rashes, skin ulcers, and other skin manifestations occur frequently in rheumatic diseases. In a few cases skin involvements are nearly pathognomonic of the underlying rheumatic disease (e.g., digital pitting scars and thickened skin of the fingers in systemic sclerosis, Gottron's nodules or sign in dermatomyositis; dilatation and dropout of the nail fold capillaries in systemic sclerosis/dermatomyositis, and the butterfly rash of lupus).

In a second group, skin manifestations often assist in making the diagnosis of a rheumatic disease by narrowing the number of the diseases in the differential (e.g., erythema nodosum, palpable purpura in the vasculitides, Keratoderma blennorrhagicum, and circinate balanitis in the spondyloarthropathies).

A third group of skin manifestations serve, along with other cutaneous/non-cutaneous manifestations, by becoming part of diagnostic or classification criteria for one or more rheumatic diseases (e.g., oral mucosal ulcers along with vulval ulcers in Behcet's, digital necrosis in a male smoker or digital necrosis in the vasculitides, discoid lesions in lupus, and salmon-colored rash of Adult Still's Disease).

The fourth and most common skin manifestations are neither specific nor pathognomonic for a single rheumatic disease but are seen with some frequency throughout rheumatic diseases (e.g., Raynaud's, alopecia, oral ulcers, skin ulcers, hyperpigmentation, and subcutaneous nodules).

The compendium that you have in your hands is the product of the collaboration of expert dermatologists with expert rheumatologists throughout the world. Dermatology is a visual specialty; as a result the skin manifestations are shown (in photographic images) as they occur in patients. In some instances the histology of the skin lesions is shown as well. The words that accompany the images are from rheumatologists, who use these figures as focal points for their discussions: epidemiologic, demographic, histological, diagnostic, and therapeutic.

This volume will allow the dermatologist and the rheumatologist to use the dermatologic manifestations to consider and narrow diagnostic probabilities. Being able to correctly identify the rash and what it means will help diagnose the rheumatic condition, and remembering that some skin manifestations may be nearly pathognomonic, may narrow the differential, may serve by being a part of the diagnostic or classification criteria, or may be a manifestation frequently seen in the rheumatic diseases. The dermatologist and the rheumatologist can then move forward with the diagnostic plan and treat the patient accordingly.

   This book exemplifies the close collaboration and relationship between dermatology and rheumatology and can be a desk reference, useful on a daily basis.

Los Angeles, USA   Philip J. Clements

Preface

Rheumatologists and internists see many patients whose disease manifestations include skin rashes, yet they often do not have expertise regarding dermatological manifestations of rheumatic diseases. Dermatologists and rheumatologists have worked together to produce this practical handbook for rheumatologists (or internists) to guide them in day-to-day practice.

The handbook is, above all else, a practical guide. Chapters are short and diagrams are frequent. The approach includes the idea that rheumatologists and others may be faced with a rash they do not understand, or, alternatively, that they would like to know the spectrum of dermatologic manifestations that can be seen in a given rheumatic disease. Thus, the early chapters examine rashes per se (e.g., erythema nodosum, malar erythema, and panniculitis) and outline how to recognize them, their histology, and their differential diagnosis. Specific emphasis for differential diagnosis is placed upon location and morphology of the skin lesions. Later chapters examine the dermatological manifestations of specific rheumatologic diseases (e.g., JIA, parvovirus, and Sjogren's syndrome), detailing the spectrum of skin manifestations in each disease.

Each chapter is brief (three to five pages), including an introduction or general background, a description of the histology, the rash distribution, and a differential diagnosis of the most common diseases which might be confused with that particular dermatological manifestation. Mannequins are used to show the distribution of the rash so that it is easy (and quick) for the examining physician. Diagrammatic algorithms for differential diagnosis are often also included. At times, images of the rashes are provided to aid in recognition.

While it is not the purpose of this handbook to outline therapies, particularly since these are a rapidly changing area, some general therapeutic approaches are included when they are judged to be particularly helpful. Only pertinent references are included, rather than an exhaustive list, again with an eye to the practical.

We hope that this handbook, easily available on the physician's desk, will be helpful when faced with rheumatologic patients with skin manifestations.

Florence, Italy   Marco Matucci-Cerinic
Los Angeles, CA, USA   Daniel Furst
Redwood City, CA, USA   David Fiorentino

Contents

Contributors

Othman Abahussein, MBBS, SSC –DERM, ABHS, DERM, Department of Dermatology and Skin Science, University of British Columbia, Vancouver, BC, Canada

Yannick Allanore, M.D., Ph.D. Rheumatology A department, Paris Descartes University, Assistance Publique-Hôpitaux de Paris, Cochin Hospital, Paris, France

Martin Aringer, M.D. Division of Rheumatology, Department of Medicine III, University Medical Centre Carl Gustav Carus at the Technical University of Dresden, Dresden, Germany

Chiara Baldini, M.D. Department of Internal Medicine, Rheumatology Unit, University of Pisa, Pisa, Italy

Can Baykal, M.D. Department of Dermatology, Istanbul University, Istanbul Medical Faculty, Istanbul, Turkey

Anna Belloni-Fortina, M.D. Pediatric Dermatology – Internal Medicine, Azienda Ospedaliera – Università di Padova, Padova, Italy

Elisabetta Bernacchi, M.D. Malattie Muscolo Scheletriche e Cutanee, Ospedale S. Chiara, Unità Operativa di Reumatologia, AOUP, Pisa, Italy

Stefano Bombardieri, M.D. Department of Internal Medicine, Rheumatology Unit, University of Pisa, Pisa, Italy

Diletta Bonciani, M.D. Area Critica Medico-Chirurgica, Dermatologia, Casa Di Cura Santa Chiara, Florence, Italy

Alain Brassard, M.D., FRCPC Division of Dermatology & Cutaneous Sciences, Department of Medicine, University of Alberta, Edmonton, AB, Canada

Rolando Cimaz, M.D. Department of Pediatric Rheumatology, AOU Meyer, Florence, Italy

M. Kari Connolly, M.D. Departments of Dermatology and Internal Medicine, University of California, San Francisco, CA, USA

Giovanna Cuomo, M.D. Department of Internal Medicine – Rheumatology Unit, Second University of Naples, Naples, Italy

Maurizio Cutolo, M.D. Department of Internal Medicine, Research Laboratory and Academic Unit of Clinical Rheumatology, University of Genova, Genoa, Italy

László Czirják, M.D., Ph.D. Department of Rheumatology and Immunology, Clinical Center, University of Pécs, Pécs, Hungary

Alessandra Della Rossa, M.D. Malattie Muscolo Scheletriche e Cutanee, Ospedale S. Chiara, Unità Operativa di Reumatologia, AOUP, Pisa, Italy

Christopher P. Denton, Ph.D., FRCP Centre for Rheumatology, Royal Free Hospital, London, UK

Ayhan Dinç, M.D. Rheumatology, Patio Clinic, Ankara, Turkey

Mehmet Tuncay Duruoz, M.D., Physical Medicine and Rehabilitation Department, Rheumatology Division, Celal Bayar University Medical School, Manisa, Turkey

Jan Peter Dutz, M.D., FRCPC Department of Dermatology and Skin Science, University of British Columbia, Vancouver, BC, Canada

Fernanda Falcini, M.D. Internal Medicine, Rheumatology Section, University of Florence, Florence, Italy

Flavia Fedeles, M.D., M.S. Department of Dermatology, Rhode Island Hospital/ Warren Alpert Medical School of Brown University, Providence, RI, USA

David Fiorentino, M.D., Ph.D. Department of Dermatology, Stanford University School of Medicine, Redwood City, CA, USA

Ivan Foeldvari, M.D. Hamburger Zentrum für Kinder- und Jugendrheumatologie, Hamburg, Germany

Anna Belloni Fortina, M.D. Department of Pediatric Dermatology – Internal Medicine, Azienda Ospedaliera – Università di Padova, Padova, Italy

Camille Francès, M.D. Department of Dermatology-Allergology, Pierre et Marie Curie University, Assistance Publique-Hôpitaux de Paris, Tenon Hospital, Paris, France

Marco Gattorno, M.D. Genoa and Department of Pediatrics, UO Pediatria, Istituto G. Gaslini, University of Genoa, Genoa, Italy

Jane M. Grant-Kels, M.D. Department of Dermatology, University of CT Health Center, Farmington, CT, USA

Antonella Greco, M.D. Department of Pediatric Dermatology, AOU Meyer, Florence, Italy

Parbeer S. Grewal, M.D., FRCPC Stratica Medical Centre for Dermatology, Edmonton, AB, Canada

Serena Guiducci, M.D., Ph.D. Department of Biomedicine Section of Rheumatology, University of Florence, Florence, Italy

Loïc Guillevin, M.D. Department of Internal Medicine, National Referral Center for Rare Systemic and Autoimmune Diseases, Necrotizing Vasculitides and Systemic Sclerosis, Hôpital Cochin, Assistance Publique–Hôpitaux de Paris, Paris, France

Peter Häusermann, M.D., FMH Department of Dermatology, University Hospital Basel, Basel, Switzerland

Gerd Horneff, M.D. Department of Pediatrics, Asklepios Clinic Sankt Augustin, Sankt Augustin, Germany

Gene G. Hunder, M.D. Emeritus Staff Center, Mayo Clinic, Rochester, MN, USA

Nicolas Hunzelmann, M.D. Department of Dermatology, University Cologne, Cologne, Germany

Murat İnanç, M.D. Department of Internal Medicine, Division of Rheumatology, Istanbul Faculty of Medicine, Istanbul University, Istanbul, Turkey

Endre Kálmán, M.D. Department of Pathology, Clinical Center, University of Pécs, Pécs, Hungary

Jonathan Kay, M.D. Rheumatology Division, Department of Medicine, University of Massachusetts School of Medicine, Worcester, MA, USA

Richard M. Keating, M.D. Section of Rheumatology, Department of Medicine, The University of Chicago, Chicago, IL, USA

Jessica S. Kim, M.D. Department of Dermatology, UC San Diego, San Diego, CA, USA

Thomas Krieg, M.D. Department of Dermatology and Venerology, University Hospital of Cologne, Cologne, Germany

Annegret Kuhn, M.D. Department of Dermatology, University of Muenster, Muenster, Germany

Min Ae Lee-Kirsch, M.D. Children's Hospital, University Medical Centre Carl Gustav Carus at the Technical University of Dresden, Dresden, Germany

Stephanie W. Liu, M.D. Department of Dermatology, Brigham and Women's Hospital/Harvard Medical School, Boston, MA, USA

Walter P. Maksymowych, M.D., FRCPC Division of Rheumatology, Department of Medicine, University of Alberta, Edmonton, AB, Canada

Mirko Manetti, Ph.D. Department of Biomedicine Section of Rheumatology, University of Florence, Florence, Italy

Lidia Ibba Manneschi, M.D., Ph.D. Department of Biomedicine Section of Rheumatology, University of Florence, Florence, Italy

Costanza Marchiani, M.D. Department of Internal Medicine, Azienda Ospedaliera Universitaria Careggi, Florence, Italy

Manuel Martínez-Lavin, M.D. Rheumatology Department, National Institute of Cardiology, Mexico City, Mexico

Stanley J. Naides, M.D. Immunology R&D, Quest Diagnostics Nichols Institute, San Juan Capistrano, CA, USA

Rosalynn M. Nazarian, M.D. Dermatopathology Unit, Department of Pathology, Massachusetts General Hospital and Harvard Medical School, Boston, MA, USA

Catherine H. Orteu, B.Sc., M.D., FRCP Department of Dermatology, Royal Free Hospital, London, UK

Nicolas Ortonne, M.D., Ph.D. Department of Pathology, Paris Est Creteil University (UPEC), Henri Mondor Hospital, Assistance Publique-Hôpitaux de Paris, Creteil, France

Christian Pagnoux, M.D., MPH Division of Rheumatology, Mount Sinai Hospital/University Health Network, The Rebecca MacDonald Centre for Arthritis and Autoimmunity, Toronto, ON, Canada

Federico Perfetto, M.D. Department of Internal Medicine, Azienda Ospedaliera Universitaria Careggi, Florence, Italy

Alberto Moggi Pignone, M.D., Ph.D. Department of Internal Medicine, University of Florence, Florence, Italy

Nicolò Pipitone, M.D., Ph.D. Department of Rheumatology, Division of Medicine, Arcispedale Santa Maria Nuova, Reggio Emilia, Italy

Carmen Pizzorni, M.D., Ph.D. Department of Internal Medicine, Research Laboratory and Academic Unit of Clinical Rheumatology, University of Genova, Genoa, Italy

Silvia Bellando Randone, M.D., Ph.D. Department of Biomedicine Section of Rheumatology, University of Florence, Florence, Italy

Kristian Reich, M.D. Dermatologikum Hamburg, Hamburg, Germany

Eloisa Romano, Ph.D. Department of Biomedicine Section of Rheumatology, University of Florence, Florence, Italy

Beth S. Ruben, M.D. Departments of Dermatology and Pathology, Dermatopathology Service, University of California, San Francisco, CA, USA

Carlo Salvarani, M.D. Department of Rheumatology, Division of Medicine, Arcispedale Santa Maria Nuova, Reggio Emilia, Italy

Noëlle S. Sherber, M.D. Johns Hopkins Scleroderma Center, Baltimore, MD, USA

Ismail Simsek, M.D. Rheumatology, Gulhane School of Medicine, Ankara, Turkey

Vanessa Smith, M.D., Ph.D. Department of Rheumatology, Ghent University Hospital, Ghent, Belgium

Richard D. Sontheimer, M.D. Department of Dermatology, University of Utah School of Medicine, Salt Lake City, UT, USA

Alberto Sulli, M.D. Department of Internal Medicine, Research Laboratory and Academic Unit of Clinical Rheumatology, University of Genova, Genoa, Italy

Kazuhiko Takehara, M.D., Ph.D. Department of Dermatology, Kanazawa University, Kanazawa, Ishikawa, Japan

Rosaria Talarico, M.D., Ph.D. Department of Internal Medicine, Rheumatology Unit, University of Pisa, Pisa, Italy

Sabina Trainito, M.D. Pediatric Rheumatology Unit, University of Padua, Padua, Italy

Alan Tyndall, Ph.D., M.D. Department of Rheumatology, Felix Platter Spital, University Hospital Basel, Basel, Switzerland

Gabriele Valentini, M.D. Department of Internal Medicine – Rheumatology Unit, Second University of Naples, Naples, Italy

Laurence Valeyrie-Allanore, M.D. Department of Dermatology, Paris XII University, Henri Mondor Hospital, Assistance Publique-Hôpitaux de Paris, Paris, France

Ruth Ann Vleugels, M.D., MPH Department of Dermatology, Brigham and Women's Hospital/Harvard Medical School, Boston, MA, USA

Victoria P. Werth, M.D. Department of Dermatology, University of Pennslyvania School of Medicine, Philadelphia, PA, USA

David A. Wetter, M.D. Department of Dermatology, Mayo Clinic, Rochester, MN, USA

Fredrick M. Wigley, M.D. Department of Rheumatology, Johns Hopkins University School of Medicine, Baltimore, MD, USA

Francesco Zulian, M.D. Pediatric Rheumatology Unit, Department of Pediatrics-Rheumatology Section, University of Padua, Padua, Italy

Part I
Presentation of Skin Manifestation

Chapter 1
Approach to Patients with Skin Manifestations

Richard D. Sontheimer

In this presentation, I will discuss a hypothetical case of subacute cutaneous lupus erythematosus (SCLE) representing a mosaic of several real-life patients for whom I have personally cared over the past three decades. The case will be discussed at three different time points in the patient's disease course to illustrate my approach to the initial evaluation and diagnosis of such patients, recognition and management of adverse effects of treatment, and management of complications resulting from the failure to recognize clinical issues related to the development of overlapping autoimmune disorders over a patient's disease course.

My Initial Interaction with Patient

When I first see the patient, I want to know what part of the body on which the skin change or rash first appeared. Some skin conditions reveal their identities by the regional skin anatomy that they prefer or tend to avoid. For example, the early inflammatory manifestations of cutaneous dermatomyositis prefer the stretch areas over the knuckles of the hands and fingers, while early cutaneous LE inflammation prefers the hair-bearing areas of skin overlying the dorsal aspects of the fingers between the knuckles. I want to know whether the skin change has been present continuously throughout the present illness or whether it waxes and wanes and whether environmental stimuli are associated with such cycles.

I then question the patient about self-treatments with over-the-counter products that may have been used for the skin problem as well as prescription treatments that have been given by physicians prior to the patient's seeing me. Adverse reactions to

R.D. Sontheimer, M.D. (✉)
Department of Dermatology, University of Utah School of Medicine,
30 North 1900 East #4A 330, Salt Lake City, UT 84132, USA
e-mail: richard.sontheimer@hsc.utah.edu

M. Matucci-Cerinic et al. (eds.), *Skin Manifestations in Rheumatic Disease*,
DOI 10.1007/978-1-4614-7849-2_1, © Springer Science+Business Media New York 2014

prior treatments can sometimes mask the underlying primary skin problem. As an example, patients typically have used several over-the-counter products for their skin problem before seeing a dermatologist. When a topical sensitizing chemical (such as topical diphenhydramine, or Benadryl) touches the skin, a poison ivy-like allergic contact dermatitis reaction will develop several days after contact. Such superimposed, self-treatment-elicited skin changes can mask the underlying primary dermatologic process.

When managing chronic multisystem autoimmune disorders such as SLE, one must always keep in mind Greenwald's Law of Lupus. In 1992, Bob Greenwald, a rheumatologist, published his Law of Lupus. That law states that if a patient is diagnosed with SLE, there is a tendency to attribute (rightly or wrongly) everything that subsequently happens to the patient to SLE [1]. Banal skin changes such as rosacea are often confused with cutaneous LE by failure to apply this law. This is likely true for many of the connective tissue diseases.

Case Presentation

History of Present Illness. The patient is a 50-year-old white female who presented with a 6-month history of a persistent, non-pruritic rash that started initially on her arms and then spread to her upper chest, upper back, and neck. By history her central face had never been involved and she had never experienced similar skin changes below her waist. She had noticed that the rash worsened by sunlight exposure but indicated that some skin areas that were affected such as her shoulders and upper back were never exposed to sunlight. The patient had tried a nonprescription topical corticosteroid without benefit. Her primary care physician prescribed a topical cream containing both clotrimazole and betamethasone with only mild improvement of the rash. However, the rash returned quickly to its original appearance after this topical combination treatment was stopped.

Personal analysis of history of present illness. A chronic eruption presenting in an anatomical distribution such as this raises the question of a photosensitive cutaneous process (Table 1.1). The absence of pruritus argues against photosensitive disorders that are characterized by pruritus including cutaneous dermatomyositis, solar urticaria, a photosensitive drug eruption, and polymorphous light eruption. Cutaneous lupus is a photosensitive disorder that characteristically does not cause significant itching, but as always in medicine there are exceptions.

Some photosensitive disorders can display skin changes in areas not directly exposed to natural (sunlight) or artificial forms of ultraviolet light (e.g., cutaneous dermatomyositis, cutaneous LE, eczematous or lichenoid photosensitive drug eruptions) as well as in photoexposed areas. Typically, the rash starts in the areas of skin directly exposed to ultraviolet light and then spreads to contiguous nonexposed

Table 1.1 Photosensitive skin disorders[a]

Those not associated with a systemic illness
Photosensitive drug eruptions
Photoallergic contact dermatitis
Polymorphous light eruption and its variants
Solar urticaria
Those that can be associated with a systemic illness
Cutaneous LE
Cutaneous dermatomyositis
Porphyria/pseudoporphyria

[a]Extremely rare causes of photosensitivity not relevant to this discussion were not included in this table (e.g., Bloom's syndrome, xeroderma pigmentosum)

areas. Other photosensitive disorders characteristically produce skin involvement limited to areas directly exposed to ultraviolet light (e.g., polymorphous light eruption, solar urticaria, photoallergic contact dermatitis).

The patient denied using any over-the-counter topical products likely to contain contact-sensitizing chemicals (neomycin, bacitracin, diphenhydramine). Therefore, it is likely that the observed skin changes are the expression of the primary disease process rather than secondary changes produced by allergic contact dermatitis.

Clinical Context. The patient's Past Medical History includes mild hypertension over the past 5 years currently controlled with medical therapy. For the past 10 years, the patient had been under medical care for gastroesophageal reflux disease. The patient has a 20-year history of hypothyroidism. Review of Systems – The patient admitted to mild joint pains predominantly in her wrists and fingers over the past 3 months. She had also recently noticed the onset of malaise and easy fatigue upon exertion. Social History – The patient has smoked one-half pack of cigarettes daily for the past 30 years. Family History – The patient's mother had a history of alopecia areata and her younger sister developed vitiligo as a youth. Current Medications – Hydrochlorothiazide, lisinopril, omeprazole, and levothyroxine. Medication Allergies – None known.

Personal analysis of clinical context findings. Medical disorders such as hypertension and acid reflux disease are often treated with drugs that have the potential to cause photosensitive adverse skin reactions. Several of the medications that this patient is taking for her other medical problems fall into this category (e.g., hydrochlorothiazide, lisinopril, and omeprazole). In addition, these same drug classes have been reported to be capable of triggering drug-induced SCLE.

Early-onset hypothyroidism often results from autoimmune thyroid disease such as Hashimoto's thyroiditis. Individuals have had one end-organ autoimmune disease like autoimmune thyroiditis that is linked to the 8.1 ancestral HLA haplotype

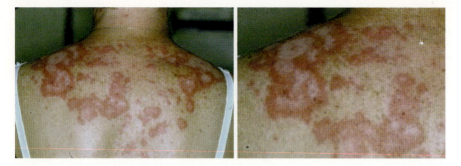

Fig. 1.1 Annular SCLE lesions. The *right panel* is an enlargement of the *left upper quadrant* of the clinical shown in the *left panel*. Note the light color of the skin within the inactive central parts of the annular lesions. Also note the polycyclic arrays resulting from the merging together of the larger annular lesions on the posterior aspects of the patient's shoulders

are at risk for developing other diseases that are linked to this haplotype (e.g., vitiligo, alopecia areata, SCLE, Sjögren's syndrome, type 1 diabetes mellitus, Addison's disease, pernicious anemia) [2].

The patient's recent onset of mild arthralgia, malaise, and easy fatigue would suggest the presence of a photosensitive skin disorder that is associated with systemic manifestations such as a cutaneous LE or cutaneous dermatomyositis rather than photosensitive skin disorders that are typically not accompanied by systemic inflammation (see Table 1.1).

If the patient proves to have a form of cutaneous LE, her history of cigarette smoking could result in a suboptimal clinical response to aminoquinoline antimalarial therapy [3].

Physical Examination. The patient was asked to disrobe and put on a hospital gown. The patient had papulosquamous skin lesions of varying size and shape distributed symmetrically on the lateral aspects of her neck, the V area of her upper chest, her shoulders, her upper back, the extensor surfaces of her distal arms, the extensor surface of her forearms, and the dorsal aspects of her hands. The smaller lesions were papulosquamous (i.e., red and scaly) papules and small plaques. However, the larger lesions were ring-shaped (i.e., annular) lesions with erythema and scale at the active edges and the absence of such changes centrally. The inactive centers of the lesions displayed a white-gray hue (i.e., leukoderma, meaning a decrease in or absence of melanin pigment) compared to the noninvolved perilesional skin (Fig. 1.1). In some areas, the annular lesions merged producing a polycyclic arrangement of lesions (Fig. 1.1).

There was no obvious dermal scarring associated with any of these skin changes. In addition, there was no periungual erythema on her fingers nor any grossly visible periungual microvascular abnormalities. Bedside capillaroscopy with a dermatoscope failed to reveal any significant periungual microvascular abnormalities. In addition, there were no grossly visible cuticular abnormalities including hypertrophy or disarray. There was no tenderness, erythema, or swelling of the small joints of her hands and fingers. The ocular and oral mucosal membranes were not involved.

Personal analysis of physical examination findings. In a patient having a chronic rash of unknown etiology, it is important to have the patient disrobe and put on an examination gown so that a complete skin evaluation can be performed. Attention should be paid to pertinent negative findings as well as pertinent positive findings during the exam. For example, our patient indicated that her rash did not occur below her waist. However, subtle skin changes of disorders that can produce changes below the waist such as cutaneous dermatomyositis can be missed if the patient is not examined completely (e.g., patchy violaceous erythema over the lateral hips [holster sign], subtle violaceous erythema over the knees and medial malleoli). Most forms of cutaneous LE do not produce changes below the waist.

In addition, inflammatory skin changes on one part of the body can at times be secondary to a focus of skin inflammation on another part of the body. As an example, patients with inflammatory skin changes on their feet resulting from dermatophyte fungal infection can develop aseptic eczematous skin changes over their upper extremities and back as a result of the dermatophytid reaction (a fungus-triggered autoeczematization reaction) [4]. One can misinterpret the cause of the rash on the arms and back in this setting if one does not examine the feet to recognize the appropriate etiologic association.

There are four dimensions to the skin examination: (1) primary lesions, (2) secondary lesions, (3) lesional arrangement, and (4) regional anatomic distribution of lesions. The starting point in diagnosing a skin rash is to identify the primary skin lesions and any secondary skin changes that might be present, recognize any patterns resulting from how primary skin lesions associate with each other, and deduce the predominant regional anatomy targeted by the primary skin lesions. Questioning the patient about what the skin lesions looked like when they first appeared can help separate the earlier primary lesions from the later appearing secondary skin changes. Some might argue that awareness of pertinent negative physical exam findings might represent a fifth dimension of the physical exam. With respect to differential diagnosis, what a skin disease does not say about itself can at times be as important as what it does say.

The patient in question here had a papulosquamous eruption presenting in an anatomic distribution suggesting that sunlight exposure may have been a precipitating or aggravating environmental trigger. A key physical finding that distinguishes the skin lesions in this patient from those of other papulosquamous disorders was the tendency of the early small papulosquamous plaques to enlarge radially and regress centrally to produce annular lesions with leukodermatous centers unaccompanied by dermal scarring. This constellation of skin changes in the appropriate regional anatomical distribution is virtually pathognomonic of SCLE. (Other cutaneous annular inflammatory disorders such tinea corporis and erythema annulare centrifugum do not display leukoderma at their inactive centers).

The type of primary lesions, their pattern of physical association with each other, and their proclivity for affecting certain anatomic regions allow an experienced clinician to recognize a diagnostic pattern or clinical gestalt. However, the missing pieces of this gestalt necessary for a specific diagnosis must be filled in with diagnostic analysis (e.g., skin biopsy, laboratory results).

Workup to Confirm a Clinical Diagnosis of SCLE

A 4 mm punch biopsy of lesional forearm skin was performed on the active red scaly border of one of the annular lesions. The reported dermatopathologic findings of biopsy sections stained with hematoxlyn and eosin included a cell-poor interface dermatitis with increased dermal mucin infiltration (the increase in dermal mucin deposition was confirmed by special stains). These findings would be consistent with both cutaneous LE and cutaneous dermatomyositis and exclude the other photosensitive skin disorders listed in Table 1.1.

In addition, a separate 4 mm lesional punch biopsy was obtained from forearm skin for direct immunofluorescent examination. Reported results included a continuous band of IgG and IgM at the dermal-epidermal junction deposited in a discrete dust-like pattern. This finding would be much more typical of SCLE than cutaneous DM.

Venous blood was sampled for a complete blood count and a serum chemistry screen. Both assays were reported to be within normal limits. Antinuclear antibodies (ANA) and individual autoantibody specificities that are associated with cutaneous and systemic LE (SLE) (Ro/SS-A, La/SS-B, URNP, Sm) were assayed. The ANA was elevated at a titer of 1:320 and Ro/SS-A autoantibodies were present. The presence of Ro/SS-A autoantibodies would be more typical of SCLE than cutaneous dermatomyositis. In addition, an erythrocyte sedimentation rate and a urinalysis were reported to be within normal limits arguing against SLE disease activity. Also, the normal complete blood count and serum chemistry screen results argue further against SLE disease activity by excluding leukopenia, thrombocytopenia, anemia, renal dysfunction, and hyperglobulinemia.

The above biopsy and lab results would confirm a diagnosis of SCLE in our patient. The annular skin lesions displayed by this patient would allow subclassification as annular SCLE. Arthralgia, malaise, and easy fatigue are not uncommon in patients with untreated SCLE skin lesions. However, clinically significant inflammation in the vital internal target organs such as the kidneys and central nervous system are very uncommon in patients presenting with SCLE.

Management Strategies

Conventional approach. As the patient had previously failed strong topical corticosteroid therapy, it was felt that systemic therapy with hydroxychloroquine would be indicated to treat both the patient's skin lesions as well as her mild musculoskeletal symptoms. The patient was started on hydroxychloroquine 200 mg by mouth twice daily following a baseline ophthalmological examination.

At follow-up in 8 weeks the patient had not substantially improved with respect to her skin inflammation. She was told that her cigarette smoking could be a factor in the failure of hydroxychloroquine to control her skin. The patient was encouraged to continue her efforts at discontinuing cigarette smoking including the possibility of starting oral varenicline (Chantix) through her primary care provider. She was then started on a compounded formulation of quinacrine at a dose of 100 mg/ day.

On follow-up 6 weeks later the patient had experienced marked reduction in her papulosquamous skin inflammation. Two months later the patient was free of skin lesions. At that time the hydroxychloroquine was decreased to 200 mg p.o. daily. The patient was told that it would be best for her to stay on antimalarial therapy for a total of 12 months before discontinuing this treatment in order to maximize the chance for an extended drug-free remission.

Alternative approach. Since the original description of SCLE, it has become increasingly clear that in addition to ultraviolet light, certain classes of medications prescribed for other medical problems can serve as environmental triggers for SCLE [5]. Discontinuing a triggering drug alone can result 6–8 weeks later in complete resolution SCLE skin disease activity without additional treatment. The representative SCLE patient described here had been on several classes of medications for other indications prior to onset of her annular SCLE lesions (a thiazide diuretic, an ACE inhibitor, and a proton pump inhibitor). However, there is no objective way to determine which of the drugs from these three classes if any might be triggering the patient's SCLE lesions. The only way to test this hypothesis is to work with the patient's other physicians to determine whether it would be possible to safely withdraw one or more of these three drugs from the patient's treatment regimen and avoid replacement with other drugs in the same class. Typically it would take to up to 2 months for the SCLE skin inflammation to respond clinically to the withdrawal of the triggering medication. However, in practice, this alternative management approach can be very difficult to coordinate and accomplish.

Interaction with the Patient One Year After My Initial Evaluation

The patient returned one year later complaining that her lupus skin disease activity was returning. About 3 months earlier she experienced a return of red scaly skin changes on her arms and upper back. These skin changes were more pruritic than they had been originally. There had been no interval change in her general medical status. She was still taking the hydroxychloroquine and quinacine. She denied starting taking any new medications over the last year.

Physical examination revealed the presence of skin lesions illustrated in Fig. 1.2. The new lesions were qualitatively different than those at the patient's initial

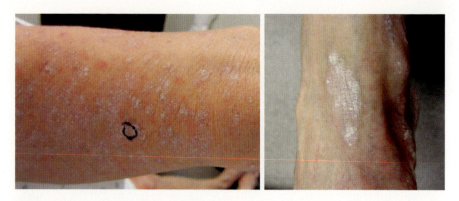

Fig. 1.2 Lichenoid drug eruption. *Left panel* – Note the small papulosquamous plaques on the extensor aspect of the patient's upper arm bearing confluent white scale (the *black circle* was drawn to indicate the location of a planned punch skin biopsy). *Right panel* – A papulosquamous plaque displaying thick adherent white surface scale on the anterior aspect of the patient's ankle

presentation 1 year earlier. In addition, the new lesions were present both above and below the waist. The new lesions were papulosquamous plaques of varied size with a thickened, adherent white scale. No annular lesions were evident.

Diagnostic possibilities for these new skin lesions included a return of SCLE disease activity with a shift from the annular to the papulosquamous clinical sub-types. However, the presence of the thickened adherent scale was not typical of any form of SCLE. In addition, SCLE lesions rarely occur below the waist. Perhaps the new lesions represented a shift from SCLE to classical discoid LE (approximately 20 % of SCLE patients will at some point in their disease course display typical discoid LE skin lesions). However, the new lesions lacked dilated, keratin plugged follicles and induration which are two hallmark clinical features of classic discoid LE skin lesions.

Another possibility for these new lesions would include precipitation of previously subclinical psoriasis, a recognized adverse reaction to antimalarial therapy. A skin biopsy could help address this possibility as the histopathology of psoriasis and LE-specific skin disease is quite different.

In addition, the patient could be suffering from a lichenoid drug reaction to one or a combination of the antimalarial drugs she is taking. The thickened hyperkera-totic nature of the new skin lesions and increased pruritus would be consistent with a hypertrophic lichen planus-like skin reaction.

A punch biopsy of the new lesions revealed a cell-rich interface dermatitis (syn. lichenoid tissue reaction). It was felt that the new skin lesions were most likely the result of a lichenoid drug reaction to the antimalarial drugs she was taking. The quinacrine was stopped but the hydroxychloroquine was continued. Over the following 2 months the new skin lesions melted away completely. On follow-up exam 3 months later, the patient's original annular SCLE skin lesions were still in remission.

Interaction with the Patient Two Years After My Initial Evaluation

At follow-up 24 months after her initial presentation, the patient was free of skin inflammation except for perlèche changes at the angles of her mouth. Over the previous 12 months she had been successfully withdrawn from hydroxychloroquine without signs of cutaneous LE recurrence. However, the patient indicated that over the past several weeks, she has been noticing progressive weakness in the muscles of her arms and legs. Within the last several days, this had gotten so severe as to make it difficult for her to get out of bed. She was brought to the clinic by her daughter in a wheelchair to have this problem evaluated. When questioned, the patient admitted experiencing increasing problems recently with dry eyes and dry mouth.

Upon exam, no cutaneous inflammation was noted other than the changes of perlèche. Muscle examination revealed flaccid weakness of the shoulder and hip girdle musculature. In addition the patient had poor control of her cervical muscles.

How might this new clinical problem be explained? One possibility would be the patient is developing an overlap syndrome with polymyositis or early dermatomyositis. However, it is quite unusual for SCLE to overlap with any form of inflammatory myositis.

Another possibility would relate to the patient's new symptoms of dry eyes and dry mouth and her new skin finding of perlèche. Perhaps she had developed an overlap with Sjögren's syndrome. It is not uncommon for patients presenting with SCLE to later developed features or Sjögren's syndrome over their disease course as both of these conditions develop in the context of the same 8.1 ancestral HLA haplotype.

The patient's muscle weakness could be explained by hypokalemia resulting from tubulointerstitial nephropathy that occurred as a result of an extraglandular autoimmune manifestation of Sjögren's syndrome. To address this possibility, the patient's blood electrolytes were measured. Her serum potassium level was 2.0 mEq/L. Upon potassium replacement and alkali therapy, the patient's muscle weakness resolved rapidly. She was then referred to a nephrologist for more definitive management of the tubulointerstitial nephropathy.

Acknowledgments The author's understanding of the diagnosis and management of rheumatologic skin disorders was built up on a foundation of knowledge and experience that was shared with him by several more senior American academic dermatologists. Those individuals include James N. Gilliam (deceased), Thomas T. Provost (deceased), Denny L. Tuffanelli (deceased), Sam L. Moschella, and Irwin M. Braverman. Several of these individuals served as mentors to the author providing him with instrumental career development guidance. The author will be eternally grateful for the support these individuals provided to him and the contributions they as a group made to our modern understanding of rheumatologic skin disease.

References

1. Greenwald RA. Greenwald's law of lupus. J Rheumatol. 1992;19:1490.
2. Candore G, Modica MA, Lio D, et al. Pathogenesis of autoimmune diseases associated with 8.1 ancestral haplotype: a genetically determined defect of C4 influences immunological parameters of healthy carriers of the haplotype. Biomed Pharmacother. 2003;57:274–7.
3. Jewell ML, McCauliffe DP. Patients with cutaneous lupus erythematosus who smoke are less responsive to antimalarial treatment. J Am Acad Dermatol. 2000;42:983–7.
4. Iglesias ME, Espana A, Idoate MA, Quintanilla E. Generalized skin reaction following tinea pedis (dermatophytids). J Dermatol. 1994;21:31–4.
5. Lowe G, Henderson CL, Grau RH, Hansen CB, Sontheimer RD. A systematic review of drug-induced subacute cutaneous lupus erythematosus. Br J Dermatol. 2011;164:465–72.

Chapter 2
Chilblain Lupus Erythematosus

Min Ae Lee-Kirsch, Martin Aringer, and Annegret Kuhn

Chilblain lupus erythematosus is clinically classified as a subtype of chronic cutaneous lupus erythematosus (CCLE) [1]. It is characterized by inflammatory, painful lesions at acral locations, which are precipitated by cold and wet exposure. Therefore, chilblain lupus erythematosus could well have found its place in Chapter 33 "Skin Manifestations of Systemic Lupus Erythematosus." However, the recent elucidation of the genetic basis of a rare familial form of chilblain lupus has provided novel insights into the molecular pathogenesis of lupus erythematosus [2–4], which have significant impact on our understanding of SLE manifestations of the skin. Therefore, this chapter will provide an overview of the molecular biology of this disease phenotype below.

Definition

Chilblain lupus erythematosus is a rare form of CCLE, characterized by painful, bluish-red, inflammatory plaques in acral locations (Fig. 2.1), including the dorsal aspects of fingers and toes, as well as heels, nose, cheeks, and ears [1]. The lesions

M.A. Lee-Kirsch, M.D.
Children's Hospital, University Medical Centre Carl Gustav Carus at the Technical University of Dresden, Fetscherstrasse 74, 01037 Dresden, Germany
e-mail: minae.lee-kirsch@uniklinikum-dresden.de

M. Aringer, M.D. (✉)
Division of Rheumatology, Department of Medicine III,
University Medical Centre Carl Gustav Carus at the Technical University of Dresden,
Fetscherstrasse 74, 01037 Dresden, Germany
e-mail: martin.aringer@uniklinikum-dresden.de

A. Kuhn, M.D.
Department of Dermatology, University of Muenster,
Von-Esmarch-Strasse 58, D-48149 Muenster, Germany
e-mail: kuhnan@uni-muenster.de

M. Matucci-Cerinic et al. (eds.), *Skin Manifestations in Rheumatic Disease*,
DOI 10.1007/978-1-4614-7849-2_2, © Springer Science+Business Media New York 2014

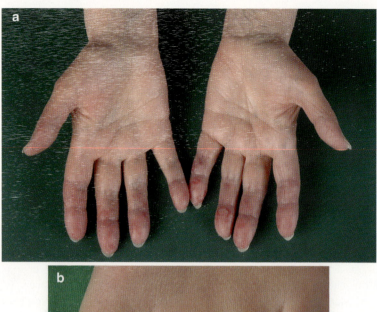

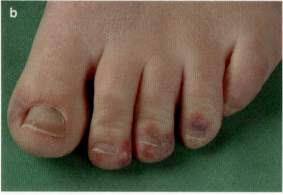

Fig. 2.1 Chilblain lupus erythematosus. (**a**) Symmetrically distributed, violet lesions with single erythematous papules and plaques involving acral locations of fingers. (**b**) Circumscribed, papulo-nodular, painful, bluish-red lesions at distal part of toes

are precipitated by cold and wet exposure and tend to improve during summer; photosensitivity is not observed. Commonly, lesions ulcerate, but usually heal without scars. Antinuclear antibodies (ANA), in particular autoantibodies to anti-Ro/SSA, may be present [5]. In the majority of cases, chilblain lupus erythematosus occurs sporadically in middle-aged women; however, a distinct form of this CLE subtype, also known as autosomal dominant familial chilblain lupus, manifests within the first years of life [2]. The clinical and histological features of familial chilblain lupus are indistinguishable from other forms of the disease. While progression to SLE is observed in up to 20 % of sporadic cases [6], it has not been described in familial cases, although arthralgia and skin lesions resembling SLE may occur [2, 7]. The treatment of chilblain lupus erythematosus is rather difficult; in addition to local corticosteroids and antimalarials, such as hydroxychloroquine and chloroquine, calcium-channel blockers may be effective [8]. However, prevention of cold exposure is highly recommended.

Differential Diagnosis

The differential diagnoses include true cold-induced perniones or chilblains as well as cryoglobulinemia [5], which are often difficult to distinguish from chilblain lupus erythematosus. In addition, erythema nodosum, lupus pernio associated with sarcoidosis, or embolic events, as well as acral vasculitis/vasculopathy may also be considered [9, 10].

Histology

While the picture will often be diagnostic in typical cases, histology may secure the diagnosis in case of doubt. Histological findings of lesional skin in chilblain lupus erythematosus consist of vacuolar degeneration of the dermoepidermal junction with occasional single-cell necrosis and broadening of the basement membrane. In addition, a superficial and deep lymphocytic and histiocytic infiltration with periadnexial and perivascular distribution along with interface dermatitis is observed. Throughout the stratum reticulare, increased mucin deposits may occur. On direct immunofluorescence, granular deposits of immunoglobulins as well as complement within the basement membrane zone can be visualized [2, 11].

Molecular Genetics of Familial Chilblain Lupus

Unlike sporadic forms of the disease, familial chilblain lupus is inherited as an autosomal dominant trait manifesting in early childhood [2]. It is caused by heterozygous mutations of the TREX1 gene encoding three prime repair exonuclease [3, 4]. Thus, familial chilblain lupus represents the first monogenic form of cutaneous lupus erythematosus (CLE). Moreover, rare variants in the TREX1 gene are also found in patients with multifactorial systemic lupus erythematosus (SLE) [12], implicating TREX1-associated defects in nucleic acid metabolism in the pathogenesis of systemic autoimmunity.

TREX1, three prime repair exonuclease 1, is a ubiquitously expressed intracellular DNase with high specificity for single-stranded DNA (ssDNA) [13].

TREX1 mutations are associated with overlapping, but distinct inflammatory phenotypes underscoring the role of nucleic acid metabolism in immune regulation. Biallelic TREX1 mutations cause autosomal recessive Aicardi-Goutières syndrome, an early-onset encephalopathy resembling congenital viral infection, which is characterized by intracranial calcification and elevated interferon-α (IFNα) in cerebrospinal fluid [14]. Remarkably, some children with Aicardi-Goutières syndrome develop lupus-like symptoms over time [15]. Heterozygous TREX1 mutations have also been described in patients with autosomal dominant retinal vasculopathy with cerebral leukodystrophy, an adult-onset disorder characterized by central nervous system degeneration, retinal vasculopathy, and nephropathy [15], and in patients with multifactorial SLE. Thus, rare variants of the TREX1 gene confer a high risk for developing SLE [12].

TREX1 has been implicated in a number of biological processes that involve degradation of intracellular DNA. Loss of TREX1 function has been shown to impair DNA degradation during granzyme A-mediated apoptosis [3]. Apoptosis is highly relevant in the pathogenesis of different forms of lupus erythematosus. First, defective apoptosis may lead to impaired antigen-mediated B cell maturation and selection of autoreactive T cells, causing loss of self-tolerance. Secondly, self-antigens displayed on cell surfaces as a result of deficient disposal of extracellular nuclear waste can induce an autoimmune response. Finally, uncontrolled apoptosis is an effector mechanism responsible for autoimmune destruction of healthy cells. Moreover, recent evidence suggests that intracellular accumulation of ssDNA in TREX1-deficient cells is also caused by defective degradation of nucleic acids derived from chronic cell cycle checkpoint activation or from endogenous retroelements [16, 17]. Retroelements including endogenous retroviruses and L1 elements account for almost half of the human genome. They replicate through retrotransposition, a copy and paste mechanism which involves reverse transcription of an RNA intermediate [18]. Interestingly, TREX1 has been shown to degrade retroelement-derived ssDNA and to prevent retrotransposition of endogenous retroelements [16].

Nucleic acids exposed in a cell by microbial infection or during tissue damage can evoke immune responses. This is accomplished by membrane-associated receptors such as Toll-like receptors and a growing number of cytosolic sensors, such as RIG-1, DAI, and AIM2, which mediate recognition of danger-associated molecular patterns and initiate innate immune responses mainly through induction of IFNα [19]. These nucleic acid-sensing systems have evolved as a first line of defense against pathogens such as bacteria and viruses. Defects in nucleic acid metabolism may lead to an inappropriate activation of nucleic acid sensors. The ensuing induction of the innate immune response may, through its stimulatory effect on the adaptive immune system, eventually result in the phenotypic expression of an autoimmune disease. In fact, nucleic acids are among the key targets of the autoimmune attack in lupus erythematosus. Moreover, the autoimmune phenotype of TREX1 deficient mice can be rescued by intercrossing with mice deficient for interferon regulatory factor 3 (IRF3) or the IFNα receptor 1 (IFNaR1), indicating that the phenotype is type 1 IFN-dependent [16]. In view of the important role of IFNα pathways for the pathogenesis of lupus erythematosus [20], the TREX1-associated phenotypic spectrum paradigmatically highlights the interplay between the innate and the adaptive immune systems in the pathogenesis of systemic autoimmunity (Fig. 2.2).

Conclusions

The nuclease TREX1 represents a novel negative regulator of the innate immune response. Although the exact molecular mechanisms underlying activation of intracellular nucleic acid sensors and signalling pathways due to TREX1 deficiency

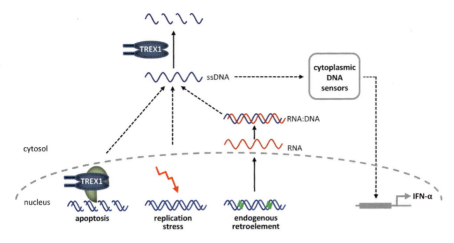

Fig. 2.2 Functional properties of TREX1 in nucleic acid metabolism. Nucleic acid species such as ssDNA generated during granzyme A-mediated apoptosis, DNA replication stress, or endogenous retroelement propagation are degraded by TREX1. Defects in TREX1 lead to accumulation of ssDNA and activation of nucleic acid sensors, which trigger an IFNα-mediated innate immune response

remain not fully understood, current data indicate that TREX1 participates in the removal of nucleic acid species produced during apoptosis, cell cycle checkpoint activation, or propagation of endogenous retroviruses [13]. Failure of any of these processes results in an inappropriate activation of the innate immune system. Thus, the elucidation of the genetic cause of chilblain lupus and associated phenotypes has revealed novel functional relationships between intracellular nucleic acid degradation, nucleic acid recognition, and the activation of an innate immune response underscoring the importance of nucleic acid metabolism for mechanisms of immune tolerance and the prevention of systemic autoimmunity.

The clinical picture of lupus erythematosus is characterized by considerable phenotypic heterogeneity. Until to date, the diagnosis and classification of patients with this disease is primarily based on clinical, histological, and immunoserological criteria. While current classification systems and disease activity scores have proven useful in the clinical setting, they do not consider molecular genetic or pathophysiological relationships. Thus, recognition of TREX1-associated forms of lupus erythematosus represents a first step towards a disease classification that incorporates molecular genetic evidence.

See Also

Skin Manifestations of Systemic Lupus Erythematosus by Martin Aringer and Annegret Kuhn.

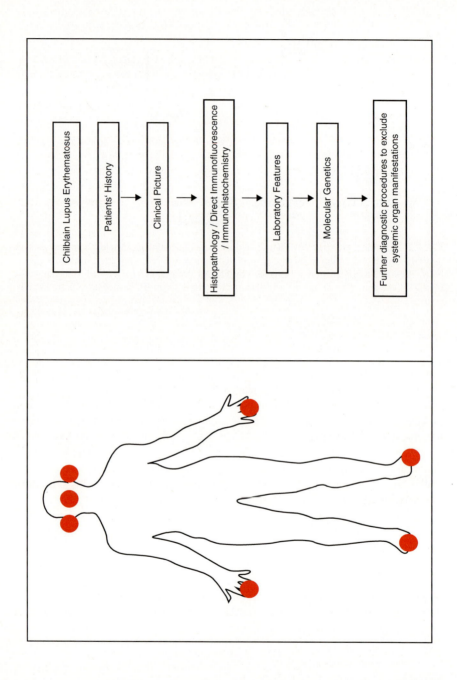

Acknowledgment We thank P. Wissel, J. Bückmann, and Professor T. A. Luger, University Muenster, Germany, for providing the clinical figures.

References

1. Kuhn A, et al. Clinical manifestations of cutaneous lupus erythematosus. In: Kuhn A, Lehmann P, Ruzicka T, editors. Cutaneous lupus erythematosus. Heidelberg: Springer 2004. pp. 59–92
2. Lee-Kirsch MA, et al. Familial chilblain lupus, a monogenic form of cutaneous lupus erythematosus, maps to chromosome 3p. Am J Hum Genet. 2006;79:731–7.
3. Lee-Kirsch MA, et al. A mutation in TREX1 that impairs susceptibility to granzyme A-mediated cell death underlies familial chilblain lupus. J Mol Med. 2007;85:531–7.
4. Rice G, et al. Heterozygous mutations in TREX1 cause familial chilblain lupus and dominant aicardi-goutières syndrome. Am J Hum Genet. 2007;80:811–5.
5. Franceschini F, et al. Chilblain lupus erythematosus is associated with antibodies to SSA/Ro. Lupus. 1999;8:215–9.
6. Millard LG, et al. Chilblain lupus erythematosus (Hutchinson). A clinical and laboratory study of 17 patients. Br J Dermatol. 1978;98:497–506.
7. Gunther C, et al. Familial chilblain lupus–a monogenic form of cutaneous lupus erythematosus due to a heterozygous mutation in TREX1. Dermatology. 2009;219:162–6.
8. Rustin MH, et al. The treatment of chilblains with nifedipine: the results of a pilot study, a double-blind placebo-controlled randomized study and a long-term open trial. Br J Dermatol. 1989;120:267–75.
9. Goette DK. Chilblains (perniosis). J Am Acad Dermatol. 1990;23:257–62.
10. Kuhn A, et al. Clinical manifestations in cutaneous lupus erythematosus. J Dtsch Dermatol Ges. 2007;5:1124–37.
11. Viguier M, et al. Clinical and histopathologic features and immunologic variables in patients with severe chilblains. A study of the relationship to lupus erythematosus. Medicine (Baltimore). 2001;80:180–8.
12. Lee-Kirsch MA, et al. Mutations in the gene encoding the 3′-5′ DNA exonuclease TREX1 are associated with systemic lupus erythematosus. Nat Genet. 2007;39:1065–7.
13. Lee-Kirsch MA. Nucleic acid metabolism and systemic autoimmunity revisited. Arthritis Rheum. 2010;62:1208–12.
14. Crow YJ, et al. Aicardi-Goutières syndrome displays genetic heterogeneity with one locus (AGS1) on chromosome 3p21. Am J Hum Genet. 2000;67:213–21.
15. Ramantani G, et al. Expanding the phenotypic spectrum of lupus erythematosus in Aicardi-Goutières syndrome. Arthritis Rheum. 2010;62:1469–77.
16. Stetson DB, et al. Trex1 prevents cell-intrinsic initiation of autoimmunity. Cell. 2008;134:587–98.
17. Yang YG, et al. Trex1 exonuclease degrades ssDNA to prevent chronic checkpoint activation and autoimmune disease. Cell. 2007;131:873–86.
18. Deininger PL, et al. Mobile elements and mammalian genome evolution. Curr Opin Genet Dev. 2003;13:651–8.
19. Yanai H, et al. Regulation of the cytosolic DNA-sensing system in innate immunity: a current view. Curr Opin Immunol. 2009;21:17–22.
20. Ronnblom L, et al. Type I interferon and lupus. Curr Opin Rheumatol. 2009;21:471–7.
21. Richards A, et al. C-terminal truncations in human 3′-5′ DNA exonuclease TREX1 cause autosomal dominant retinal vasculopathy with cerebral leukodystrophy. Nat Genet. 2007;39:1068–70.

Chapter 3
Erythema Nodosum

Yannick Allanore, Nicolas Ortonne, and Laurence Valeyrie-Allanore

Definition

Erythema nodosum (EN) is a painful nodular syndrome, most likely of immunologic origin, which involves dermis and subcutaneous tissue. It is the most frequent clinicopathologic variant of panniculitis. Its pathologic process is reflected by inflammation of fat lobules' septa, and in fully developed lesions, a delayed hypersensitivity mechanism can be suggested. The disorder usually exhibits a sudden onset of symmetrical, erythematous, tender, rounded or oval nodules and raised plaques predominantly located on the extensors of lower extremities, mainly the shins, ankles or knees and more rarely the forearm. Usually the size of the nodules is over 1 cm. At the initial stages, the nodules show a bright red colour evolving toward red or purplish lesions (Fig. 3.1) and finally exhibit a yellow or greenish appearance (biligenin colour). The lesions show spontaneous regression (usually in 3–6 weeks), without ulceration, and with time, the nodules heal without atrophy or scarring but recurrent episodes are not uncommon.

Y. Allanore, M.D., Ph.D. (✉)
Rheumatology A department, Paris Descartes University, Assistance Publique-Hôpitaux de Paris, Cochin Hospital, 27 rue du faubourg, Saint Jacques, 75014, Paris, France
e-mail: yannick.allanore@cch.aphp.fr

N. Ortonne, M.D., Ph.D.
Department of Pathology, Paris Est Creteil University (UPEC), Henri Mondor Hospital, Assistance Publique-Hôpitaux de Paris, Creteil, France
e-mail: nicolas.ortonne@hmn.aphp.fr

L. Valeyrie-Allanore, M.D.
Department of Dermatology, Paris XII University, Henri Mondor Hospital, Assistance Publique-Hôpitaux de Paris, Paris, France
e-mail: laurence.allanore@hmn.aphp.fr

M. Matucci-Cerinic et al. (eds.), *Skin Manifestations in Rheumatic Disease*,
DOI 10.1007/978-1-4614-7849-2_3, © Springer Science+Business Media New York 2014

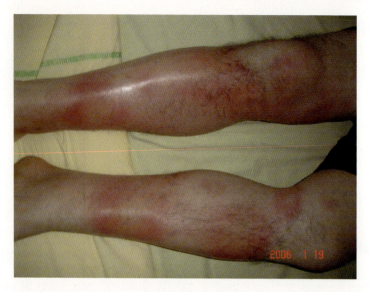

Fig. 3.1 Erythema nodosum of limbs: symmetrical, erythematous, tender, rounded and oval nodules

The peak incidence is closed to the 20–30 years of age and the sex ratio favours females (3–6 times). The clinical picture is always that of a nonspecific systemic illness with mild-grade fever (in 60 % of cases with 38–39 °C), arthralgias (60 %), sometimes arthritis (30 %) and fatigue, while associated illness, in case of any, may prevail the presentation. It is consensually agreed that EN is a hypersensitive reaction to different antigenic stimuli and can therefore occur within the course of many diseases including infections, inflammatory and immune disorders, malignancies or drug therapy. However, an underlying aetiology cannot be found in about half of cases [1].

Differential Diagnosis

Differential diagnoses: insect bites, erysipelas, erythema induratum (nodular vasculitis), urticaria, thrombophlebitis.

Biopsy

In the large majority of cases, which exhibit typical EN, there is no indication to perform a skin biopsy. The dermatological diagnosis is based on clinical features. However, in very few atypical cases of unusual presentation, a skin biopsy can be

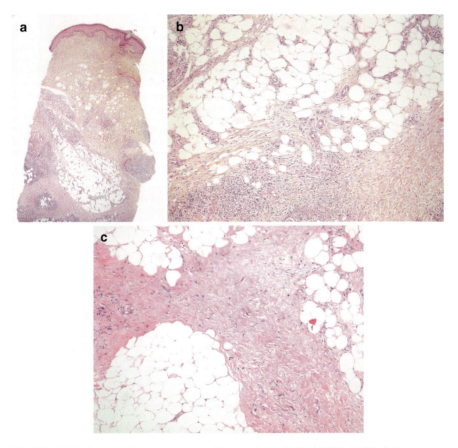

Fig. 3.2 (**a**) Erythema nodosum characterised by septal panniculitis (X50). (**b**) The inflammatory infiltrate is made of lymphocytes admixed with few neutrophils, and extends in the periseptal part of the fat lobules (X100). (**c**) A septal fibrosis without inflammation is seen in this late lesion of erythema nodosum (X100)

performed to rule out other diagnoses. Histopathologically, erythema nodosum is a septal panniculitis (Fig. 3.2a), which is characterised by inflammation of fibrous septa between fat lobules variably spreading into the lobules, septa being thickened [2, 3]. Inflammatory cells often extend to the periseptal areas of the fat lobules. Direct immunofluorescence studies have shown deposits of immunoglobulins in the blood vessel walls of the septa of subcutaneous fat. At early stages, lymphocytes and macrophages dominate but neutrophils are often present (Fig. 3.2b). Oedema, fibrin deposition and foci of vasculitis may also be seen; at later stages, fibrosis dominates (Fig. 3.2c). In some cases, giant cells may be present, located around

Table 3.1 Aetiologies

Bacterial infections	Streptococcal infections are one of the most common causes
	Mycobacteries: Tuberculosis (primo infection) is still an important cause, atypical mycobacterial infections and erythema nodosum leprosum (histologic picture is that of leukocytoclastic vasculitis)
	Gut infection: *Yersinia enterocolitica*, Salmonella, Shigella, Campylobacter
	Mycoplasma pneumonia, *Chlamydia psittaci*, *Klebsiella pneumoniae*
	Lymphogranuloma venereum (*Chlamydia trachomatis*)
	Syphilis
Fungal infections	Coccidioidomycosis (San Joaquin Valley fever) is the most common cause of erythema nodosum in the American Southwest
	Histoplasmosis
	Blastomycosis
	Aspergillosis
Viral infections	Herpes viruses
	Hepatitis B and C
	HIV
	Parvovirus B19
Inflammatory, autoimmune disorders	Sarcoidosis: the most common cause of EN, in its acute subset termed Löfgren syndrome that includes the association of EN, hilar lymphadenopathy, fever, arthritis
	Behçet disease (pathological variant of EN with presence of vasculitis)
	Inflammatory bowel diseases: ulcerative colitis and Crohn (EN may precede the bowel disease)
	Adult Still disease, lupus erythematosus, vasculitis
Malignancies	Hodgkin disease and non-Hodgkin's lymphoma
	Acute leukaemia
	Mycosis fungoides
	Solid tumours (stomach, pancreatic, colon, lung, uterine, cervix)
Drugs	Sulphonamides including sulphasalazine
	Amoxicillin and other penicillins
	Quinolone antibiotics
	Tetracyclines
	Azathioprine, D-penicillamine, gold salts
	Nonsteroidal anti-inflammatory drugs (ibuprofen, indomethacin, diclofenac, acetaminophen, naproxen)
	Oral contraceptive pills
	Thalidomide
	Verapamil, nifedipine

Based on data from Refs. [1–5]

clefts in collagen. *Miescher's granuloma* is unconstant but prototypical of EN and is formed by more or less radially arranged macrophages, often around cleft-like defects of septal collagen.

Some series have reported the characteristic of EN patients seen in rheumatology (Table 3.1). A series from Greece included 110 patients (83 % women, mean age

41.0 ± 14.0 years) [4]. Sarcoidosis was diagnosed in 28 % of the patients, infections in 17.3 % and tuberculosis in 1.5 %. Other aetiologic factors were Adamantiadis-Behçet's syndrome (3.8 %), pregnancy (6 %), oral contraceptives (3.8 %) and other drugs (3.8 %). The aetiology of EN was not found in 35 % of the patients. Among 100 Turkish patients [2], the leading aetiology was poststreptococcal (11 %), followed by primary tuberculosis (10 %), sarcoidosis (10 %), Behçet's syndrome (6 %), drugs (5 %), inflammatory bowel diseases (IBD) (3 %) and pregnancy (2 %), but nearly half (53 %) of the cases had undetermined aetiology. Recurrences occurred in patients having primary EN in 62 % (33/53) of patients. The outcomes were usually favourable within 7 days, patients being at bed rest and receiving non-steroidal anti-inflammatory drugs, together with specific treatment for patients with an underlying disease.

As stated above, usually, nodules of EN regress spontaneously within a few weeks. The course is benign and self-limited, and the prognosis is excellent. Bed rest and restriction of physical activities is encouraged during the active phase. Aspirin, nonsteroidal anti-inflammatory drugs, such as indomethacin or naproxen, but also colchicine may be helpful to enhance analgesia and resolution. Systemic corticosteroids are very rarely indicated in EN because of the benign nature of EN. In addition, an underlying infection or other disease that may be masked after treatment should be ruled out before any administration.

See Also

Behcet disease
Sarcoidosis
Inflammatory enteropathies
Hemopathies

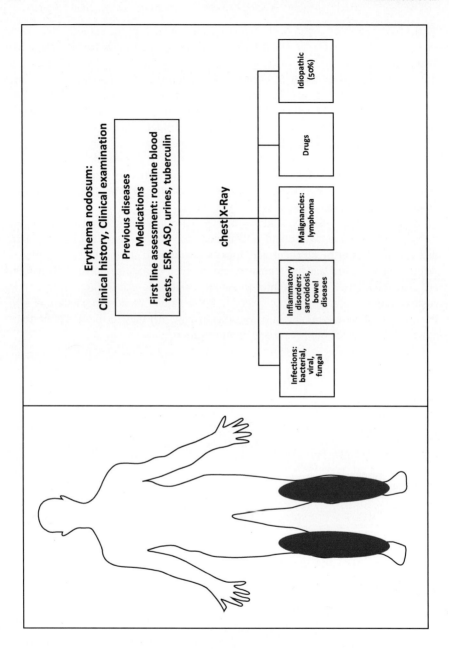

References

1. Albrecht J, Atzeni F, Baldini C, Bombardieri S, Dalakas MC, Demirkesen C, Yazici H, Mat C, Werth VP, Sarzi-Puttini P. Skin involvement and outcome measures in systemic autoimmune diseases. Clin Exp Rheumatol. 2006;24(1 Suppl 40):S52–9. Review.
2. Mert A, Kumbasar H, Ozaras R, Erten S, Tasli L, Tabak F, Ozturk R. Erythema nodosum: an evaluation of 100 cases. Clin Exp Rheumatol. 2007;25:563–70.
3. Requena L, Yus ES. Erythema nodosum. Dermatol Clin. 2008;26:425–38.
4. Psychos DN, Voulgari PV, Skopouli FN, Drosos AA, Moutsopoulos HM. Erythema nodosum: the underlying conditions. Clin Rheumatol. 2000;19:212–6.
5. Tavarela VF. Review article: skin complications associated with inflammatory bowel disease. Aliment Pharmacol Ther. 2004;20 Suppl 4:50–3.

Chapter 4
Livedo Reticularis

Stephanie W. Liu and Ruth Ann Vleugels

Definition

Livedo reticularis (LR) is a common physical finding consisting of a mottled, reticulated vascular pattern resulting from alterations in blood flow through the cutaneous microvasculature system. It most commonly occurs on the extremities, with the legs usually more affected than the arms (Fig. 4.1). Livedo reticularis can be benign, occurring in healthy individuals without systemic associations, or it may be secondary, occurring in association with underlying disease. The appearance of LR reflects the anatomy of the cutaneous microvascular system, which consists of perpendicularly oriented arterioles that divide into capillary beds and then drain into the venous plexus. Livedo reticularis can manifest by any process that reduces arteriole blood flow (vasospasm, hyperviscosity, inflammation, thromboemboli) or venous outflow, leading to accumulation of deoxygenated venous blood.

It is important to distinguish LR from livedo racemosa, a distinct entity characterized by a violaceous, irregular net-like pattern that is often annular or polycyclic. Livedo racemosa is always secondary to a pathologic process, such as SLE, antiphospholipid antibody syndrome, Sneddon's syndrome, or polycythemia vera, among others, and classically remains present on rewarming of the skin. It is typically asymmetrically distributed and is often more widespread than LR, involving the extremities, buttocks, and trunk.

LR without systemic associations: There are three types of LR without systemic associations: (1) physiologic, which occurs in response to cold and resolves with warming; (2) primary, in which the appearance and resolution are independent of temperature; and (3) idiopathic, which is persistent LR without an underlying cause. Both primary and idiopathic LR are diagnoses of exclusion.

S.W. Liu, M.D. (✉) • R.A. Vleugels, M.D., MPH
Department of Dermatology, Brigham and Women's Hospital/Harvard Medical School,
221 Longwood Avenue, Boston, MA 02115, USA
e-mail: swliu@partners.org; rvleugels@partners.org

M. Matucci-Cerinic et al. (eds.), *Skin Manifestations in Rheumatic Disease*,
DOI 10.1007/978-1-4614-7849-2_4, © Springer Science+Business Media New York 2014

Fig. 4.1 Livedo reticularis of
the bilateral lower extremities

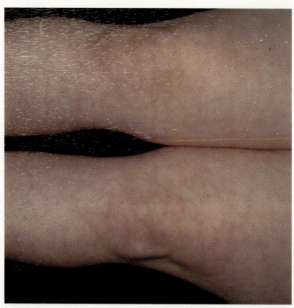

LR with systemic associations: Systemic associations with LR can occur in several broad categories, as outlined in Table 4.1.

Differential Diagnosis

Erythema ab igne is a heat-induced skin condition that begins as reversible LR and may become fixed with a reticulated pattern.

Reticulated erythematous mucinosis may look similar to LR, but the primary morphology is of papules and plaques. It usually favors the mid trunk and is pruritic.

Poikilodermatous conditions (e.g., dermatomyositis, graft-versus-host disease, mycosis fungoides) can be confused with LR, but there will typically be epidermal change.

Workup

1. Complete history and physical exam: Ask about location of LR, precipitating or alleviating factors (including temperature and leg elevation), duration of LR, and associated symptoms. Pain with LR may be more suggestive of LR due to vasculitis, emboli, or calciphylaxis. Questions about pertinent medical history should also be included, with focus on autoimmune connective tissue diseases, history of hypercoagulable states, thrombosis, or recent infections. Ask about medications. Physical exam should note the presence of ulcerations or nodules, which

Table 4.1 LR with systemic associations

Congential	In infants, cutis marmorata is physiologic LR which responds to rewarming and may be localized or generalized. Cutis marmorata telangiectatica cutis (CMTC) is LR that appears at birth, may not respond to rewarming, and may have associated abnormalities
Vasospasm	The most common cause of LR, which is often seen in association with autoimmune connective tissue diseases. It occurs commonly in patients with Raynaud's phenomenon
Hematologic/ hypercoaguability	Any process that results in hyperviscosity may produce LR. Increased quantities of normal blood products, as occurs in polycythemia vera and thrombocytosis, as well as accumulation of abnormal proteins including cryoglobulins, cryofibrinogens, cold agglutinins, and paraproteins may cause intravascular sludging [1, 2]
	Hypercoaguable states such as antiphospholipid syndrome (APS), Sneddon's syndrome (SS), protein C and S deficiency, antithrombin III deficiency, factor V Leiden mutation, homocysteinemia, disseminated intravascular coagulation, thrombotic thrombocytopenia purpura, and deep vein thromboses are other examples. In particular, antiphospholipid syndrome, characterized by thrombosis and/or recurrent fetal loss with circulating antiphospholipids, is an important cause of LR to consider. LR may be the initial presenting symptom in 25–40 % of APS patients [3, 4]. It is even more frequent in patients with APS and underlying systemic lupus erythematosus (SLE) than in patients with APS alone and can signify an increased likelihood for neuropsychiatric SLE [5]. Sneddon's syndrome, characterized by cerebrovascular events and LR and/or livedo racemosa, typically affects young to middle-aged women. The LR in Sneddon's syndrome is widespread, almost always involving the trunk and buttocks, and often predates cerebrovascular events by years [6]
Vasculitis, autoimmune connective tissue diseases	Vasculitis, particularly of the small- or medium-sized arterioles, is associated with LR. Cutaneous polyarteritis nodosa is a classic example (Fig. 4.2). Other vasculitides to consider are Churg-Strauss syndrome, Wegener's granulomatosis, microscopic polyangiitis, nodular vasculitis, rheumatoid vasculitis, and giant cell arteritis [7–9]. Autoimmune connective tissue diseases including SLE, rheumatoid arthritis, Sjörgen's syndrome, dermatomyositis, and systemic sclerosis may present with large network pattern LR
Vessel obstruction	Embolic events or thromboses can obstruct the vessel lumen. Cholesterol emboli syndrome, seen in patients with atherosclerotic disease, results when a cholesterol plaque is dislodged from the vessel wall. It may be spontaneous or precipitated by catheter procedures and intraluminal operations. Usually, LR will present distal to the dislodged plaque [10]. Similarly, septic emboli, most commonly from *Staphylococcus aureus*, may produce LR [11]
	Deposition disorders can also present with LR. Calciphylaxis, typically seen in the setting of end-stage renal disease, features calcium deposition within the vessel walls. Primary hyperoxalurias, rare autosomal recessive metabolic disorders associated with abnormal overproduction of serum oxalate and subsequent deposition in tissue, can manifest as LR. The deposition of these crystals results in intravascular obstruction, end-organ damage, and LR associated with ulceration and necrosis [12]

(continued)

Table 4.1 (continued)

	Livedoid vasculopathy is a combination of intraluminal obstruction and vessel wall pathology. The blood vessel lumina are filled with hyaline thrombi and fibrinoid material collects in the walls. It presents as distal lower extremity LR and recurrent painful purpuric ulcerations that heal with stellate, white atrophie blanche scars (Fig. 4.3) [13]
Medications	Thrombolytics, anticoagulants, and any drug that causes vasoconstriction can present with LR. One of the most well-known medications associated with LR is amantadine. Used in multiple sclerosis and Parkinson's disease, amantadine can cause LR in up to 40 % of patients [14]. Other drugs that have been reported include minocycline, norepinephrine, heparin, and interferon [15]
Infections	Associated infections causing LR are often seen in the setting hypercoagulable states. Hepatitis C, causing mixed cryoglobulinemia, and *mycoplasma* pneumonia, causing cold hemagglutinin disease, are known causes. Other infections reported to be associated with LR include syphilis, streptococcemia, rheumatic fever, meningococcemia, rickettsial disease, endocarditis, and viral infections [16]
Neoplasms	Malignancies (renal cell carcinoma, breast cancer) resulting in vascular obstruction have been reported to cause LR in a few cases [17, 18]
Neurologic	Any disorder with dysautonomia can present with LR due to vasospasm and venodilation. Reflex sympathetic dystrophy, characterized by pain, dysautonomia, and somatosensory and somatomotor dysfunction, can present with LR. Stroke, paraplegia, and multiple sclerosis are other disorders associated with LR

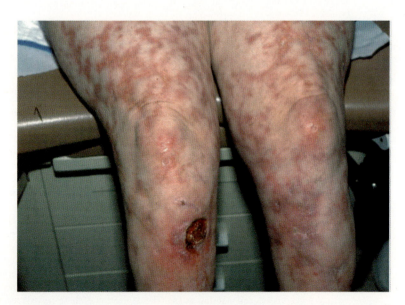

Fig. 4.2 Cutaneous polyarteritis nodosa presenting with livedo reticularis on the bilateral lower extremities (Photo courtesy of Dr. Samuel Moschella)

Fig. 4.3 Livedoid vasculopathy on the lower extremity with characteristic stellate, white atrophie blanche scarring (Photo courtesy of Dr. Laura Winterfield)

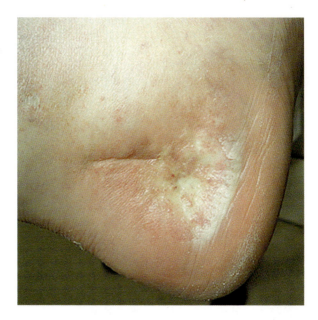

can suggest vasculitis. Areas of necrosis may suggest calciphylaxis or LR due to intraluminal obstruction. The pattern of LR can also be useful. An evenly distributed, fine pattern can be seen with intraluminal pathology, whereas a larger network with a patchy distribution is more characteristic of vasculitis or vessel wall pathology-associated LR.

2. Laboratory studies: The lupus anticoagulant panel should be considered in all patients with LR, given the common association and implications. Additional screening studies should be chosen based on history and physical exam (e.g., vasculitis, autoimmune or hematologic directed serologies).

3. Skin biopsy: Livedo reticularis without systemic associations does not require a skin biopsy. If an associated systemic condition is suspected, a skin biopsy can help differentiate the cause of LR, distinguishing between vasculitis, vasculopathy, etc. The goal of the biopsy is to obtain samples of the medium vessels found in the deep reticular dermis. Therefore, a wedge excision or large punch biopsy is preferred. If this is not possible, several biopsies should be taken from different areas of LR, including the central blanched area and the outer, bluish area, but avoiding the vessel itself. If there is evidence of purpura, nodules, ulcerations, or necrosis, these areas should be biopsied as well.

Treatment

For primary LR, no treatment is needed. For physiologic or idiopathic LR, avoidance of cold and tobacco is recommended. LR associated with systemic conditions is treated based on the underlying cause.

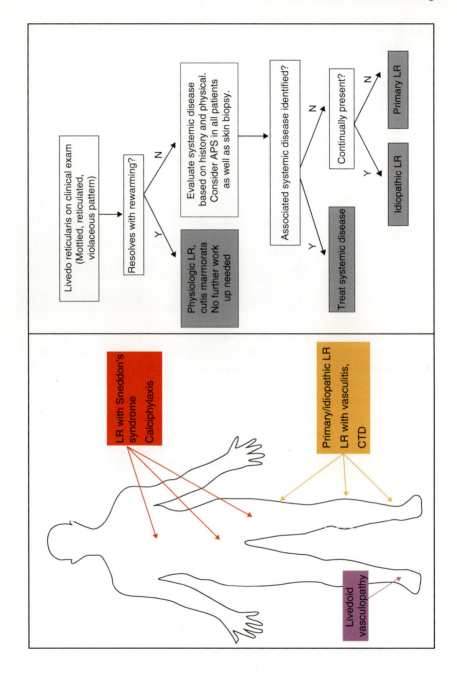

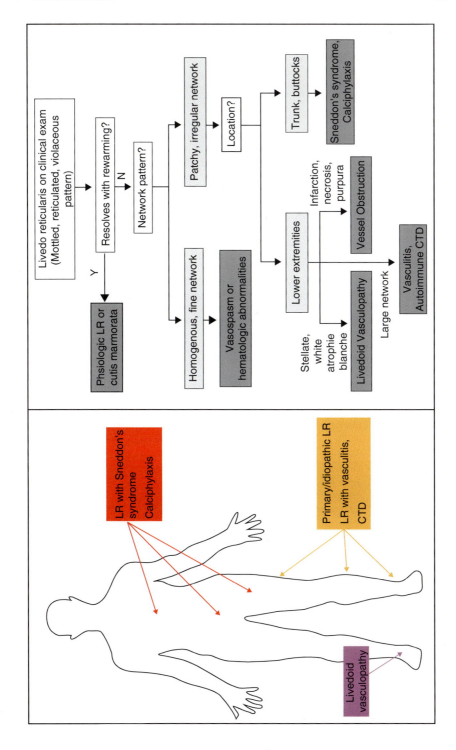

Acknowledgments Diagnostic Flow Chart 1 based on data from Gibbs MB, English JC, Zirwas MJ. Livedo reticularis: an update. J Am Acad Dermatol. 2005;Jun;52(6):1009–1019.

References

1. Speight EL, Lawrence CM. Reticulate purpura, cryoglobulinaemia and livedo reticularis. Br J Dermatol. 1993;129(3):319–23.
2. Filo V, Brezova D, Hlavcak P, Filova A. Livedo reticularis as a presenting symptom of polycythaemia vera. Clin Exp Dermatol. 1999;24(5):428.
3. Frances C, Niang S, Laffitte E, Pelletier F, Costedoat N, Piette JC. Dermatologic manifestations of the antiphospholipid syndrome: two hundred consecutive cases. Arthritis Rheum. 2005;52(6):1785–93.
4. Kriseman YL, Nash JW, Hsu S. Criteria for the diagnosis of antiphospholipid syndrome in patients presenting with dermatologic symptoms. J Am Acad Dermatol. 2007;57(1):112–5.
5. Frances C. Dermatological manifestations of Hughes' antiphospholipid antibody syndrome. Lupus. 2010;19(9):1071–7.
6. Kraemer M, Linden D, Berlit P. The spectrum of differential diagnosis in neurological patients with livedo reticularis and livedo racemosa. A literature review. J Neurol. 2005;252(10):1155–66.
7. Bosco L, Peroni A, Schena D, Colato C, Girolomoni G. Cutaneous manifestations of Churg-Strauss syndrome: report of two cases and review of the literature. Clin Rheumatol. 2011;30(4):573–80.
8. Dion J, Bachmeyer C, Moguelet P, Lescure FX, Pagnoux C. Livedo reticularis and erythematous macules of the forearms indicating cutaneous microscopic polyangiitis. Am J Med. 2010;123(11):e5–6.
9. Gunderson CG, Federman DG. Web of confusion. Am J Med. 2011;124(6):501–4.
10. Chaudhary K, Wall BM, Rasberry RD. Livedo reticularis: an underutilized diagnostic clue in cholesterol embolization syndrome. Am J Med Sci. 2001;321(5):348–51.
11. Izumi AK, Samlaska CP, Hew DW, Bruno PP. Septic embolization arising from infected pseudoaneurysms following percutaneous transluminal coronary angioplasty: a report of 2 cases and review of the literature. Cutis Cutan Med Pract. 2000;66(6):447–52.
12. Blackmon JA, Jeffy BG, Malone JC, Knable Jr AL. Oxalosis involving the skin: case report and literature review. Arch Dermatol. 2011;147:1302–5.
13. Dean SM. Livedo reticularis and related disorders. Curr Treat Options Cardiovasc Med. 2011;13(2):179–91.
14. Vollum DI, Parkes JD, Doyle D. Livedo reticularis during amantadine treatment. Br Med J. 1971;2(5762):627–8.
15. Elkayam O, Yaron M, Caspi D. Minocycline induced arthritis associated with fever, livedo reticularis, and pANCA. Ann Rheum Dis. 1996;55(10):769–71.
16. Gibbs MB, English 3rd JC, Zirwas MJ. Livedo reticularis: an update. J Am Acad Dermatol. 2005;52(6):1009–19.
17. Erel A, Ozsoy E, University G. Livedo reticularis associated with renal cell carcinoma. Int J Dermatol. 2001;40(4):299–300.
18. Spiers EM, Fakharzadeh SS. Livedo reticularis and inflammatory carcinoma of the breast. J Am Acad Dermatol. 1994;31(4):689–90.

Chapter 5
Malar Erythema

Jessica S. Kim and Victoria P. Werth

Definition

Malar erythema is defined as redness symmetrically involving the bilateral cheeks as well as the skin on the bridge of the nose. This erythema might be associated with scaling or other findings, such as papules or pustules. The clinical diagnosis of malar erythema is straightforward. The etiology is often due to photosensitivity, but other causes can be associated. Malar erythema has many causes, and differentiation is important for diagnosis and management.

The classic "butterfly rash" of ACLE presents as a confluent erythema with edema over the malar eminences with sparing of the nasolabial folds. The acute-onset transient eruption typically follows sun exposure in a photodistribution and is seen almost exclusively in patients with SLE whose illness is active in other organ systems. SCLE manifests as photoexacerbated, non-indurated papulosquamous or annular skin lesions that may develop on the face as well as the neck, dorsal upper extremities, and upper trunk. An eruption similar to ACLE but with targeting of the nasolabial folds and perioral sparing can be seen in association with the skin, cuticular and muscle changes of dermatomyositis. Rosacea, in contrast, is confined to the face and generally more persistent by history, with flushing exacerbated by heat, hot drinks, alcohol, spicy foods, menstruation, or exercise [1]. SCLE can involve the face and approximate a malar erythema, but there tend to be discrete lesions, and the lesions show more epidermal changes such as scale or even vesiculation and crusting.

J.S. Kim, M.D.
Department of Dermatology, UC San Diego, 8899 University Center Lane,
Suite 350, San Diego, CA 92122, USA
e-mail: JessicaSKim@gmail.com

V.P. Werth, M.D. (✉)
Department of Dermatology, University of Pennsylvania School of Medicine,
2 Maloney Bldg, 36th and Spruce Sts, Philadelphia, PA 19104, USA
e-mail: werth@mail.med.upenn.edu

M. Matucci-Cerinic et al. (eds.), *Skin Manifestations in Rheumatic Disease*,
DOI 10.1007/978-1-4614-7849-2_5, © Springer Science+Business Media New York 2014

ANA testing may be useful in the evaluation of a rheumatologic cause, as more than 95 % of ACLE patients and 80 % of SCLE patients will have significant ANA titers. However, these can be elevated even when the patient does not have lupus, and a lesional biopsy should be done to confirm or rule out the diagnosis of LE if the patient does not have classic SLE with systemic features, or if the eruption is somewhat unusual or unresponsive to SLE therapies.

Differential Diagnosis

Genetic disorders: Certain heritable disorders are associated with photosensitivity and a resultant secondary erythema of the face. These include Bloom's syndrome or Rothmund-Thompson syndrome, which can be identified by childhood onset and other associated features.

Vitamin deficiency: Pellagra (deficiency of niacin) can cause a photodistributed erythema that can result in a malar rash. There is often characteristic hyperpigmentation as well. In addition, systemic features such as diarrhea, dementia, and even death are associated.

Infection: Bacterial cellulitis (erysipelas) can cause a well-demarcated facial erythema. This is often unilateral, however, and associated with fever and sudden onset. Many viral infections (including erythema infectiosum, parvovirus B19, primary HIV). Toxin-mediated infectious disorders such as toxic shock syndrome or scarlet fever, as well as viral infections, such as erythema infectiosum, parvovirus B19, and primary HIV can be associated with this finding as well. Differentiation can be made by history and other signs of infection.

Polymorphous light eruption (PMLE): PMLE can result in a photodistributed erythema than can sometimes be difficult to distinguish from connective tissue disorders. Typically, the photosensitivity of polymorphic light eruption tends to be more immediate (e.g., hours) following sun exposure, while classic lupus lesions may take up to 1–2 weeks to develop following sun exposure. In addition, the lesions of PMLE tend to occur only at selected times of the year, usually following a sun exposure that is atypically intense compared to that over the preceding months.

Flushing: Many medications can cause flushing, such as niacin. In addition, exposure to heat or drinking alcohol can result in malar erythema. Scomboid fish poisoning (caused by eating decayed fish) can also result in intense flushing and erythema. These exposures can usually be easily detected by history. Some people inherently have an exaggerated vasomotor flushing response. This can be identified as it typically is associated with intense feeling of burning, heat, and discomfort, and it has a typical short and episodic course. These patients often admit to the use of fans or other means to cool down the face. Finally, rare tumors, such as carcinoid, can be associated with flushing. These patients will often have associated diarrhea, cramping, or wheezing.

Allergic or photoallergic disorders: An allergy to an airborne contactant can result in erythema of the exposed areas of skin that can resemble a malar erythema. Close inspection of the skin often reveals involvement of certain areas of the skin that are typically not involved in a photodistributed malar erythema (e.g., eyelids and

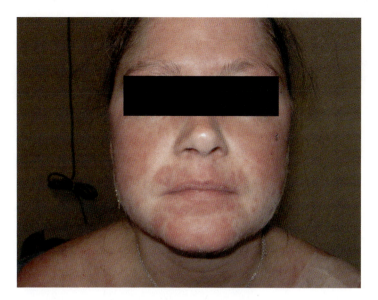

Fig. 5.1 Malar erythema from rosacea with characteristic papules and pustules

behind the ears). The erythema in these disorders is typically confluent across the entire skin of the face, unlike a true malar erythema. Certain medications can cause a photoallergic or phototoxic reaction that can result in a malar erythema that can be very difficult to distinguish from connective tissue diseases. A history can be helpful; however, further testing may be required to make this diagnosis. Photo-patch testing can be helpful as well as a skin biopsy that would not show other findings (e.g., increased mucin deposition) that are more typical of connective tissue diseases.

Inflammatory skin disorders: Acne rosacea can be associated with a malar erythema that is often confused with lupus erythematosus or other related diseases. The presence of papules or pustules helps to make this diagnosis (Fig. 5.1), as does frank rhinophyma. In addition, these patients typically have triggers such as alcohol use, heat, or spicy foods. Seborrheic dermatitis can cause facial erythema. Typically this is associated with a waxy, yellow scale that is characteristic and has a predilection for the nasolabial folds (which are not typically involved in lupus) and hair-bearing areas. The color of seborrheic dermatitis is more orange-red than the violaceous color of connective tissue disorders. In addition, the eyebrows, scalp, ears, and chest are often involved and can be helpful in making this diagnosis. Atopic dermatitis is another common disorder that can have facial erythema. These patients typically give a family history of atopy and often have involvement of more classic areas, such as the antecubital and popliteal fossae and hands. There is often an associated "hyperlinearity" of the palms, in which the number of skin creases on the palms is greatly increased. Pemphigus erythematosus is a photodistributed autoimmune blistering disorder that can cause a facial erythema. Typically, however, this disorder will be associated with erosions and vesicles as the primary lesions.

Fig. 5.2 Malar erythema
from acute LE demonstrates
confluent erythema with
edema and sparing of the
nasolabial folds

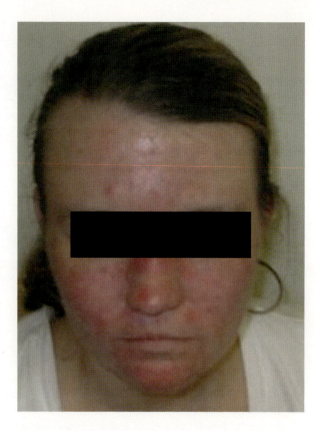

Lupus erythematosus: The malar rash is classically associated with acute cutaneous lupus erythematosus (ACLE) or subacute cutaneous lupus erythematosus (SCLE). The malar rash of ACLE does not tend to show very much epidermal change (other than perhaps minimal scaling), thus, the presence of crusting or erosions is more indicative of other disorders. This rash typically involves the nasal bridge but spares the nasolabial folds (Fig. 5.2). As mentioned, there are no pustules, although papules can occasionally be found. These patients can also have involvement of other photodistributed areas, such as the chest and arms. Typically, these patients are experiencing a flare of their SLE and thus have other LE-related symptoms. The malar erythema of SCLE is associated with more scale, and usually there is associated involvement of the chest, back, or arms. One can typically find more classical annular or psoriasiform configured lesions, and they are characteristically associated with hypopigmentation. The erythema of SCLE has a telangiectatic quality not typically seen in other causes of malar erythema.

Dermatomyositis (DM): Patients with DM can have a malar erythema that is indistinguishable from LE-related erythema. Clues for DM include involvement of the eyelids, edema, predilection to involve the nasolabial folds (Fig. 5.3), associated involvement of other areas (especially the scalp), and a dysesthetic burning and itch. The rash of DM also has a characteristic violaceous color.

Fig. 5.3 Malar erythema
from dermatomyositis
targeting nasolabial fold with
perioral sparing; note the
associated periorbital
heliotrope erythema

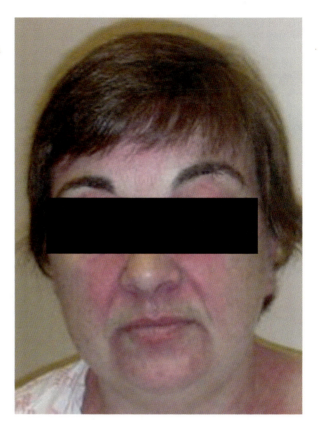

Biopsy

The histopathology of the lesional skin can be critical to differentiate rheumatic
diseases from nonrheumatic such as rosacea. LE and DM lesions share features of
hyperkeratosis or epidermal atrophy, orthohyperkeratosis or parakeratosis, vacuolar
alteration of basal keratinocytes, and a sparse-to-moderate mononuclear cell infiltrate focused at the dermal-epidermal junction (Fig. 5.4) and perivascularly [2].
Mucinous dermal deposition and thickening of the epidermal basement membrane
are also present (Fig. 5.5). Direct immunofluorescence staining in ACLE may show
a fluorescent band of granular deposits at the dermal-epidermal junction in both
involved and uninvolved skin, although this same pattern may also be found in non-
LE skin disease, in actinically damaged skin, and in normal skin as well. In acne
rosacea, a dense inflammatory infiltrate comprised of lymphocytes, histiocytes, and
multinucleated giant cells is seen around hair follicles. Hyperplasia of the sebaceous glands is also seen. Drug eruptions may show lymphocytic inflammation at
the dermal-epidermal junction, but the presence of eosinophils allows consideration
of a drug eruption as a clinical mimicker of cutaneous lupus.

A diagnostic algorithmic approach to the patient with malar erythema is given in
Fig. 5.6

Fig. 5.4 Skin biopsy of acute LE showing a lymphocytic perivascular and band-like, lichenoid infiltrate (H&E staining)

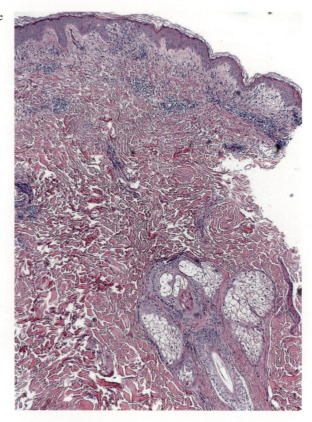

Fig. 5.5 Skin biopsy of acute LE showing increased dermal accumulation of mucin (*blue*) (Hale stain)

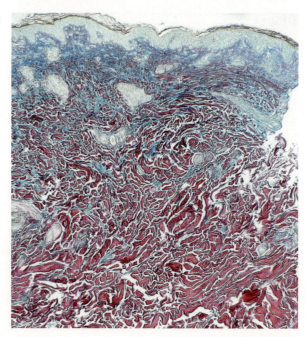

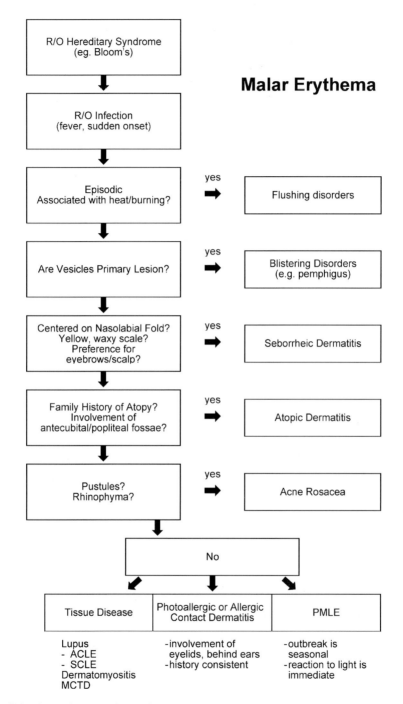

Fig. 5.6 Diagnostic approach to malar erythema

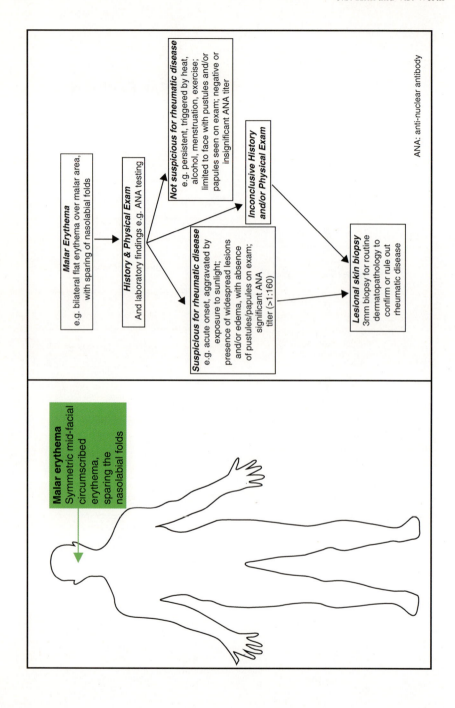

Malar Erythema
e.g. bilateral flat erythema over malar area, with sparing of nasolabial folds

History & Physical Exam
And laboratory findings e.g. ANA testing

Not suspicious for rheumatic disease
e.g. persistent, triggered by heat, alcohol, menstruation, exercise; limited to face with pustules and/or papules seen on exam; negative or insignificant ANA titer

Suspicious for rheumatic disease
e.g. acute onset, aggravated by exposure to sunlight; presence of widespread lesions and/or edema, with absence of pustules/papules on exam; significant ANA titer (>1:160)

Inconclusive History and/or Physical Exam

Lesional skin biopsy
3mm biopsy for routine dermatopathology to confirm or rule out rheumatic disease

ANA: anti-nuclear antibody

Malar erythema
Symmetric mid-facial circumscribed erythema, sparing the nasolabial folds

References

1. Black A, McCauliffe D, Sontheimer R. Prevalence of acne rosacea in a rheumatic skin disease subspecialty clinic. Lupus. 1992;1:229–37.
2. Costner M, Jacobe H. Dermatopathology of connective tissue disease. Adv Dermatol. 2000;16:323–59.

Chapter 6
Purpura

David A. Wetter

Definition

Purpura is visible hemorrhage in the skin or mucous membranes [1–3]. The color of purpura is due to hemoglobin (bright red for fully oxygenated; reddish blue, blue-black, or purple for less saturated; and blue-black to black for hemorrhage due to hemorrhagic tissue necrosis) [3]. Primary purpura means that the mechanism of lesion production is the same mechanism that produced the hemorrhage (as opposed to secondary purpura which represents hemorrhage into lesions occurring from another primary process, for example, hemorrhage occurring into areas of stasis dermatitis on the lower extremities due to increased intravascular pressures) [1, 3].

By definition, a lesion of purpura must have a color characteristic of hemorrhage, and some of the color must remain despite the application of direct pressure to the lesion with a glass slide (diascopy) [1, 3]. The direct pressure compresses the dermal vessels in the lesion and displaces any blood that is free to move [1, 3]. In contrast, if blood is external to the lesional vessels or if the vessels are occluded by clot, then some color will remain (i.e., purpura) [1, 3].

Purpuric lesions can have varying degrees of associated inflammation. This can be assessed by evaluating how much of the color of the lesion is blanchable via diascopy. The blanchable component of the color (i.e., that which is displaced with application of direct pressure with a glass slide) represents erythema and is a surrogate marker for the degree of inflammation present [3]. The residual color that does not blanch represents hemorrhage (purpura) [3]. The ratio of erythema (inflammation) to purpura (hemorrhage) can help the clinician to determine the relative role of inflammation and hemorrhage contributing to the lesion [1].

Purpura can be either macular (flat) or palpable (raised or indurated). The palpability of a lesion is due to edema, extravasated fibrin, and inflammation present

D.A. Wetter, M.D. (✉)
Department of Dermatology, Mayo Clinic, 200 First Street SW, Rochester, MN 55905, USA
e-mail: wetter.david@mayo.edu

M. Matucci-Cerinic et al. (eds.), *Skin Manifestations in Rheumatic Disease*,
DOI 10.1007/978-1-4614-7849-2_6, © Springer Science+Business Media New York 2014

within the lesion [1, 2]. Retiform purpura describes a subset of lesions that have a branched or reticulated shape (either to the entire lesion or of its edges) [3, 4]; other lesions of purpura may assume a stellate shape (consisting of peripheral radiating extensions like a star) [2].

Differential Diagnosis

There are three main pathogenic mechanisms of purpura: simple hemorrhage, inflammatory hemorrhage (i.e., inflammation directed at the blood vessels), and occlusive hemorrhage with minimal inflammation [3]. The morphology of purpura at the bedside can be used to help a clinician determine the most likely mechanism for the purpura. The following six morphologic subsets of purpura can be used to generate an abbreviated differential diagnosis [1–3]:

1. *Macular petechiae* (**≤4 mm in diameter, flat, noninflammatory, type of "simple hemorrhage"**): Thrombocytopenia (due to numerous causes), abnormal platelet function (hereditary or acquired), pigmented purpuric dermatoses (Fig. 6.1), and elevated intravascular pressure spikes (e.g., Valsalva-like maneuvers).

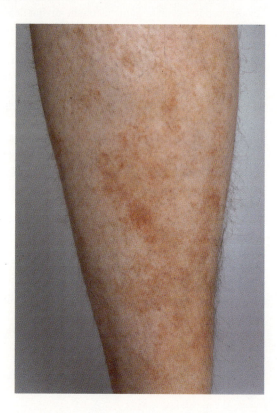

Fig. 6.1 Pigmented purpuric dermatosis (progressive pigmentary dermatosis [Schamberg disease]) occurring on the leg as reddish-brown patches with superimposed pinpoint petechiae

Fig. 6.2 Macular ecchymoses of the dorsal hand and forearm. These were due to long-term systemic corticosteroid therapy for rheumatoid arthritis

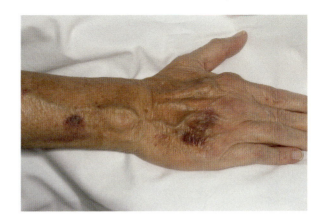

2. *Intermediate macular purpura* **(5–9 mm in diameter, flat, noninflammatory, type of "simple hemorrhage")**: Hypergammaglobulinemic purpura of Waldenström and other causes of macular petechiae and macular ecchymoses.

3. *Macular ecchymoses* **(≥1 cm in diameter, flat, noninflammatory, type of "simple hemorrhage")**: Hemophilia, anticoagulants, vitamin K deficiency, hepatic insufficiency, actinic purpura, corticosteroid therapy (topical or systemic; Fig. 6.2), vitamin C deficiency (scurvy), systemic amyloidosis, and Ehlers-Danlos syndrome.

4. *Palpable purpura* **(inflammatory purpura with prominent early erythema; round, port-wine color; partially blanches with diascopy indicating the presence of both inflammation and hemorrhage)**: The most important consideration in this category is cutaneous small-vessel vasculitis (e.g., leukocytoclastic vasculitis; Figs. 6.3 and 6.4). ANCA-associated vasculitides and vasculitides that affect both small- and medium-sized vessels can also present with palpable purpura. Targetoid lesions with a central purpuric component can be seen with IgA vasculitis and erythema multiforme. Pityriasis lichenoides et varioliformis acuta (PLEVA) can also manifest palpable purpura.

5. *Noninflammatory retiform purpura* **(minimal early erythema; some lesions are palpable; typically due to microvascular occlusion)**: Calciphylaxis (Figs. 6.5 and 6.6), heparin necrosis, warfarin necrosis, antiphospholipid antibody syndrome, cryoglobulinemia (monoclonal type only; mixed cryoglobulinemia usually presents with palpable purpura and demonstrates leukocytoclastic vasculitis on histology), hypercoagulable disorders (e.g., protein C or S deficiency), disseminated intravascular coagulation, cocaine use (levamisole-tainted), oxalosis, cholesterol emboli, livedoid vasculopathy, vessel-invasive infection (e.g., Aspergillus, ecthyma gangrenosum), malignant atrophic papulosis (Degos' disease), and marantic endocarditis.

6. *Inflammatory retiform purpura* **(early lesions have prominent erythema; some lesions are palpable)**: IgA cutaneous small-vessel vasculitis, vasculitis affecting both small- and medium-sized vessels (such as ANCA-associated and connective tissue disease-associated vasculitides), and chilblains (perniosis).

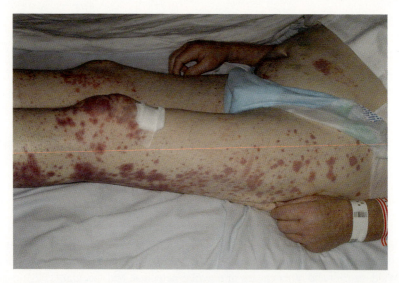

Fig. 6.3 Palpable purpura in a patient with cutaneous small-vessel vasculitis manifesting as purpuric papules and plaques on the lower extremities. Note the presence of both hemorrhage (purpura) and erythema (inflammation). Skin biopsy demonstrated leukocytoclastic vasculitis

Fig. 6.4 Palpable purpura manifesting as purpuric papules and plaques (some with overlying necrosis) on the lower extremities. Skin biopsy demonstrated leukocytoclastic vasculitis, and direct immunofluorescence microscopy of lesional skin revealed the presence of IgA within superficial dermal blood vessels. Evaluation for associated causes of this patient's IgA vasculitis revealed the presence of renal cell carcinoma

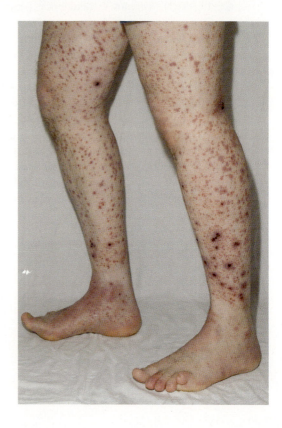

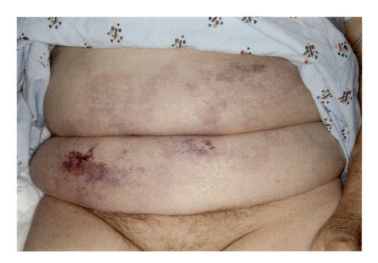

Fig. 6.5 Noninflammatory, retiform purpura manifesting as purpuric patches and indurated, exquisitely tender plaques on the abdomen. Skin biopsy demonstrated findings consistent with calciphylaxis

Fig. 6.6 Noninflammatory retiform purpura. Necrotic, stellate ulceration of the hip in a patient with calciphylaxis

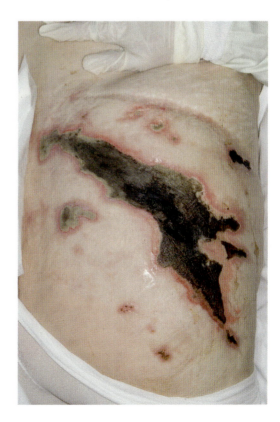

Typical Locations of Purpura

Acral predominant (e.g., hands, feet, ears) can be due to various causes, including cryoglobulinemia, embolic phenomena (e.g., cholesterol emboli, endocarditis), antiphospholipid antibody syndrome, perniosis, cocaine use (particularly the ears), disseminated intravascular coagulation, systemic amyloidosis ("pinch purpura" around eyes), and cutaneous small-vessel vasculitis (associated with drug, infection, connective tissue disease, malignancy, ANCA-associated vasculitis).

Dependent areas (typically lower extremities, also sacral back and buttocks in a hospitalized patient lying down): Cutaneous small-vessel vasculitis (i.e., leukocytoclastic vasculitis), pigmented purpuric dermatosis, and secondary purpura (e.g., due to hemorrhage into stasis dermatitis or hemorrhage into an area of drug eruption due to thrombocytopenia [1]).

Areas of extensive subcutaneous fat (e.g., breasts, hips, buttocks, thighs): Warfarin necrosis and calciphylaxis (this typically also occurs on the lower extremities).

Common sites of trauma (dorsal hands and forearms): Actinic purpura and corticosteroid-induced purpura.

Site of subcutaneous injection (e.g., abdomen): Heparin necrosis (may also occur at sites distant from this).

Approach to the Diagnosis of Purpura (Fig. 6.7) [1–3]

(A) First determine if the lesion is:

> *Purpura?* (via diascopy)
> *Primary purpura?*

(B) Determine if the lesions are *palpable* (exclude major trauma-induced hemorrhagic contusions):

1. If none are palpable – represents "**simple hemorrhage**" – classify by size (**macular petechiae, ≤4 mm; intermediate macular purpura, 5-9 mm; macular ecchymoses, ≥1 cm**).

2. If some are palpable, classify as one of the following:

   (a) Early lesions are round, port-wine colored, and have prominent erythema (partially blanch with diascopy) – represents **palpable purpura** (often due to cutaneous small-vessel vasculitis).

   (b) Early lesions lack erythema and demonstrate a retiform, branched appearance – represents **noninflammatory retiform purpura** (usually due to conditions associated with microvascular occlusion).

   (c) Early lesions have prominent erythema and demonstrate a retiform, branched appearance – represents **inflammatory retiform purpura** (usually due to IgA vasculitis or other subtypes of vasculitis).

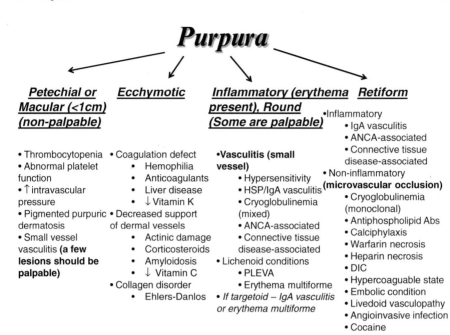

Fig. 6.7 Algorithm for approaching the patient with purpura (Adapted from Refs. [1–3])

(C) Perform history and review of systems to identify factors that may be contributing to purpura, guided by the differential diagnosis of the morphology of the purpura (e.g., preexisting medical conditions or medications that may affect coagulation and hemostasis).

(D) Pursue skin biopsy when the cause of purpura is uncertain.

1. *It is imperative to know the age of the lesion chosen for biopsy,* since late lesions of noninflammatory retiform purpura (due to microvascular occlusion) develop erythema (inflammation) as a wound healing response to ischemic injury or necrosis [3]. Thus, a late lesion of noninflammatory retiform purpura could appear clinically (and histologically) similar to an early lesion of palpable purpura (e.g., inflammatory hemorrhage due to cutaneous small-vessel vasculitis) [1–3].

2. Routine histopathology of palpable purpura should be from a lesion no more than 24–48 h old.

3. When the morphology of purpura is concerning for vasculitis, direct immunofluorescence studies should be performed on the skin biopsy (to rule out IgA vasculitis). Direct immunofluorescence in this setting should ideally be performed on an early lesion (less than 24 h old) to ensure the presence of the immune complex deposits.

(E) Targeted laboratory studies can be performed based upon the morphology of the purpura and its accompanying differential diagnosis (See section "Differential Diagnosis").

References

1. Piette WW. The differential diagnosis of purpura from a morphologic perspective. Adv Dermatol. 1994;9:3–23. Discussion 24.
2. Piette WW. Purpura: mechanisms and differential diagnosis. In: Bolognia JL, Jorizzo JL, Rapini RP, editors. Dermatology. 2nd ed. London: Mosby; 2008. p. 321–30.
3. Piette WW. Purpura. In: Callen JP, Jorizzo JL, Bolognia JL, Piette WW, Zone JJ, editors. Dermatologic signs of internal disease. 4th ed. London: Saunders Elsevier; 2009. p. 85–92.
4. Wysong A, Venkatesan P. An approach to the patient with retiform purpura. Dermatol Ther. 2011;24:151–72.

Chapter 7
Telangiectasias

David Fiorentino

Definition

Mucocutaneous telangiectasias are dilatation of the capillaries, arterioles, and/or venules of the dermis. They appear as erythematous or bluish macules (that can be confluent into patches) that are blanchable on diascopy. They can be linear, lacy, or matted. If the blood vessels involved are deep (and thus not as compressible from external forces), they can sometimes appear as non-blanching lesions and should still be considered in the differential diagnosis of purpura. They can occur almost anywhere on the surface of the skin and mucous membranes. Telangiectasias can be simply a cosmetic nuisance or they can be a sign of underlying disease. Their distribution, configuration, associated signs and symptoms, and the medical history of the patient are all important clues to being able to distinguish between isolated lesions and those which require consideration for underlying systemic pathology. It should be noted that telangiectasias can also be secondary findings in a number of dermatologic lesions (e.g., basal cell carcinoma), but those will not be discussed here.

Differential Diagnosis

Primary Telangiectasia Syndromes

Certain hereditary syndromes (e.g., genodermatoses) are associated with telangiectasias. These include ataxia telangiectasia, Bloom's syndrome, xeroderma pigmentosum, Sturge-Weber disease, Rothmund-Thompson syndrome, and Klippel-Trénaunay

D. Fiorentino, M.D., Ph.D. (✉)
Department of Dermatology, Stanford University School of Medicine, 450 Broadway Street, Pavilion C-234, Redwood City, CA 94063, USA
e-mail: Fiorentino@stanford.edu

syndrome. The most common hereditary telangiectasia is actually a capillary malformation—the nevus flammeus. Also known as the port-wine stain, these lesions typically present as confluent patches (1–5 cm) on the posterior neck or occipital scalp. Hereditary hemorrhagic telangiectasia (Osler-Weber-Rendu) usually presents in the third or fourth decade with discrete, round telangiectatic macules on the face, lips, oral mucosa, trunk, arms, and fingers [1]. Palmar erythema can also be seen. The lesions are actually small arteriovenous shunts that can also occur in the liver, gastrointestinal tract, lungs, and brain. Clues to this diagnosis include a family history (with autosomal dominant pattern), mucous membrane lesions, recurrent epistaxis, and visceral involvement.

Generalized essential telangiectasia is one of the most common forms of idiopathic generalized telangiectasia [2]. In this disorder, lesions most commonly begin on the feet, ankles, and distal legs but are characterized by slow extension to other areas. The lesions can be associated with numbness or burning. Patients typically present in the fourth or fifth decade of life. Typically the lesions are bright red, and individual, discrete capillaries can be seen that often form lacy, syncytial networks. Less commonly the lesions can be "matted" (e.g., present as a nearly confluent macule). Histopathology demonstrates only dilatation of the superficial dermal vasculature with no inflammation or abnormality in the surrounding connective tissue.

Cutaneous collagenous vasculopathy is a rare disorder that can clinically be confused with generalized essential telangiectasia [3]. Histologically, however, the lesions are characterized by a thick perivascular wall of collagen surrounding the dermal capillaries.

Unilateral nevoid telangiectasia syndrome (UNTS) is a rare disorder (both congenital and acquired) that can occur at any age (peak onset in the third decade of life) characterized by focal telangiectasias in a dermatomal distribution most commonly in the distribution of the trigeminal, cervical, or upper thoracic nerves [4]. A possible etiologic relationship to estrogens has been debated, as it occurs frequently in pregnancy and with liver disease.

Secondary Telangiectasias

Venous hypertension can be a common cause of telangiectasias on the legs and feet. These lesions are secondary to high pressure in the venous system that is most commonly due to poor valve function, but any chronic impairment of venous return can result in these lesions. Because they are dilations in the venous system, the lesions are typically more bluish than the erythematous capillary dilations that are seen in other disorders. There will often be associated, palpable bluish venous varicosities and a history of leg edema.

Telangiectasia can be the natural result of response to many types of trauma, including ulceration. Chronic UV exposure can result in telangiectasias, as can radiation. These irradiation-driven telangiectasias can be identified as they are often associated with pigmentation abnormalities and/or epidermal atrophy and usually are bound by the limits of the exposure (e.g., photodistributed or in the field of radiation), and this can be helpful in the diagnosis.

Telangiectasias can also be induced by certain medications. The most commonly associated oral medications include lithium, oral contraceptives, thiotixene, interferon alpha, and isotretinoin. These can occur anywhere on the body. Calcium channel blockers (namely, amlodipine and nifedipine) can induce telangiectasias with a photodistribution, as can rarely other medications such as bosentan or venlafaxine [5]. Chronic use of topical corticosteroids can result in telangiectasia—helpful associated findings include epidermal atrophy, striae, and/or acneiform lesions. Exposure to aluminum has been associated with the appearance of characteristic, asymptomatic, erythematous, matted, 0.2–3 cm telangiectatic lesions primarily on the upper chest and back [6]. Lesions are characterized histologically by elastic degeneration of the stroma and a mononuclear cell infiltrate.

Telangiectasias are seen in certain systemic or metabolic diseases. Liver disease or pregnancy can commonly be associated with cutaneous telangiectasias, due to the effects of high levels of estrogen. Palmar erythema is often seen, as are discrete, lacy, red telangiectasias, often found over the chest and back. Other metabolic abnormalities including thyroid disease can also result in telangiectasias.

Red fingers syndrome is characterized by painless erythema and telangiectasia of the dorsal tips of the fingers and toes and is classically associated with HIV, HBV, or HCV [7]. It is thought that the association with these viruses might be ultimately due to the liver dysfunction that ensues in these patients.

Certain neoplasms can result in the appearance of telangiectasias. Atrial myxomata have been reported in association with telangiectasias of the chest [8]. The most common malignancies that are associated with telangiectasias are carcinoid, intravascular (angiotropic) lymphoma, and mycosis fungoides—however, they have also been reported in association with ovarian, bronchogenic, and breast carcinoma.

Telangiectasias are associated with certain inflammatory diseases that are not necessarily autoimmune in nature. Cutaneous mastocytosis can present with telangiectatic macules, mostly commonly with the subtype known as telangiectasia macularis eruptiva perstans (TMEP). These lesions are usually hyperpigmented, pruritic, truncal, and often urticate (become raised) when rubbed. Acne rosacea is associated with telangiectasias of the face, especially the cheeks and nose. The presence of inflammatory papules or pustules helps the clinician make this diagnosis, although these are often absent (in the so-called erythrotelangiectatic form of acne rosacea), and can often be confused with the malar rash of acute cutaneous lupus erythematosus or dermatomyositis (see below).

Finally, telangiectasias can be a sign of underlying rheumatic disease. The erythema of dermatomyositis and cutaneous lupus erythematosus is often telangiectatic on close examination (Fig. 7.1). Violaceous color, photodistribution (e.g., face, upper back, chest, upper arms), and itch or burning (especially in the case of dermatomyositis) are all clues to an underlying autoimmune inflammatory disease. The inflammatory lesions of dermatomyositis and cutaneous lupus often resolve with lacy telangiectasia (Fig. 7.2). Dermatomyositis patients can also present with telangiectatic patches adjacent to white, avascular appearing macules that are often found in a

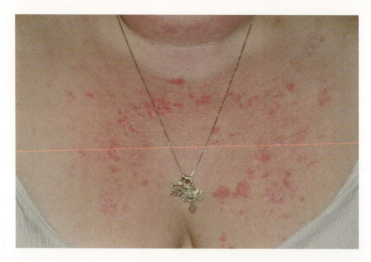

Fig. 7.1 Telangiectatic papules and plaques in a patient with subacute cutaneous erythematosus

Fig. 7.2 Postinflammatory telangiectasia in a patient with dermatomyositis

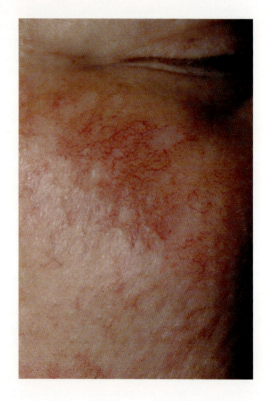

Fig. 7.3 Telangiectatic and avascular patches typical of dermatomyositis

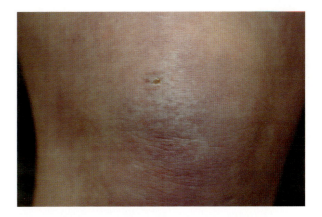

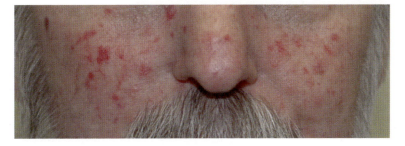

Fig. 7.4 Matted telangiectasias of systemic sclerosis

reticulate pattern (Fig. 7.3). In contrast, the telangiectasias seen in patients with systemic sclerosis are typically matted, discrete 1–5 mm lesions (Fig. 7.4). These typically occur on the hands and digits (palmar greater than dorsal surface) and the face and lips but can also be found on the chest and arms. Some data suggest that the presence of these lesions might correlate with the risk of developing pulmonary hypertension [9]. Patients with systemic sclerosis can also have discrete (non-matted) telangiectasias over the interphalangeal and metacarpophalangeal joints (Fig. 7.5), which are usually associated with prior digital ischemic ulcerations in these regions. Patients with SLE, dermatomyositis, and systemic sclerosis all can present with periungual capillary telangiectasias, which are often visible to the naked eye (Fig. 7.6). The periungual lesions of dermatomyositis are often associated with tenderness, while those of systemic sclerosis are associated with acrosclerosis or puffy fingers as well as Raynaud's. Periungual telangiectasias are considered to have high specificity for the presence (or future development) of connective tissue disease.

Fig. 7.5 Lacy telangiectasias overlying the proximal interphalangeal joints in a patient with systemic sclerosis. Note active digital ischemic lesion which is associated with this pattern of telangiectasia

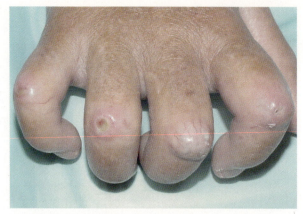

Fig. 7.6 Typical periungual telangiectasias in this patient with lupus erythematosus

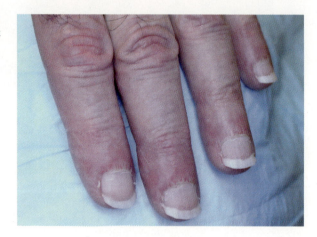

Approach to the Patient

In summary, when presented with a patient with mucocutaneous telangiectasias, one should first rule out a primary, congenital syndrome as well as possible secondary causes such as medication or malignancy. The associated cause of the telangiectasias is then decided upon by both configuration and distribution of the lesions.

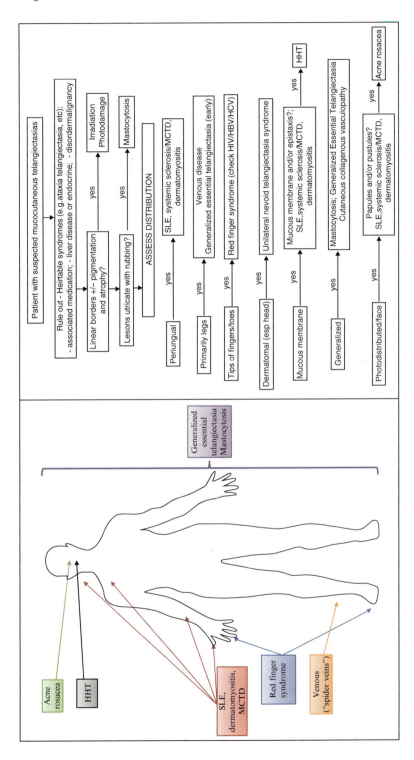

References

1. Grand'Maison A. Hereditary hemorrhagic telangiectasia. CMAJ. 2009;180(8):833–5.
2. Karen JK, et al. Generalized essential telangiectasia. Dermatol Online J. 2008;14(5):9.
3. Perez A, et al. Cutaneous collagenous vasculopathy with generalized telangiectasia in two female patients. J Am Acad Dermatol. 2010;63(5):882–5.
4. Wenson SF, Jan F, Sepehr A. Unilateral nevoid telangiectasia syndrome: a case report and review of the literature. Dermatol Online J. 2011;17(5):2.
5. Basarab T, Yu R, Jones RR. Calcium antagonist-induced photo-exposed telangiectasia. Br J Dermatol. 1997;136(6):974–5.
6. Theriault G, Cordier S, Harvey R. Skin telangiectases in workers at an aluminum plant. N Engl J Med. 1980;303(22):1278–81.
7. Pechere M, et al. Red fingers syndrome in patients with HIV and hepatitis C infection. Lancet. 1996;348(9021):196–7.
8. Bridges BF, Hector DA. Possible association of cutaneous telangiectasia with cardiac myxoma. Am J Med. 1989;87(4):483–5.
9. Shah AA, Wigley FM, Hummers LK. Telangiectases in scleroderma: a potential clinical marker of pulmonary arterial hypertension. J Rheumatol. 2010;37(1):98–104.

Chapter 8
Ulceration in Rheumatic Disease

Othman Abahussein and Jan Peter Dutz

Definition

Skin breakdown results in ulceration or erosion. An **erosion** is a superficial skin breakdown that involves the epidermis only and is most often traumatic. An **ulcer** is loss of cutaneous tissue that extends into the dermis and sometimes reaches subcutaneous fat. The causes of ulceration include trauma, inflammation, vasculopathy, and vasculitis. Inflammation, vasculopathy, and vasculitis may be the result of a connective tissue disease or an adverse effect of drug use.

Cutaneous or Mucocutaneous Ulceration Due to Connective Tissue Disease (CTD)

Several CTDs are associated with characteristic patterns of skin ulceration and are listed here:

Behçet's disease (BD) is characterized by recurrent oral or genital aphthous ulcers. Oral ulcers occur on the soft palate, tongue, and gingival or buccal mucosa; have a white, fibrinous base; and heal without scarring (Fig. 8.1). Pyoderma gangrenosum (PG) is another cutaneous manifestation of BD. It has a characteristic cribriform (grate-like) appearance with undermined ulcer and purple edges (Fig. 8.2).

Reactive arthritis or Reiter's syndrome (RS) is triad of reactive arthritis and conjunctivitis following urogenital or gastrointestinal tract infection. Patients with

O. Abahussein, MBBS, SSC – DERM, ABHS- DERM • J.P. Dutz, M.D., FRCPC (⊠)
Department of Dermatology and Skin Science, University of British Columbia,
835 West 10th Avenue, Vancouver, BC V5Z 4E8, Canada
e-mail: UTH1234@yahoo.com; dutz@interchange.ubc.ca

M. Matucci-Cerinic et al. (eds.), *Skin Manifestations in Rheumatic Disease*,
DOI 10.1007/978-1-4614-7849-2_8, © Springer Science+Business Media New York 2014

Fig. 8.1 Aphthous ulcer on
the *lower lip* shows a
fibrinous base

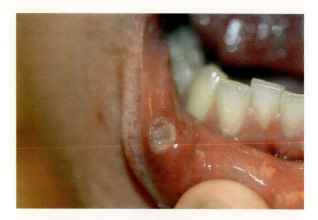

Fig. 8.2 Right leg image
shows pyoderma
gangrenosum with an
undermined ulcer

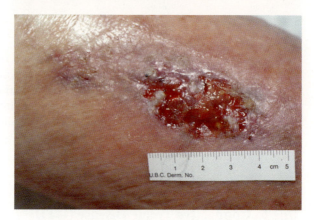

RS may have superficial painless oral and genital ulcers. The genital ulcers in the
male have a characteristic of circinate white plaques that grow centrifugally on
the uncircumcised glans penis (circinate balanitis).

Systemic lupus erythematosus (SLE). Digital ulceration is a rare manifestation of SLE.
It occurs most commonly in patients with disease of long duration and may be the
result of vasculitis, the presence of antiphospholipid antibody, or atherosclerosis. In
addition to digital ulcers, sometimes panniculitis and vasculitis can lead to ulceration.
Lupus panniculitis occurs on the face, the breast, the abdomen, and thighs and is seen
in 2–5 % of SLE patients. Vasculitis may cause lower leg ulceration.

Systemic sclerosis (SSc). The most common type of ulceration in SSc is the digital
ischemic lesion (DIL). These ulcerations occur in up to 40 % of patients with
SSc and can be extremely debilitating due to pain. The lesions come in two
forms: those occurring on the digital pulp and those occurring overlying extensor
joints (such as the interphalangeal joints or metacarpophalangeal joints). The
digital pulp lesions usually occur on the digital tips, although they can occur at

Fig. 8.3 Right hand in dermatomyositis patient. Note the ulceration on the digit pulp and the lateral erythema

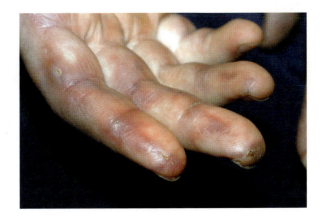

the hyponychium (the junction of the free edge of the nail plate and the fingertip) or on the lateral tips of the digit. They present as punctate ulcerations filled with a hyperkeratotic inclusion without surrounding erythema and are usually quite tender. They resolve with a pitted scar. The other type of lesion overlying the extensor joints typically presents as true ulcerations, which can often be associated with some crust and/or eschar. They often heal with lacy telangiectasias. In addition to being found on the hands, they are also seen overlying the elbows, knees, and malleoli. These lesions are likely the result of a combination of trauma and poor blood supply.

Another cause of ulceration in the SSc patient is pyoderma gangrenosum. These commonly present as ulcers on the leg with a rolled, inflammatory border and they can change in size quickly.

Dermatomyositis (DM). An ulcer in DM can be the result of calcinosis or vasculopathy. In general, ulcers can indicate one of three scenarios: first, necrotic skin ulceration, especially in non-acral regions and regions without surrounding rash, is considered a predictive factor for the presence of underlying cancer; second, ulceration of Gottron's papules can occur following DMARD therapy, especially methotrexate or mycophenolate mofetil; and third, patients with melanoma differentiation-associated gene 5 antibodies (MDA5) have a higher incidence of ulcerative cutaneous lesions on the digital pulp and periungual areas, within Gottron's papules, and over the elbows (Fig. 8.3) [1]. In addition diffuse punched-out ulcerations and ischemic digital necrosis have been described in literature. These patients may be at higher risk of interstitial lung disease. It should be noted that ulcers can also occur in areas of intense inflammation and may be of no particular prognostic significance.

Rheumatoid arthritis (RA): Pyoderma gangrenosum (PG), rheumatoid vasculitis, venous insufficiency, peripheral arterial disease, peripheral neuropathy, and Felty's syndrome are causes of skin ulcers in RA. The most common location of ulceration is on the lower leg. Leg ulcers in RA patients usually are chronic and occur in patients with seropositive and erosive disease. PG presents as a painful necrotic

Fig. 8.4 Left leg with ulcers in a patient with rheumatoid arthritis

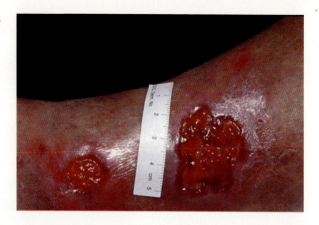

ulcer with undermined border. Felty's syndrome is characterized by RA, spleno-megaly, leg ulcers, and granulocytopenia. Leg ulcers secondary to rheumatoid vas-culitis are usually painful, deep, and punched-out in appearance (Fig. 8.4) [2].

Superficial ulcerating rheumatoid necrobiosis is a chronic, superficial ulceration, commonly on the limbs and most frequently on the lower legs, that histologically shows features of necrobiotic palisading granulomas. It occurs in association with RA but also other CTDs.

Ulceration of the psoriatic plaques secondary to methotrexate toxicity is rare. It can occur within psoriatic plaques during the first month of starting therapy. The pso-riatic plaques become red and painful and then develop a superficial ulceration [3].

Ulcers in vasculitis/vasculopathy can be seen in **granulomatous vasculitis** like Wegener's granulomatosis (WG) and Churg–Strauss syndrome (CSS) where they tend to occur on the elbows. In **necrotizing inflammation** of small to medium arteries in polyarteritis nodosa (PAN), leg ulceration is more common. Vasculopathic diseases include livedoid vasculopathy, thrombophilic disorders, and cryoglobulinemia.

Differential Diagnosis of Ulcers in the Setting of CTD

Cutaneous Ulcers

From the discussion above, it is clear that ulcer location is an important factor in deter-mining etiology – involvement of the nose and ears is suggestive of vasculopathy, often in the setting of cryoproteins, although forms of vasculitis (such as Wegener's) should be considered. In general, extreme pain and/or the presence of necrosis often indicates a vasculopathy of some kind – here, the clinician should be considering vasculopathy related to certain known CTDs (systemic sclerosis, dermatomyositis,

Fig. 8.5 Left leg ulcers in a patient with medium-vessel vasculitis; note the irregularity of the ulcer and the retiform purpura

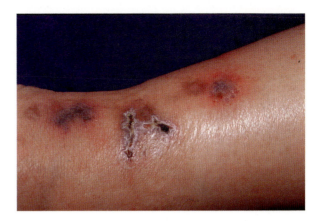

lupus) versus other vasculopathies mentioned above. Irregular borders, angulation in ulcers, and presence of livedo reticularis are suggestive of underlying vasculitis or vasculopathy (Fig. 8.5). Violaceous, elevated, and undermined borders that follow minor trauma are often indicative of pyoderma gangrenosum, which can occur most often in the setting of rheumatoid arthritis, Behçet's disease, and systemic sclerosis.

In addition to ulcers secondary to CTD, common causes of skin ulceration should be excluded. These include arterial ischemia (clues include persistent pain, claudication, diminished pulses, and capillary refill), venous stasis (edema and varicosities), and neuropathy (decreased sensation). A diagnosis of PG is a diagnosis of exclusion that requires clinicopathologic correlation. Biopsy is required for histology, special stains, and culture to exclude other infectious causes such as ecthyma gangrenosum, ecthyma, chronic herpes simplex, sporotrichosis, and mycobacterial, parasitic, or deep fungal infections. Finally, one should consider the possibility of neoplasm or factitial causes of ulceration.

Mucosal Ulcers

Aphthous ulcers can be differentiated from intraoral herpes simplex by location as herpetic ulcers affect the hard palate and attached gingiva, while aphthous ulcers affect nonkeratinized mucosa only. Varicella is characterized by widespread cutaneous vesicular eruption with fever. Hand–foot–mouth disease, caused by coxsackievirus, presents with elliptical vesicles surrounded by an erythematous halo on hands, feet, and buttocks. In herpangina the ulcers affect soft palate and tonsillar pillar areas with lymphadenopathy. Oral ulcerations secondary to inflammatory bowel disease are associated with recurrent bloody or mucous diarrhea and oral ulcerations due to cyclic neutropenia present with fever, cervical lymphadenopathy, and neutropenia [4].

Drugs That Have Been Associated with Ulceration

Methotrexate, hydroxyurea, penicillamine, and cocaine/levamisole have all been associated with skin ulceration. NSAIDs may induce aphthous stomatitis.

Biopsy

A biopsy is useful to confirm the diagnosis histologically, to obtain tissue for culture, and to rule out malignancy. Generally any ulcer that does not heal over 4 months requires a biopsy to exclude underlying malignant changes either primary or secondary, e.g., Marjolin's ulcer (squamous cell carcinoma arising in a preexisting chronic ulcer). The specimen should include subcutaneous tissue from the periphery of the ulcer and the area near the ulcer center. This is achieved by incisional biopsy perpendicular to ulcer edge or multiple punch biopsies. The ulcer tissue specimen needs to be stained with hematoxylin and eosin (routine histology), PAS or silver for fungi, Ziehl–Neelsen for mycobacteria, and Giemsa for leishmaniasis.

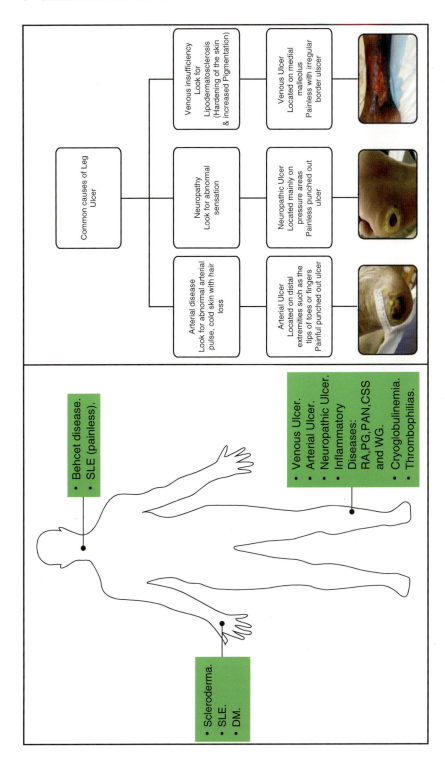

References

1. Fiorentino D, Chung L, Zwerner J, Rosen A, Casciola-Rosen L. The mucocutaneous and systemic phenotype of dermatomyositis patients with antibodies to MDA5 (CADM-140): a retrospective study. J Am Acad Dermatol. 2011;65(1):25–34.
2. McRorie ER, Jobanputra P, Ruckley CV, Nuki G. Leg ulceration in rheumatoid arthritis. Br J Rheumatol. 1994;33(11):1078–84.
3. Pearce HP, Wilson BB. Erosion of psoriatic plaques: an early sign of methotrexate toxicity. J Am Acad Dermatol. 1996;35(5 Pt 2):835–8.
4. McBride DR. Management of aphthous ulcers. Am Fam Physician. 2000;62(1):149–154, 160.

Chapter 9
Panniculitis

Alan Tyndall and Peter Häusermann

Definition

Panniculitis is a nonseptic inflammation of the subcutaneous adipose tissue often reflecting another disorder. It is divided into four histological subgroups, mostly lobular or mostly septal, each one being either with or without vasculitis.

Originally described in 30 patients by Weber and Christian over 60 years ago as a syndrome of recurrent episodes of fever, arthralgia, fatigue, and nodular panniculitis, 30 such cases were later reclassified as erythema nodosum (12 cases), thrombophlebitis (6 cases), fictitial (5 cases), trauma (3 cases), or other lymphoma, leukemia, etc.) [1].

Differential Diagnosis

The diagnosis of panniculitis and the exclusion of other conditions are dependent on an adequately deep biopsy.

Conditions mimicking panniculitis include thrombophlebitis, fictitial lesions, trauma, local sepsis, and infiltrative lesions, e.g., lymphoma.

Within the classification of panniculitis itself, the histological subgrouping into mostly septal or mostly lobular ± vasculitis will guide the clinician as to which

A. Tyndall, Ph.D., M.D. (✉)
Department of Rheumatology, Felix Platter Spital, University Hospital Basel,
Burgfelderstrasse 101, Basel, Switzerland
e-mail: alan.tyndall@usb.ch

P. Häusermann, M.D., FMH
Department of Dermatology, University Hospital Basel, Petersgraben 4,
Basel 4031, Switzerland
e-mail: phaeusermann@uhbs.ch

M. Matucci-Cerinic et al. (eds.), *Skin Manifestations in Rheumatic Disease*,
DOI 10.1007/978-1-4614-7849-2_9, © Springer Science+Business Media New York 2014

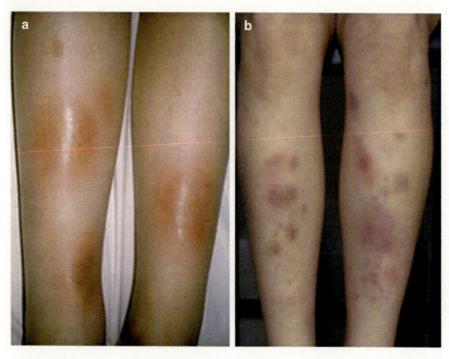

Fig. 9.1 Typical erythema nodosum of the lower legs (**a**) and an atypical macular form (**b**)

condition may be associated. On many occasions the diagnosis of panniculitis may remain as idiopathic.

The commonest panniculitis seen by a rheumatologist is erythema nodosum [2], a painful nonvasculitic, mostly septal form seen on the anterior surface of the lower legs (Fig. 9.1a).

However, erythema nodosum may be atypical, being either widespread small, macular mimicking cutaneous vasculitis or the neutrophilic dermatoses such as Sweet's syndrome (Fig. 9.1b) or diffuse periarticular and mimicking arthritis (Fig. 9.2). Involvement of the upper extremities alone is very rare for erythema nodosum. Known associations and triggers of erythema nodosum include intercurrent viral illnesses; streptococcal, mycobacterial, and yersinia infection; oral contraceptives; antibiotics; SLE and other connective tissue diseases; Crohn's disease; and primary biliary cirrhosis. In many cases of erythema nodosum, an associated trigger or disease will not be identified, up to 20 % in one series [3].

Another nonvasculitic, mostly lobular panniculitis is the rheumatoid nodule. Typically occurring on pressure areas such as the elbows (Fig. 9.3a) with a distinct histology (Fig. 9.4), they may occur anywhere and mimic gouty tophi.

Two other lesions have a similar histology to the rheumatoid nodule: granuloma annulare [4] and necrobiosis lipoidica diabeticorum. The former may be referred to a rheumatologist following biopsy of isolated nodular skin lesions, usually on the dorsum of the foot in a young patient following an intercurrent viral respiratory infection (Fig. 9.3b). Awareness of this self-limiting benign condition will avoid unnecessary biopsies and other investigations.

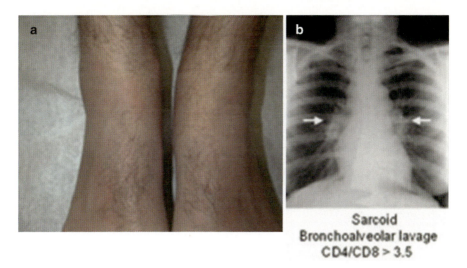

Sarcoid
Bronchoalveolar lavage
CD4/CD8 > 3.5

Fig. 9.2 Diffuse periarticular erythema nodosum on the right ankle – a chest X-ray showed large, bilateral adenopathy (*arrows*) consistent with Loeffler's syndrome (sarcoidosis)

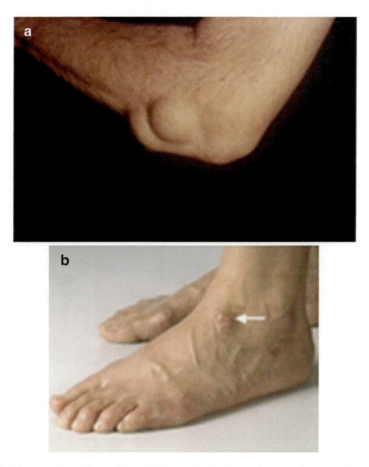

Fig. 9.3 Rheumatoid nodule on elbow (**a**), histologically identical to granuloma annulare on dorsum of foot in another patient (**b**)

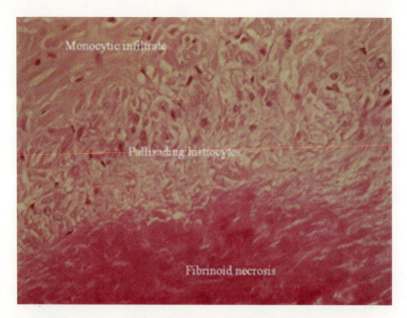

Fig. 9.4 Histology of a rheumatoid nodule

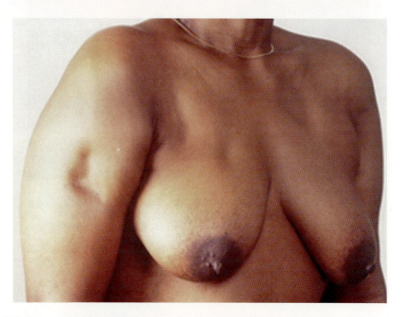

Fig. 9.5 Lupus profundus. Initially inflammatory nodules evolving to atrophy

An unusual form of panniculitis seen in <2 % of SLE patients is lupus profundus [5]. Occurring on the trunk and proximal extremities, this nonvasculitic, painless lesion is mostly lobular and evolves to atrophy (Fig. 9.5).

Fig. 9.6 Cryoglobulin-induced palpable purpura (**a**) after "cold pack" knee pain treatment. The cryoglobulins may precipitate at room temperature and be lost to assay (**b**)

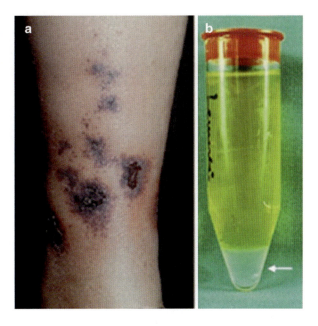

The vasculitides may either mimic or induce a panniculitis. Vasculitides may be classified according to size or etiology. Large-vessel vasculitis is rarely associated with panniculitis. Cutaneous polyarteritis nodosa and the palpable purpura such as Henoch-Schönlein purpura and cryoglobulinemia (Fig. 9.6a) may all be confused with panniculitis. Cutaneous PAN is often seen in younger patients and children and, like HSP, may follow a streptococcal throat infection. HSP is associated with IgA deposition in the vessel wall. In cases of suspected cryoglobulinemia, serum should be kept at 37 °C before testing; otherwise, the cryoprotein may precipitate (Fig. 9.6b). Rheumatoid factor, antibodies to HCV, and paraproteins should be sought.

Behçet's disease may be associated with erythema nodosus-like lesions which differ from classical erythema nodosum in that the backs of the lower legs are involved, and the biopsy shows a vasculitic, mostly lobular histology. This is similar to the nonseptic panniculitis associated with TB called Bazin disease [6].

Biopsy

Figure 9.4 Rheumatoid nodule. Central fibrinoid necrosis surrounded by palisading histiocytes and an outer zone of monocytic infiltrate.

Figure 9.7. The mostly septal, nonvasculitic panniculitis of erythema nodosum (a) showing mixed inflammatory cells extending into the adjacent lobular fat. Small nodules composed of spindle to oval histiocytes arranged around a minute slit may be found (Miescher's radial granulomas). This is compared with the mostly lobular,

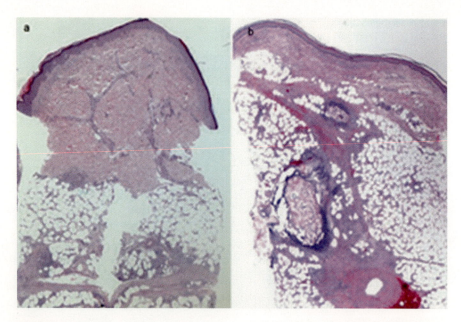

Fig. 9.7 Comparison of mostly septal (**a**) in erythema nodosum and mostly lobular (**b**) in pancreatitis-induced panniculitis. Neither have vasculitis

nonvasculitic panniculitis induced by pancreatitis (b) showing enzymatic fat necrosis, with the ghostlike outline of fat cells remaining. At the margins of the necrotic fat, there is a variable neutrophilic infiltrate with fine basophilic calcium deposits and some hemorrhage.

See Also

SLE, Vasculitis, sarcoidosis,

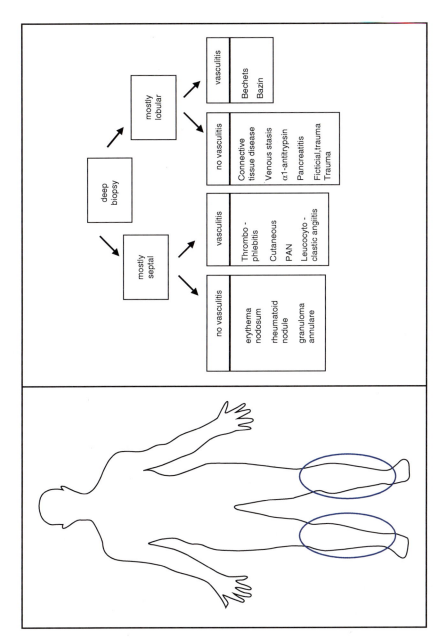

References

1. White Jr JW, Winkelmann RK. Weber-Christian panniculitis: a review of 30 cases with this diagnosis. J Am Acad Dermatol. 1998;39:56–62.
2. Requena L, Yus ES. Erythema nodosum. Dermatol Clin. 2008;26:425–38.
3. Bohn S, Buchner S, Itin P. Erythema nodosum: 112 cases. Epidemiology, clinical aspects and histopathology. Schweiz Med Wochenschr. 1997;127:1168–76.
4. Cyr PR. Diagnosis and management of granuloma annulare. Am Fam Physician. 2006;74: 1729–34.
5. Fraga J, Garcia-Diez A. Lupus erythematosus panniculitis. Dermatol Clin. 2008;26:453–63.
6. Mascaro Jr JM, Baselga E. Erythema induratum of bazin. Dermatol Clin. 2008;26:439–45.

Chapter 10
Diagnosing Puffy Fingers in the Rheumatic Patient

Kazuhiko Takehara

Introduction

In the literature, a clear definition of puffy fingers is not found, but patients with many different rheumatic disorders complain of this sign. Herein, the diseases that may present with puffy fingers are presented.

Differential Diagnosis

Systemic Sclerosis (SSc)

Recently it has been shown that very early SSc may be suspected on the basis of Raynaud's phenomenon, puffy fingers, autoantibodies, and SSc capillaroscopic pattern [1]. We previously reported that patients with both Raynaud's phenomenon and positive anticentromere antibody (ACA) developed the symptoms of SSc after several years of observation. In contrast, patients with ACA without Raynaud's phenomenon did not develop SSc [2].

lcSSc with ACA

In many cases of limited cutaneous SSc (lcSSc), Raynaud's phenomenon, puffy fingers, and SSc abnormal capillaroscopic pattern precede skin sclerosis. ACA is also

K. Takehara, M.D., Ph.D. (✉)
Department of Dermatology, Kanazawa University, 13-1 Takaramachi,
Kanazawa, Ishikawa 920-8641, Japan
e-mail: takehara@med.kanazawa-u.ac.jp

M. Matucci-Cerinic et al. (eds.), *Skin Manifestations in Rheumatic Disease*,
DOI 10.1007/978-1-4614-7849-2_10, © Springer Science+Business Media New York 2014

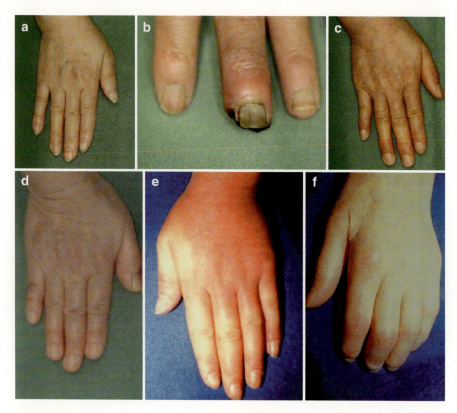

Fig. 10.1 Puffy fingers in SSc. (**a**) lcSSc with ACA, which may tend towards sclerodactyly. (**b**) lcSSc with ACA, associated with skin gangrenous ulcers but not sclerosis. (**c**) lcSSc with ACA exhibiting sclerodactyly. (**d**) lcSSc with anti-Th/To antibody; only puffy fingers without tendency towards sclerodactyly. (**e**) SSc with anti-topo. Puffy fingers with skin sclerosis. (**f**) Sclerodactyly following puffy fingers in patients with anti-RNAP

detected in the very early stage of SSc [3]. Figure 10.1a shows the early puffy fingers of lcSSc, which may tend towards sclerodactyly. Figure 10.1b shows fingers with gangrenous ulcers, which do not exhibit skin sclerosis; our diagnosis was early lcSSc with ACA and prominent vascular disturbance. Figure 10.1c shows fingers of a late stage of lcSSc with ACA, which should be expressed as "sclerodactyly."

lcSSc with Anti-Th/To Antibody

Autoantibody against Th/To antigen is well known as a serological marker of SSc sine scleroderma [4, 5], meaning that many of the patients with anti-Th/To antibody exhibit only puffy fingers without a tendency to exhibit sclerodactyly. Figure 10.1d shows typical fingers of patients with lcSSc and Th/To antibody.

Early SSc with Anti-Topoisomerase I Antibody (Anti-Topo)

In general, SSc patients with anti-topo develop rapidly progressing skin sclerosis, and most of them are eventually diagnosed with diffuse cutaneous SSc (dcSSc). These patients exhibit puffy fingers tending towards sclerodactyly from an early stage of the disease. Figure 10.1e shows the typical puffy fingers associated with skin sclerosis. Histological examination also showed dermal fibrosis.

Sclerodactyly in dcSSc with Anti-RNA Polymerase Antibody (Anti-RNAP)

The patients with anti-RNAP develop rapid progression of skin sclerosis. Therefore, puffy fingers in this subset accompany development of sclerodactyly with joint contracture. Figure 10.1f shows typical sclerodactyly following puffy fingers.

Anti-u1 RNP Antibody Syndrome

Mixed connective tissue disease (MCTD) was first described by Sharp et al. in 1972 [6]; subsequently, this disease was characterized by the presence of anti-u1 RNP antibody. The clinical entity includes mixed features of different rheumatic diseases such as SSc, systemic lupus erythematosus, and/or dermatomyositis/polymyositis. However, in 1980 LeRoy et al. claimed that this syndrome includes ongoing rheumatic disorders and should be expressed as "undifferentiated connective tissue syndrome (UCTS)" [7].

As described above, a consensus has not yet been reached, and the debate over whether MCTD constitutes a distinct clinical entity has yet to be resolved. However, patients with anti-u1 RNP antibody almost always also exhibit Raynaud's phenomenon, abnormal capillaroscopic findings, and puffy fingers. In this condition, edematous fingers are generally expressed as "sausage-like fingers." Therefore, I include above disorders as anti-u1 RNP antibody syndrome in this chapter.

Figure 10.2 shows typical sausage-like fingers in a case of MCTD that we previously observed. Such patients also exhibit mild overlapping clinical features such as low number of WBC, elevated CPK, arthralgia, and mild interstitial pneumonia. Most of these features were improved by oral treatment of low-dosage corticosteroid, with the exception of interstitial pneumonia. Edematous fingers were also improved but not completely cured.

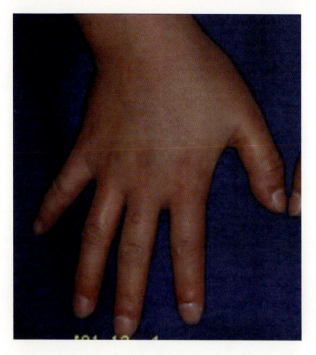

Fig. 10.2 Puffy fingers in MCTD, usually expressed as "sausage-like fingers"

SSc-Like Disorders

Many other conditions present with skin fibrosis and may be confused with SSc. SSc-like disorders include immune-mediated diseases (eosinophilic fasciitis, graft-versus-host disease), deposition disorders (scleromyxedema, nephrogenic systemic fibrosis, systemic amyloidosis), toxic exposures (toxic oil, ʟ-tryptophan, bleomycin, polyvinyl chloride), and genetic syndromes (progeria, stiff skin syndrome) [8]. Some of the above patients may seldom complain of puffy fingers. Figure 10.3 shows nephrogenic systemic fibrosis with slight contracture.

Anti-aminoacyl-tRNA Synthetase Antibody Syndrome (ARS Syndrome)

ARS is one of the myositis-specific autoantibodies, and patients with ARS frequently exhibit interstitial lung disease [9]. Some cases of ARS syndrome also exhibit Raynaud's phenomenon and abnormal capillaroscopic findings. Figure 10.4 shows puffy fingers with typical mechanic's hand. "Mechanic's hand" is frequently observed in ARS syndrome.

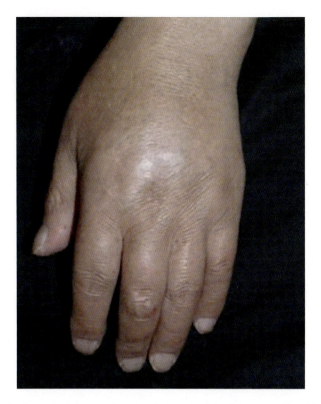

Fig. 10.3 Puffy fingers in nephrogenic systemic fibrosis with slight contracture (This figure was kindly provided by Dr. Nagai of Gunma University, Department of Dermatology)

Rheumatoid Arthritis (RA)

Patients with RA also complain of puffy fingers as well as morning stiffness, joint pain, and joint swelling. For the early diagnosis of RA, X-ray analysis, serological investigations including anti-cyclic citrullinated peptide antibody [10], and MRI examinations among others are required. Figure 10.5 shows puffy fingers in RA with PIP joint swelling.

Overlapping Syndromes

Some patients with rheumatic diseases may have multiple disorders, and the clinical features of these patients are complicated. Figure 10.6a shows puffy fingers with SSc and SLE, as well as some erythematous lesions of LE. Figure 10.6b shows puffy fingers with SSc and RA with joint swelling.

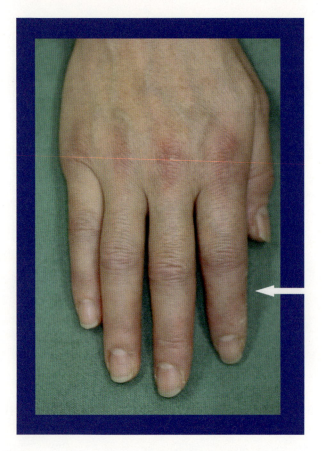

Fig. 10.4 Puffy fingers in ARS syndrome with mechanic's hand (*arrow*)

Erythema Pernio

We recently observed a case for which it was very difficult to reach a final diagnosis. As shown in Fig. 10.7, the patient exhibited swollen fingers with possible sclerodactyly. However, intensive investigation showed no evidence of rheumatic disorders. Antinuclear antibody was negative and capillaroscopy normal. Skin biopsy from fingertip erythema allowed the diagnosis of erythema pernio. By treatment with topical corticosteroid, erythematous lesions disappeared and the swollen fingers improved.

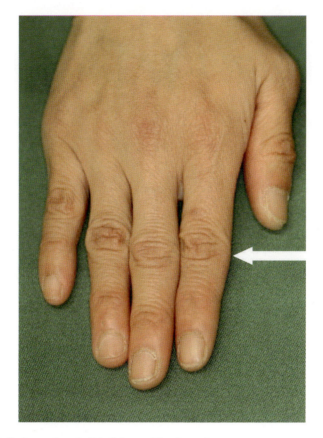

Fig. 10.5 Puffy fingers in early RA. Joint swelling (*arrow*)

Other Conditions

The patients with other conditions as thyroiditis/hypothyroidism, acromegalia, primary Raynaud's disease, dermatomyositis, etc. may complain puffy fingers, and these conditions should be kept in mind for differential diagnosis.

Differential Diagnosis Between Systemic Sclerosis and Other Rheumatic Disease Based on Histological Observation from Skin Biopsy

The typical histological findings of systemic sclerosis are shown in Fig. 10.8a, c. At the early edematous stage when a patient complains of puffy fingers, only edematous findings between collagen bundles and a small number of infiltrating lymphocytes

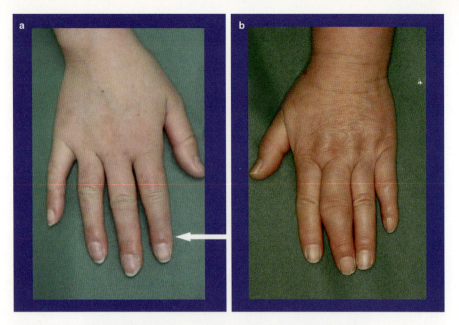

Fig. 10.6 (**a**) Puffy fingers in overlapping syndrome with SLE and SSc. LE lesion (*arrow*). (**b**) Puffy fingers in overlapping syndrome with SSc and RA

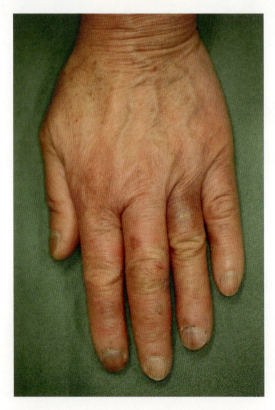

Fig. 10.7 Puffy fingers in pernio. Negative antinuclear antibody and normal capillaroscopic findings

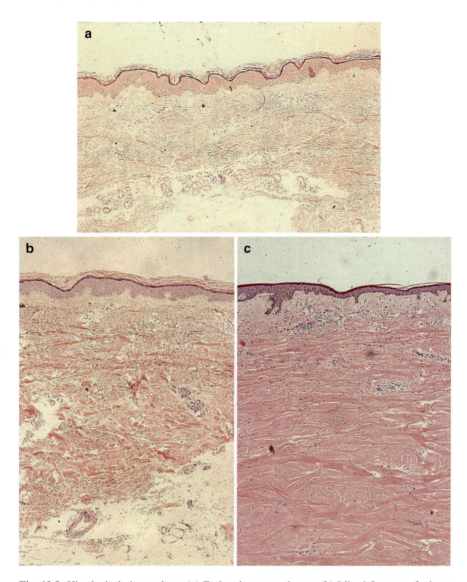

Fig. 10.8 Histological observations. (**a**) Early edematous change. (**b**) Mixed features of edema and fibrosis. (**c**) Fibrosis in the entire dermis

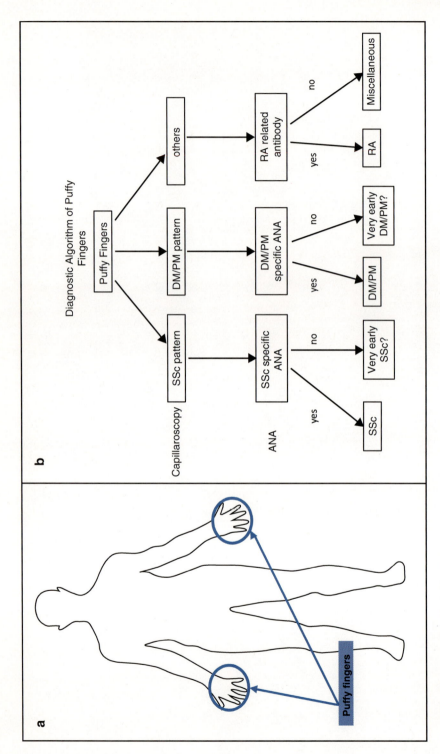

Fig. 10.9 Diagnostic algorithm of puffy fingers

are observed (Fig. 10.8a). A patient with puffy fingers tending towards sclerodactyly shows mixed features with edema and collagen accumulation in lower dermis, as shown in Fig. 10.8b. A patient with clear sclerodactyly demonstrates abundant collagen accumulations in the entire dermis, as shown in Fig. 10.8c. Thus, histological examination of skin biopsy is often useful for the detection of early systemic sclerosis.

Conclusion

Clearly, there remains some difficulty in describing puffy fingers as evidenced by this chapter. I am convinced that future EUSTAR efforts will resolve this difficult issue.

References

1. Matucci-Cerinic M, Allanore Y, Czirjá L, et al. The challenge of early systemic sclerosis for the EULAR Scleroderma Trial and Research Group (EUSTAR) community. It is time to cut the Gordian knot and develop a prevention or rescue strategy. Ann Rheum Dis. 2009;68: 1377–80.
2. Takehara K, Soma Y, Igarashi A, et al. Longitudinal study of patients with anticentromere antibody. Dermatologica. 1991;181:202–6.
3. Hamaguchi Y, Hasegawa M, Fujimoto M, et al. The clinical relevance of serum antinuclear antibodies in Japanese patients with systemic sclerosis. Br J Dermatol. 2008;158:487–95.
4. Fischer A, Meehan RT, Feghali-Bostwick CA, et al. Unique characteristics of systemic sclerosis sine scleroderma-associated interstitial lung disease. Chest. 2006;130:976–81.
5. Fischer A, Pfalzgraf FJ, Feghali-Bostwick CA, et al. Anti-th/to-positivity in a cohort of patients with idiopathic pulmonary fibrosis. J Rheumatol. 2006;33:1600–5.
6. Sharp GC, Irvin WS, Tan EM, et al. Mixed connective tissue disease–an apparently distinct rheumatic disease syndrome associated with a specific antibody to an extractable nuclear antigen (ENA). Am J Med. 1972;52:148–59.
7. LeRoy EC, Maricq HR, Kahaleh MB. Undifferentiated connective tissue syndromes. Arthritis Rheum. 1980;23:341–3.
8. Khurana A, Runge VM, Narayanan M, et al. Nephrogenic systemic fibrosis: a review of 6 cases temporally related to gadodiamide injection (omniscan). Invest Radiol. 2007;42:139–45.
9. Targoff IN. Myositis specific autoantibodies. Curr Rheumatol Rep. 2006;8:196–203.
10. Shidara K, Inoue E, Tanaka E, et al. Comparison of the second and third generation anti-cyclic citrullinated peptide antibody assays in the diagnosis of Japanese patients with rheumatoid arthritis. Rheumatol Int. 2010;31(5):617–22.

Part II
Methodology

Chapter 11
Capillaroscopy

Maurizio Cutolo, Alberto Sulli, Carmen Pizzorni, and Vanessa Smith

Capillaroscopy

Capillaroscopy is a noninvasive imaging technique that is used for the *in vivo* assessment of the microcirculation. Its principal role in rheumatology and dermatology is to differentiate the primary and secondary forms of Raynaud's phenomenon (RP) associated with connective tissue disease [1]. Capillary microscopy can be performed with various optical instruments such as the ophthalmoscope, dermatoscope, photomacrography system, stereomicroscope, conventional optical microscope, and the videocapillaroscope. The nailfold videocapillaroscope (NVC) with handheld device has the advantages that it is easy to learn and is a handheld device (=probe) which can be used in situations in which the use of the traditional microscope may be less convenient (such as in patients with finger flexion contractures) and its relatively high magnification (200–500x) is advantageous compared to the older widefield technique (Fig. 11.1).

M. Cutolo, M.D. (✉) •A. Sulli, M.D.• C. Pizzorni, M.D., Ph.D.
Department of Internal Medicine, Research Laboratory and Academic
Unit of Clinical Rheumatology, University of Genova, Viale Benedetto XV 6,
16132 Genoa, Italy
e-mail: mcutolo@unige.it; albertosulli@unige.it; carmcarmenpizzorni@virgilio.it

V. Smith, M.D., Ph.D.
Department of Rheumatology, Ghent University Hospital, De pintelaan 185,
9000 Ghent, Belgium
e-mail: Vanessa.Smith@UGent.be

M. Matucci-Cerinic et al. (eds.), *Skin Manifestations in Rheumatic Disease*,
DOI 10.1007/978-1-4614-7849-2_11, © Springer Science+Business Media New York 2014

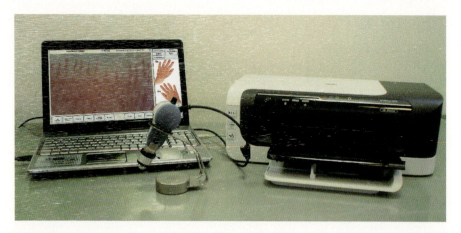

Fig. 11.1 A videocapillaroscope that is used in detecting the microcirculation at the level of the nailfold bed

Capillaroscopic Detection of the Early Microvascular Alterations That Are Markers of Secondary Raynaud's Phenomenon

The morphologic changes that characterize the microvasculature in the scleroderma-spectrum diseases at the level of the nailfold have been extensively described – giant capillaries, microhemorrhages, loss of capillaries, neovascularization, and avascular areas (Fig. 11.2) [2].

The microvascular alterations have been recently reclassified in systemic sclerosis (SSc) into three defined and different NVC patterns:

1. An "early pattern" (few giant capillaries, few capillary microhemorrhages, no evident loss of capillaries, and relatively well-preserved capillary distribution)
2. An "active pattern" (frequent giant capillaries, frequent capillary microhemorrhages, moderate loss of capillaries, absence or mild ramified capillaries with mild disorganization of the capillary architecture)
3. A "late pattern" (almost absent giant capillaries and microhemorrhages, severe loss of capillaries with extensive avascular areas, ramified/bushy capillaries, and intense disorganization of the normal capillary array) [3] (Fig. 11.3)

The marked increase in capillary size is the most characteristic feature of the nailfold capillary bed (giant capillary) in early secondary RP. In particular, the detection of enlarged and giant capillaries, together with microextravasation (hemorrhage) of the red blood cells in the nailfold, most likely represents the first morphologic sign of the altered microcirculation in systemic sclerosis.

The shape of the widened capillaries is largely heterogeneous, but giant capillaries with a homogeneous enlargement (diameter over 50 μm) are an absolute marker

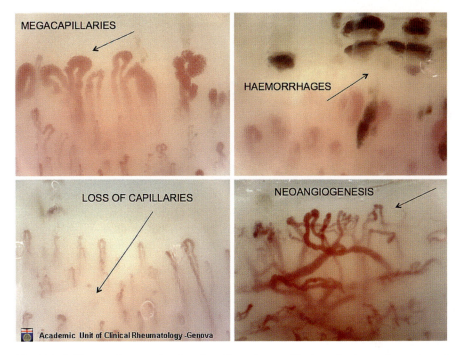

Fig. 11.2 Different microvascular alterations (i.e., *giant capillaries, microhemorrhages, loss of capillaries,* and *neovascularization*) that characterize the secondary Raynaud's phenomenon

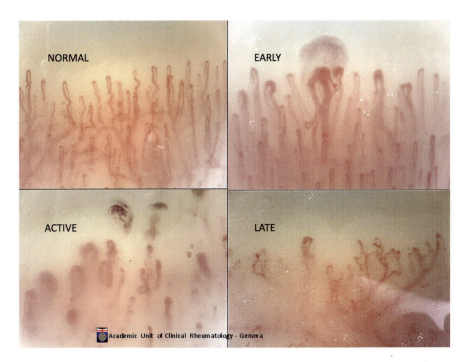

Fig. 11.3 The three scleroderma patters (*early, active, late*) compared to the microvasculature in a normal health control subject

of the scleroderma capillaroscopic pattern. This picture characterizes the "early" (initial) SSc capillaroscopic pattern (Fig. 11.3) [4]. As the pathophysiological process of SSc progresses into fibrosis, the capillaroscopic analysis most likely reflects the effects of tissue hypoxia/massive capillary destruction, then increased loss of capillaries and avascular areas are observed, together with bushy capillaries indicating neoangiogenesis. This advanced stage of the systemic sclerosis is characterized by the "late" capillaroscopic pattern (Fig. 11.3). We know that patients with the "early" capillaroscopic pattern may have had RP for many years, and a transition from primary to secondary RP may be expected in almost 15 % of subjects in an average time of 29 months [5].

To quantify the microvascular changes, a practical system to score these capillaroscopic alterations in systemic sclerosis patients has been proposed recently and validated [6, 7]. Studies on nailfold capillary changes over time or in response to therapy are currently ongoing.

Learning to Use Capillaroscopy

Recent preliminary experience indicates that technical and operative skills in capillaroscopy, using a videomicroscopy system, can be achieved in approximately five nonconsecutive hours by an untrained specialist, in the context of a self-teaching program under expert supervision [8]. The beginner's performances show that self-efficacy increases with practical experience, and image quality is reached in up to 70 % of learners by the third session [8].

Scleroderma Capillaroscopic Patterns and Serum Autoantibodies in Systemic Sclerosis

Regarding the anti-endothelial cell antibodies (AECA), these have been detected significantly more frequent in SSc patients with the "late" capillaroscopic pattern compared to the "early" and "active" patterns ($p < 0.05$) [9]. Concerning the anti-topoisomerase I (anti-Scl70) and anticentromere (ACA) antibodies, anti-Scl70 were found more frequent again in SSc patients showing the "active" and "late" patterns, whereas ACA especially in patients with the "early" pattern [10].

In a large prospective study, enlarged/giant capillaries, capillary loss, and more SSc-specific autoantibodies independently predicted definite SSc [11]. The authors reported associations between certain patterns of capillary abnormality and different specific autoantibodies. Anti-CENP-B and anti-Th/To antibodies predicted enlarged/giant capillaries; these autoantibodies and anti-RNAP III predicted capillary loss. Interestingly, each autoantibody was associated with a distinct time course of microvascular damage, as gauged by capillary enlargement or capillary loss.

At follow-up, 79.5 % of patients with one of these autoantibodies and abnormal findings on nailfold capillary microscopy at baseline had developed definite SSc. Patients with both baseline predictors (abnormal capillaroscopy and an SSc-specific autoantibody) were 60 times more likely to develop definite SSc.

Finally, the association of specific antinuclear antibodies positivity and the presence of the NVC scleroderma pattern have been proposed as biomarkers for the very early diagnosis of SSc together with clinical symptoms (i.e., Raynaud's phenomenon and/or puffy fingers) [12].

Possible Predictive Value of Capillaroscopy for Clinical Outcome in Systemic Sclerosis Patients

Systemic sclerosis microangiopathy correlates with disease subsets and the severity of peripheral vascular, skin, and lung involvement; in particular, patients with the "late" pattern showed an increased risk to have active disease and have moderate/severe skin or visceral involvement compared to patients with "early" and "active" capillaroscopic patterns [13].

Skin ulcers are a common vascular complication of SSc and seem now recognized in association with rapidly progressive capillary loss and the "late" NVC pattern, characterized by progressive avascular areas. An association with trophic lesions and loss of capillaries, as assessed by semiquantitative scoring, has also been reported [14]. Very recently, in 130 SSc patients examined at entry and after 20 months of follow-up, the diffuse cutaneous SSc phenotype with avascular areas on capillaroscopy represented, among other factors (e.g., increased IL-6), the major risk factor for ulcer development [15].

A recent study developed a capillaroscopic skin ulcer risk index (CSURI) that might predict the onset of new digital ulcers by using NVC analysis in patients with SSc [16]. However, this index is complex and time consuming, and the authors found that also the simple decrease of capillary number alone is sufficient as marker. A more recent simple capillaroscopic index (day-to-day DU index), prognostic for digital trophic skin lesions and based just on loss of capillaries alone, has been published showing high sensitivity and specificity [17].

Digital ulcers have been associated with significantly reduced blood flow at fingertips; in addition, SSc patients with the scleroderma "active" and "late" NVC patterns showed decreased blood flow velocity (65.5 % and 66.2 % reduction, respectively), and in particular, the reduced blood flow velocity was significantly associated with capillary ramification and capillary loss [18].

Ideally, future studies examining associations between digital ulceration and nailfold capillaroscopic patterns should consider digital tip ulcers and extensor surface ulcers. Recent studies showed that nailfold capillary density and its decrease are associated with the presence of lung involvement and severity of pulmonary arterial hypertension in systemic sclerosis patients [19, 20].

Conclusions

Videocapillaroscopy is considered fundamental for differentiating between primary and secondary Raynaud's phenomenon [1–3, 5]. The validated scoring of the capillaroscopic markers of the scleroderma patterns is supported for follow-up of systemic sclerosis patients, at least already in some centers [6, 7]. The prognostic and predictive value of capillary density is becoming an index of outcome in patients affected by systemic sclerosis [21, 22]. As with specific autoantibodies, further larger-scale studies, both cross-sectional and longitudinal, are required and are ongoing to examine further the associations between capillaroscopic findings and other parameters/biomarkers of disease.

References

1. Cutolo M, Sulli A, Smith V. Assessing microvascular changes in systemic sclerosis diagnosis and management. Nature Rev Rheumatol. 2010;6:578.
2. Herrick AL, Cutolo M. Clinical implications from capillaroscopic analysis in patients with Raynaud's phenomenon and systemic sclerosis. Arthritis Rheum. 2010;62:2595.
3. Cutolo M, Sulli A, Pizzorni C, et al. Nailfold videocapillaroscopy assessment of microvascular damage in systemic sclerosis. J Rheumatol. 2000;27:155.
4. Cutolo M, Sulli A, Secchi ME, et al. The contribution of capillaroscopy to the differential diagnosis of connective autoimmune diseases. Best Pract Res Clin Rheumatol. 2007;21:1093.
5. Cutolo M, Pizzorni C, Sulli A. Identification of transition from primary Raynaud's phenomenon to secondary Raynaud's phenomenon by nailfold videocapillaroscopy. Arthritis Rheum. 2007;56:2102.
6. Sulli A, Secchi ME, Pizzorni C, Cutolo M. Scoring the nailfold microvascular changes during the capillaroscopic analysis in systemic sclerosis patients. Ann Rheum Dis. 2008;67:885.
7. Smith V, Pizzorni C, De Keyser F, et al. Reliability of the qualitative and semiquantitative nailfold videocapillaroscopy assessment in a systemic sclerosis cohort: a two-centre study. Ann Rheum Dis. 2010;69:1092.
8. De Angelis R, Cutolo M, Salaffi F, Restrepo JP, Grassi W. Quantitative and qualitative assessment of onc rheumatology trainee's experience with a self-teaching programme in videocapillaroscopy. Clin Exp Rheumatol. 2009;27:651.
9. Riccieri V, Germano V, Alessandri C, et al. More severe nailfold capillaroscopy findings and anti-endothelial cell antibodies. Are they useful tools for prognostic use in systemic sclerosis? Clin Exp Rheumatol. 2008;26:992.
10. Cutolo M, Pizzorni C, Tuccio M, et al. Nailfold videocapillaroscopic patterns and serum autoantibodies in systemic sclerosis. Rheumatology (Oxford). 2004;43:719.
11. Koenig M, Joyal F, Fritzler MJ, et al. Autoantibodies and microvascular damage are independent predictive factors for the progression of Raynaud's phenomenon to systemic sclerosis: a twenty-year prospective study of 586 patients, with validation of proposed criteria for early systemic sclerosis. Arthritis Rheum. 2008;58:3902.
12. Avouac J, Fransen J, Walker UA, et al. Preliminary criteria for the very early diagnosis of systemic sclerosis: results of a Delphi consensus study from EULAR scleroderma trials and research group. Ann Rheum Dis. 2011;70:476.
13. Caramaschi P, Canestrini S, Martinelli N, et al. Scleroderma patients nailfold videocapillaroscopic patterns are associated with disease subset and disease severity. Rheumatology (Oxford). 2007;46:1566.

14. Smith V, Pizzorni C, De Keyser F, et al. Validation of the qualitative and semiquantitative assessment of the scleroderma spectrum patterns by nailfold videocapillaroscopy: preliminary results. Arthritis Rheum. 2009;60:S164.
15. Alivernini S, De Santis M, Tolusso B, et al. Skin ulcers in systemic sclerosis: determinants of presence and predictive factors of healing. J Am Acad Dermatol. 2009;60:426.
16. Sebastiani M, Manfredi A, Colaci M, et al. Capillaroscopic skin ulcer risk index: a new prognostic tool for digital skin ulcer development in systemic sclerosis patients. Arthritis Rheum. 2009;61:688.
17. Smith V, De Keyser F, Pizzorni C, et al. Nailfold capillaroscopy for day-to-day clinical use: construction of a simple scoring modality as a clinical prognostic index for digital trophic lesions. Ann Rheum Dis. 2011;70:180.
18. Cutolo M, Ferrone C, Pizzorni C, et al. Peripheral blood perfusion correlates with microvascular abnormalities in systemic sclerosis: a laser-Doppler and nailfold videocapillaroscopy study. J Rheumatol. 2010;37:1174.
19. Ong YY, Nikoloutsopoulos T, Bond CP, et al. Decreased nailfold capillary density in limited scleroderma with pulmonary hypertension. Asian Pac J Allergy Immunol. 1998;16:8.
20. Hofstee HM, Noordegraaf AV, Voskuyl AE, et al. Nailfold capillary density is associated with the presence and severity of pulmonary arterial hypertension in systemic sclerosis. Ann Rheum Dis. 2009;68:19.
21. Sulli A, Pizzorni C, Smith V, et al. Timing of transition between capillaroscopic patterns in systemic sclerosis. Arthritis Rheum. 2012;64:821–5.
22. Smith V, Decuman S, Sulli A, et al. Do worsening scleroderma capillaroscopic patterns predict future severe organ involvement? A pilot study. Ann Rheum Dis. 2012;71(10):1636–9.

Chapter 12
Use of Biopsy

Flavia Fedeles and Jane M. Grant-Kels

Introduction

Abnormalities of the skin can frequently be found in rheumatic diseases. The skin is easily accessible to biopsy and can serve as an important diagnostic and prognostic marker. A variety of lesions may be present such as papulosquamous rashes, vesicles and bullae, nodules, purpura, and ulcers. Not all skin lesions require biopsy but given the variability of the cutaneous clinical manifestations of rheumatologic diseases, a properly performed skin biopsy can be a powerful diagnostic tool. Correlation of histological findings with the clinical presentation is often necessary to arrive at the correct diagnosis.

Site Selection

Anatomical Region

In choosing a site of biopsy, one should avoid as much as possible cosmetically important areas (such as the face) and areas with poor healing (such as the lower legs). Also, one should avoid areas that are infected or areas that have a high

F. Fedeles, M.D., M.S.
Department of Dermatology, Rhode Island Hospital/Warren Alpert Medical School
of Brown University, 593 Eddy St, APC 10, Providence, RI 02903, USA
e-mail: ffedeles@gmail.com

J.M. Grant-Kels, M.D. (⊠)
Dermatology Department, University of CT Health Center, 21 South Road,
Farmington, CT 06032, USA
e-mail: grant@uchc.edu

M. Matucci-Cerinic et al. (eds.), *Skin Manifestations in Rheumatic Disease*,   101
DOI 10.1007/978-1-4614-7849-2_12, © Springer Science+Business Media New York 2014

incidence of secondary infection (such as the groin and axillae). In addition, regions of the body with marked sun exposure or areas exposed to constant friction may be difficult for the dermatopathologist to interpret due to secondary changes.

Type of Lesion

Choosing a proper lesion to biopsy is critical to get accurate results, especially when further studies are required, such as immunofluorescence. The clinical presentation and the type of lesion characteristic for a certain disorder as a whole are important when determining the biopsy technique and the site of biopsy (Table 12.1). Generally, an untreated, well-formed skin lesion in an early stage should be chosen for biopsy [1]. Small lesions can be biopsied in the center, while large lesions should be biopsied in the area that is most abnormal or the advancing edge. When blisters, vesicles, ulcers, or necrosis are present, the edge of the lesion should be biopsied so that both the affected and adjacent normal skin can be examined [1]. Lesions with secondary changes (excoriations, fissures, erosions) should be avoided since they may show only nonspecific features. When direct immunofluorescence is needed, one should also biopsy perilesional normal-looking skin in addition to lesional skin [1].

Lupus Band Test – When lupus erythematosus (LE) is suspected, three biopsies can be done: lesional skin, non-lesional sun-exposed skin, and non-lesional sun-protected skin [2, 3]. A band-like deposition of immunoglobulin/complement at the dermal-epidermal junction is present in lesional skin in a majority of LE patients. This band may be seen in non-lesional skin of LE patients and may help to distinguish between cutaneous LE and systemic LE [3]. The presence of three or more immunoreactants at the dermal-epidermal junction in sun-protected non-lesional skin correlates with high diagnostic specificity for systemic LE [3]. Controversy about the diagnostic and prognostic significance of the non-lesional lupus band test still persists however.

Biopsy Techniques

Various techniques can be used to perform a skin biopsy based on the type of lesion, the site of lesion, the differential diagnosis, and the purpose of the biopsy. In the case of connective tissue diseases, the punch biopsy which samples both the epidermis and the dermis is most commonly used [1, 4]. Other useful techniques include incisional (wedge) biopsy, excisional biopsy, and punch within a punch biopsy (Fig. 12.1) for the purpose of sampling an adequate amount of subcutaneous tissue [4]. Shave biopsies are not recommended when biopsying inflammatory lesions of the skin.

Table 12.1 Selection of biopsy technique and biopsy site based on clinical presentation

Clinical presentation	Biopsy technique	Biopsy site	Direct immunofluorescence biopsy site	Comments
Blisters/bullae	Punch biopsy	Edge of the blister or entire blister	Punch biopsy of perilesional skin or normal skin adjacent to the lesion	Keep the roof of the blister attached
Necrosis/ulceration	Punch biopsy	Edge of the ulcer or the necrotic area	Edge of the ulcer or the necrotic area or adjacent skin	
Rash/dermatitis	Punch biopsy	New lesion	Lesional skin and non-lesional skin	Multiple punches required if multiple morphologies present
Connective tissue diseases	Punch biopsy	Lesional skin	Lesional skin Lupus band test – Lesional skin for DLE, SLE, and SCLE – Non-lesional sun-exposed skin for SLE and SCLE – Non-lesional, nonsun-exposed skin for SLE	Older lesions may show negative DIF Avoid ulcerations and facial lesions if possible Lupus profundus may have negative lupus band test
Vasculitis	Punch biopsy	Lesional skin of less than 48 h duration Non-ulcerated lesions	Lesional skin of less than 48 h duration or adjacent normal skin	DIF is helpful to rule out Henoch-Schönlein purpura
Panniculitis	Wedge incisional biopsy Punch within a punch biopsy	Lesional skin	Lesional skin	Adequate sampling of subcutaneous fat is required for diagnosis
Nodules	Punch biopsy	Lesional skin	Lesional skin	

DLE discoid lupus erythematosus, *SLE* systemic lupus erythematosus, *SCLE* subacute cutaneous lupus erythematosus, *DIF* direct immunofluorescence (Based on data from Refs. [2, 3, 9])

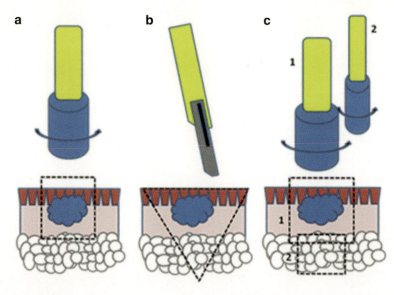

Fig. 12.1 Biopsy techniques: (**a**) punch biopsy, (**b**) incisional (wedge) or excisional biopsy, (**c**) punch within a punch biopsy

Punch Biopsy

The punch biopsy [5, 6] is the primary technique to obtain full-thickness specimens and is suitable for inflammatory lesions especially those with deep components such as lupus erythematosus and vasculitis. A disposable punch biopsy instrument is used which consists of a circular blade attached to a pencillike handle. The diameter varies from 2 to 8 mm, but in most cases a 3–4 mm instrument is adequate. The selected biopsy site is cleaned with a skin antiseptic such as isopropyl alcohol or povidone-iodine. A surgical marker can be used to mark the intended biopsy site. A local anesthetic, usually 1 % or 2 % lidocaine with epinephrine, is administered adjacent to or into the lesion by raising a skin wheal to decrease discomfort and bleeding. Epinephrine should be avoided for distal acral lesions. The skin surrounding the biopsy site is stretched perpendicular to the lines of least skin tension to obtain an oval-shaped wound. The punch is placed perpendicular to the skin and rotated downward using a twirling motion with constant pressure. Once the instrument reaches the subcutaneous fat and resistance lessens, the instrument is removed. The specimen is gently elevated with forceps or a needle tip, and scissors are used to free it from the subcutaneous tissue by cutting below the dermis or if possible below the subcutaneous tissue when fat needs to be sampled. Care is required in removing the specimen to prevent crushing artifacts. The specimen should be immediately placed in fixative (10 % formalin) or Michel's medium for immunofluorescence. The wound can be closed with one or two nylon sutures. Small wounds can be allowed to heal by secondary intention. On the scalp, best results are achieved by holding the instrument along the axis of the hair follicle. When different fixatives are required, two specimens should be taken rather than cutting one specimen into two parts. Care must be taken on the areas where the skin is thin or overlying the bone to decrease the possibility of hitting the periosteum or the nerves and arteries below the skin. Post procedure, Vaseline or antibiotic ointment can be applied, followed by a dry dressing.

Wedge Biopsy

When the primary pathologic process is in the subcutaneous fat, a punch biopsy may be inadequate since it usually does not provide sufficient adipose tissue for histopathologic diagnosis. In these cases, a wedge biopsy [7] should be performed. This technique is also useful when the lesions are large (nodules) or very fragile (bullae). The biopsy site is prepped in a similar fashion to the punch biopsy site. A scalpel blade is used to make an incision in a V down to and occasionally through the subcutaneous fat. The wedge is usually oriented at right angles to the perimeter of the lesion, and the incision may extend from the center of the lesion into the surrounding normal skin. Once the specimen is removed, the wound is closed with sutures.

Punch Within a Punch Biopsy

Alternatively, when a deep biopsy is needed, a "punch within punch" approach can be employed [8]. A larger punch biopsy is initially performed (5–6 mm) followed by a smaller punch (3–4 mm) in the same site once the first specimen is removed. This allows for sampling of the subcutaneous fat in suspected cases of panniculitis.

Potential Outcomes

Many cutaneous manifestations have nonspecific histopathology, and therefore a combination of clinical impression and biopsy results is required for diagnosis. A negative biopsy cannot always exclude a particular disease. Failure to perform a prompt biopsy is often the reason for nonspecific findings since treated lesions or secondary lesions may not show the characteristic findings of a particular disease process.

Rheumatoid Arthritis (RA) – Granulomatous and neutrophilic skin lesions are typical skin manifestations in rheumatoid arthritis. Rheumatoid nodules, while characteristic features, are not specific to RA, and clinically other entities may be considered in the differential diagnosis. Biopsy of a nodule may be helpful in establishing the diagnosis since nodules may show specific histopathologic characteristics. Skin biopsy may also be helpful in establishing the diagnosis of vasculitis in RA patients although histologically rheumatoid vasculitis may be similar to other causes of small-vessel vasculitis [9]. In the case of ulcerations or neutrophilic dermatoses that may be associated with RA, a skin biopsy may help narrow the differential diagnosis or provide supportive evidence for a classical clinical presentation (e.g., in the case of pyoderma gangrenosum).

Lupus Erythematosus (LE) – Skin biopsy and direct immunofluorescence analysis can be very helpful in diagnosis. Lesions specific and nonspecific for lupus may occur in LE patients, sometimes overlapping, and therefore diagnosis can be difficult [3]. An accurate subtyping of LE is not possible based on histological analysis alone, and lesions in different stages usually show different features on histology.
 A band-like deposition of immunoglobulin/complement at the dermal-epidermal junction is present in lesional skin in a majority of LE patients (lupus band) [3]. The presence of this deposition in non-lesional skin, especially from nonsun-exposed skin, can help confirm a diagnosis of systemic LE, especially when there are insufficient clinical criteria for a diagnosis of LE. A negative direct immunofluorescence analysis of lesional skin usually excludes a diagnosis of systemic or discoid LE.

Scleroderma – Skin biopsy may confirm a clinical diagnosis of scleroderma [1]. In addition, histological analysis may help distinguish between scleroderma and other scleroderma-like cutaneous syndromes such as eosinophilic fasciitis, scleromyxedema, scleredema, graft-versus-host disease, nephrogenic fibrosing dermopathy, and porphyria cutanea tarda.

Dermatomyositis – The histopathology of biopsy specimens from cutaneous lesions of dermatomyositis is not specific and may be seen in other connective tissue diseases such as LE. The diagnosis is made by clinical-pathologic correlation.

Psoriasis with Psoriatic Arthritis – Skin biopsy is useful in cases where diagnosis cannot be made based on clinical presentation alone. Since the differential diagnosis is extensive, a biopsy may either narrow down the possibilities or be consistent with psoriasis.

Vasculitis – Skin biopsy can help in diagnosing small-vessel vasculitis [9]. IgA-predominant vasculitis such as Henoch-Schönlein purpura can be reliably diagnosed by a biopsy for direct immunofluorescence [9]. Granulomatous vasculitis can sometimes be diagnosed by skin biopsy, but generally the findings are nonspecific. Clinical conditions that mimic vasculitis including some drug eruptions and the pigmented purpuric dermatoses can be distinguished via a skin biopsy.

Panniculitis – Adequate sampling of subcutaneous fat by biopsy is required to distinguish between different kinds of panniculitis (septal, lobular, mixed) and identify the kind of associated inflammatory infiltrate as well as absence or presence of associated vasculitis. The biopsy helps to narrow the differential diagnosis, but a specific diagnosis cannot usually be made without clinical correlation.

Contraindications

Patients with bleeding disorders, on anticoagulant drugs, or with thrombocytopenia should be referred to a dermatologist or surgeon, while patients on aspirin can be managed with the use of a pressure dressing. Biopsy of lesions on the face or palms and soles may be referred to a dermatologist or plastic surgeon.

Complications

The most common complications include bleeding and infection [5]. The risk of bleeding is higher for lesions on the scalp, face, and genitals. Bleeding can be minimized using cautery if needed, a topical hemostatic agent, and/or a pressure dressing over the wound. Infections are uncommon but may occur especially in patients taking systemic glucocorticoids, smokers, diabetics, or hospitalized patients. Patients with scleroderma may have impaired wound healing [4]. Wound infections may require oral antibiotics if severe. An allergic contact dermatitis may develop secondary to the topical antibiotic or Band-Aid in which case these should be discontinued.

Practical Considerations

Universal precautions (gloves and eye guards or face masks) should always be observed to decrease the risk of blood-borne infections. Storing the biopsy supplies in a biopsy kit can be useful to increase efficiency. Sterile gloves are not required for punch biopsy procedures since they are clean but not sterile procedures. All patients should be asked about allergies to local anesthetics, antiseptics, and topical antibiotics before the procedure.

Excess blood around the biopsy specimen should be washed with normal saline to prevent the false impression of extravasation of red blood cells [5]. The biopsy tissue should be handled carefully, and use of forceps with teeth should be avoided to prevent crush artifacts. Excess infiltration anesthesia may give the false impression of dermal edema and should be avoided as well.

References

1. Ton E, Kruize AA. How to perform and analyse biopsies in relation to connective tissue diseases. Best Pract Res Clin Rheumatol. 2009;23(2):233–55.
2. SBaH KM. How to maximize information from a skin biopsy. In: Smaller BR, Hiatt KM, editors. Dermatopathology: the basics. New York: Springer; 2009. p. 37–61.
3. SRaPT CMI. Lupus erythematosus. In: Sontheimer RD, Provost TT, editors. Cutaneous manifestations of rheumatic diseases. Philadelphia: Lippincott Williams & Wilkins; 2004.

4. Kruize AA, Bijlsma JW. Procedures related to connective tissue disease. Best Pract Res Clin Rheumatol. Jun 2005;19(3):417–36.
5. Nischal U, Nischal K, Khopkar U. Techniques of skin biopsy and practical considerations. J Cutan Aesthet Surg. 2008;1(2):107–11.
6. Alguire PC, Mathes BM. Skin biopsy techniques for the internist. J Gen Intern Med. 1998;13(1):46–54.
7. Neitzel CD. Biopsy techniques for skin disease and skin cancer. Oral Maxillofac Surg Clin North Am. 2005;17(2):143–6.
8. Ha CT, Nousari HC. Surgical pearl: double-trephine punch biopsy technique for sampling subcutaneous tissue. J Am Acad Dermatol. 2003;48(4):609–10.
9. Carlson JA. The histological assessment of cutaneous vasculitis. Histopathology. 2010;56(1):3–23.

Part III
Inflammatory Joint Diseases

Chapter 13
Skin Manifestations of Juvenile Idiopathic Arthritis

Rolando Cimaz and Antonella Greco

Definition

Juvenile idiopathic arthritis (JIA) refers to a group of disorders characterized by chronic arthritis of unknown cause. It begins before the age of 16 years and by definition lasts longer than 6 weeks. Skin manifestation is evident only in systemic-onset disease and in psoriatic arthritis [1–7].

Clinical Picture and Differential Diagnosis

Systemic JIA rash. Systemic juvenile idiopathic arthritis is peculiar with respect to the other forms of JIA. Thus, apart from arthritis, extra-articular manifestations may dominate the clinical picture. Its etiopathogenesis and response to treatment are also different from oligoarticular and polyarticular JIA.

The second most common characteristic feature of systemic juvenile idiopathic arthritis, after the presence of fever (which is part of the definition and is thus mandatory), is the rash. Present in the vast majority of patients, it is almost diagnostic when it occurs together with the fever spike. Therefore, if the diagnosis is uncertain, it is critically important that the patient be examined at the time of a fever spike in order to look for the rash, which may not be apparent during the rest of the day. The rash is typically a pink, evanescent, salmon-colored macular rash (Fig. 13.1),

R. Cimaz, M.D. (✉)
Department of Pediatric Rheumatology, AOU Meyer, Viale Pieraccini 24,
Florence 50139, Italy
e-mail: r.cimaz@meyer.it

A. Greco, M.D.
Department of Pediatric Dermatology, AOU Meyer, Viale Pieraccini 24,
Florence 50139, Italy

M. Matucci-Cerinic et al. (eds.), *Skin Manifestations in Rheumatic Disease*,
DOI 10.1007/978-1-4614-7849-2_13, © Springer Science+Business Media New York 2014

Fig. 13.1 Typical
maculopapular rash of
systemic-onset JIA

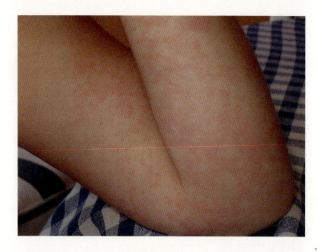

characteristically concentrated in the warmer areas of the body (thigh, axilla, and trunk). Only occasionally does it occur on the face, hands, and feet. Macules may have areas of central clearing and sometimes coalesce to form larger lesions. It may also appear as linear streaks in areas of pressure and may be elicited by stroking the skin (Koebner phenomenon). Sometimes the rash can appear as a striking urticarial and pruritic eruption and may persist even in the absence of fever.

Differential diagnosis of systemic JIA rash is wide. It is usually, however, rather nonspecific, except that it is seen within an overall clinical picture that can help in excluding other diseases (note, of course, that, by definition, JIA is a diagnosis of exclusion). The three conditions most frequently mistaken for systemic JIA are infection, malignancy, and inflammatory bowel disease. The latter condition can have mucocutaneous manifestations as well, but they occur in the form of erythema nodosum, pyoderma gangrenosum, or oral ulcerations. Malignancies can also have multiple types of rashes, but are usually diagnosed on the background of typical laboratory abnormalities. The most difficult situation from a diagnostic point of view is therefore represented by infection or post-infectious illnesses. Rheumatic fever is rare in our climate, and its cutaneous manifestations are erythema marginatum and subcutaneous nodules. This makes the rash of rheumatic fever quite easy to recognize. Particularly difficult to recognize are viral infections such as those caused by adenovirus, parvovirus, and cytomegalovirus; all these infections can mimic systemic JIA with a similar rash accompanied by fever. The course and, occasionally, laboratory features can help distinguish these illnesses.

Psoriatic arthritis occurs in 10–15 % of patients affected with psoriasis. In about half the cases, psoriasis appears years before arthritis although the arthritis can occur, occasionally, before the skin disease. The simultaneous presence of both

Fig. 13.2 The matrix of nails is often interested. Almost 70–80 % of the patients with psoriatic arthritis show alterations of nails such as nail pitting

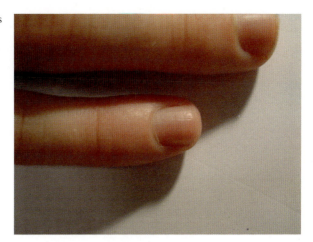

Fig. 13.3 Dactylitis in young patients with psoriatic arthritis

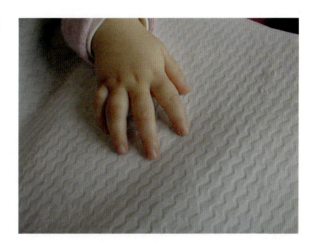

psoriasis and arthritis is more frequent in children than in adults. The severity of arthritis is not considered to be correlated to any particular type of psoriasis or to the severity/extension of the skin disease. Some clinical features are associated with the psoriatic arthritis, such as nail pitting (Fig. 13.2), dactylitis (Fig. 13.3), a psoriasis-like rash, and a family history of psoriasis. In patients with such a suspected diagnosis, since the rash can be minimal and overlooked, a careful examination of scalp, skin, and nails is necessary. Frequently children affected with psoriatic arthritis have a family history of psoriasis.

The classic lesions of psoriasis consist of round, well-demarcated, red areas of skin inflammation with characteristic grayish or silvery scales (Fig. 13.4). The disorder may present a single plaque or multiple plaques distributed over the

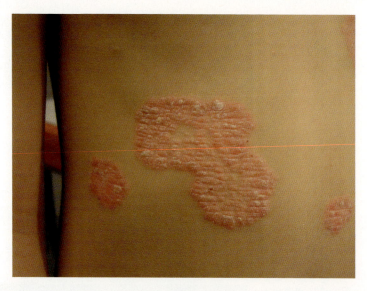

Fig. 13.4 The classic lesions of psoriasis consist of round, well-demarcated, *red* areas of skin inflammation with a characteristic *grayish* or *silvery* scales

whole body. Papules can coalesce and form patches of diameter of >1 cm over very small or wide areas of the body. Psoriatic lesions tend to appear as symmetric eruptions on the elbows, knees, lumbosacral region, the scalp, buttocks, and around genital areas. The distribution on axilla, groin, perineum, central chest, and umbilical region is called inverse psoriasis. The scalp and nails are often involved conjointly. Scalp psoriasis is frequently the earliest presentation, and it is characterized by well-demarcated erythematous plaques with thick, adherent silvery scales. Very small plaques can be confused with seborrheic dermatitis. However, while seborrhea usually remains within the hairline, psoriasis extends to the preauricular, postauricular, and nuchal regions. Onycholysis, transverse ridging, and uniform nail pitting are the three main features of nail involvement. When the diagnosis is based only on nail changes, it is important to distinguish them from trauma or fungal infection (a suspect nail clipping should be sent for microscopic examination).

Biopsy

Systemic arthritis is not usually biopsied since the clinical picture is often quite characteristic. Psoriasis, per se, is also seldom biopsied although the histological picture of psoriasis vulgaris varies according to the stage of the lesion and the site of the biopsy. Biopsy sections show epidermal thickening (slight acanthosis with

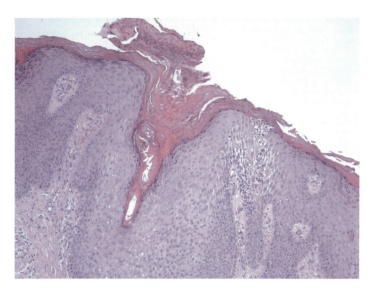

Fig. 13.5 Biopsy sections show epidermal thickening (slightly acanthosis with elongation of the netlike ridges); granular cells become vacuolated and eventually disappear. Retention of nuclei in the stratum corneum (parakeratosis) is also present

elongation of the netlike ridges), granular cell vacuolization, and retention of nuclei in the stratum corneum (parakeratosis). Parakeratosis with neutrophils in the stratum corneum or subcorneal represent the first manifestation of Munro microabscesses that are more frequent in early lesions. Typical histological changes of psoriasis are shown in Fig. 13.5.

Another lesion that may be biopsied and that can, rarely, be seen in JIA is represented by **rheumatoid nodules**. These are the classic cutaneous manifestations of adult rheumatoid arthritis (RA). In pediatrics, such a finding is extremely rare and often corresponds to RF-positive polyarticular JIA (no more 5 % of all forms of JIA). These are firm, skin-colored nodules typically located within the subcutaneous tissue in or around pressure areas such as elbows, finger joints, occiput, and extensor surface of the forearms. They are mobile and non-tender; frequently they adhere to the underlying periosteum. When biopsied, they exhibit three characteristic layers: (i) an inner necrotic zone, (ii) a surrounding zone of predominantly macrophages that form palisading granulomas, and (iii) an outer zone of perivascular infiltration with chronic inflammatory cells. The granulomas are surrounded by a zone of reactive tissue containing fibroblasts, plasma cells, and lymphocytes. There may be a small vessel vasculitis with fibrinoid necrosis due to proteolytic activity by specific enzymes.

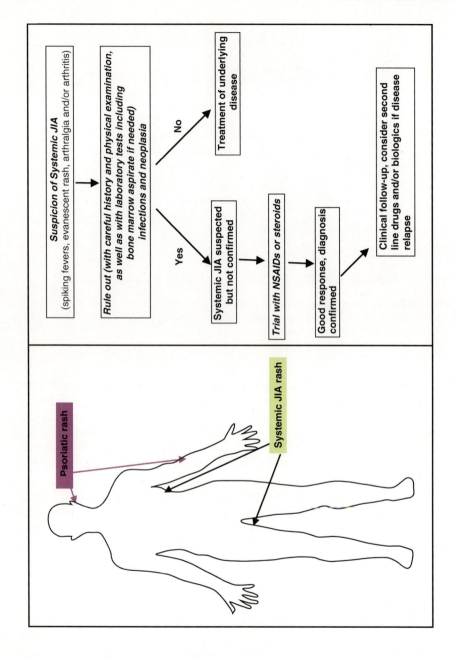

Suspicion of Systemic JIA
(spiking fevers, evanescent rash, arthralgia and/or arthritis)

Rule out (with careful history and physical examination, as well as with laboratory tests including bone marrow aspirate if needed) infections and neoplasia

No → Treatment of underlying disease

Yes → Systemic JIA suspected but not confirmed → *Trial with NSAIDs or steroids* → Good response, diagnosis confirmed → Clinical follow-up, consider second line drugs and/or biologics if disease relapse

Psoriatic rash

Systemic JIA rash

References

1. Bowyer S, Roettcher P. Pediatric rheumatology clinic populations in the United States: results of a 3 year survey. Pediatric Rheumatology Database Research Group. J Rheumatol. 1996; 23:1968.
2. Lambert JR, et al. Psoriatic arthritis in childhood. Clin Rheum Dis. 1976;2:339.
3. Petty RE, Cassidy JT. Systemic arthritis. In: Cassidy JT, Petty RE, Laxer R, Lindsley C, editors. Textbook of pediatric rheumatology. Philadelphia: Elsevier; 2005. p. 291–303.
4. Robertson DM, et al. Juvenile psoriatic arthritis: followup and evaluation of diagnostic criteria. J Rheumatol. 1996;23:1466.
5. Shore A, et al. Juvenile psoriatic arthritis-an analysis of 60 cases. J Pediatr. 1982;100:529.
6. Southwood TR, et al. Psoriatic arthritis in children. Arthritis Rheum. 1989;32:1007.
7. Stoll ML, et al. Comparison of Vancouver and International League of Associations for rheumatology classification criteria for juvenile psoriatic arthritis. Arthritis Rheum. 2008;59:51.

Chapter 14
Psoriasis and Psoriatic Arthritis

Parbeer S. Grewal, Walter P. Maksymowych, and Alain Brassard

Psoriasis is a chronic, polygenic, papulosquamous disorder associated with a variety of environmental triggers, including trauma, infections and/or medications. The prevalence varies based on geographic location and approximates 4.6 % in North America. Psoriatic arthritis occurs in approximately 5–30 % of patients affected by psoriasis. Usually, the skin manifestations of psoriasis are apparent before the joint involvement. However, 10–15 % of patients diagnosed with psoriatic arthritis develop joint symptomatology before the characteristic skin eruption [1].

Psoriasis can present with many different cutaneous manifestations. The most characteristic lesion of psoriasis vulgaris is the psoriatic plaque, which is a well-demarcated, erythematous, round or oval, sharply bordered lesion with a non-coherent, silvery-white scale (Fig. 14.1). The most typical locations of psoriasis vulgaris include the knees, elbows, scalp, umbilicus and lumbosacral regions. However, any cutaneous surface can be potentially involved with plaques of psoriasis. Auspitz sign and the Koebner phenomenon are two other clinical signs that also help to confirm the diagnosis of psoriasis. Auspitz sign is the development of pin-point bleeding following the mechanical removal of the scale from a psoriatic plaque. The Koebner phenomenon is an isomorphic reaction in which psoriatic lesions develop in areas of cutaneous trauma [2].

P.S. Grewal, M.D., FRCPC (✉)
Stratica Medical Centre for Dermatology, 10140-117 Street, Suite 200, Edmonton, AB T5K1X3, Canada
e-mail: psgrewal@ualberta.ca

W.P. Maksymowych, M.D., FRCPC
Division of Rheumatology, Department of Medicine, University of Alberta, 8440-112 Street, Edmonton, AB T6G 2G3, Canada

A. Brassard, M.D., FRCPC
Division of Dermatology & Cutaneous Sciences, Department of Medicine, University of Alberta, 2-125 Clinical Sciences Building, Edmonton, AB T6G 2G3, Canada

M. Matucci-Cerinic et al. (eds.), *Skin Manifestations in Rheumatic Disease*, DOI 10.1007/978-1-4614-7849-2_14, © Springer Science+Business Media New York 2014

Fig. 14.1 Image of a patient with typical thick and white scaling psoriatic plaques

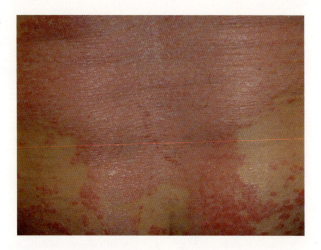

Other forms of psoriasis include guttate, inverse, seborrheic, erythrodermic, pustular and nail psoriasis.

Guttate psoriasis is an eruptive form of psoriasis commonly seen in children and young adults, classically preceded by a streptococcal throat infection. It is characterized by an eruption of dozens to hundreds of 'drop-like', 0.5–1 cm, well-defined psoriatic papules. It is often a self-limiting condition. However, individuals are more prone to the development of chronic psoriasis vulgaris in the future.

Inverse psoriasis is distinguished by its predilection for the intertriginous areas of the body – axilla, groin and neck. Inverse psoriasis can be found in the gluteal cleft and genital mucosa. It is characterized by well-demarcated, erythematous plaques, but they are usually non-scaly due to maceration from heat and moisture.

Sebopsoriasis is characterized by erythematous plaques and greasy, yellow scale in the scalp, nasolabial folds and presternal areas.

Erythrodermic psoriasis is an acute, generalized form of psoriasis characterized by erythema and superficial scale that covers more than 90 % of the total body surface area. Individuals are predisposed to the loss of heat and electrolytes, and this condition can be complicated by secondary infection, high-output cardiac failure and even impairment of renal and hepatic function [3].

Pustular psoriasis also has several different variants that can be seen on the skin. The Von Zumbusch pattern occurs as an acute-onset, generalized, erythematous and pustular eruption. It is often accompanied by systemic symptoms, including fever, chills, headaches and malaise. The annular pattern occurs when small

Fig. 14.2 Palm of patient with dozens of pustules and red scaly patches commonly seen in pustular and palmoplantar psoriasis

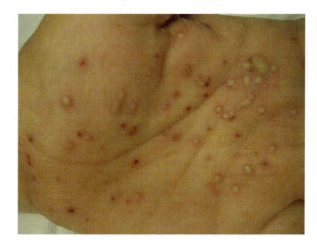

pustules surround an erythematous, scaly plaque of psoriasis. This type of reaction pattern is occasionally accompanied by systemic symptoms. The exanthematous pattern is an acute eruption of small pustules following a recent infection or medication exposure. Localized pustulosis of the palms and hands is also a very common psoriatic eruption characterized by dozens of small, sterile, yellow-brown pustules on the palms and soles. This condition can be both chronic and debilitating, and these individuals can also have coexistent plaques of psoriasis vulgaris as well (Fig. 14.2).

Nail changes in psoriasis are also very common and seen in up to 40 % of patients. Because it is so common, nail involvement is not an accurate predictor of the future development of psoriatic arthritis. However, the frequency of nail involvement is higher in those individuals that are older, have a longer history of psoriasis and have psoriatic arthritis. The most common nail findings include nail pitting (0.5–2 mm, asymmetric depressions in the nail plate), oil spots and salmon patches (translucent, yellow-brown discoloration beneath the nail plate), onycholysis (lifting of the nail plate) and subungual hyperkeratosis (crumbling debris underneath the distal edge of the nail plate). Other potential findings include leukonychia (a white nail plate), crumbling nails, splinter haemorrhages and anonychia (total loss of nail plate) [4] (Fig. 14.3).

Rare to infrequent forms: There are few mucosal manifestations of psoriasis and psoriatic arthritis. Geographic tongue, also known as benign migratory glossitis, is an idiopathic inflammatory disorder that results in the localized loss of the

Fig. 14.3 Typical presentation of a psoriatic nail with onycholysis, pitting and discoloration

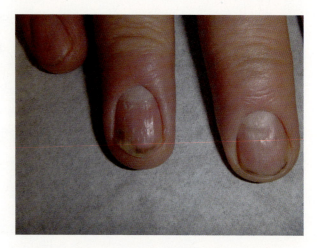

Fig. 14.4 Deep fissures and grooves in the tongue of a patient with psoriasis

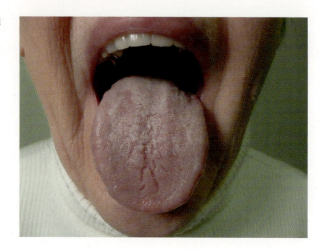

filiform papillae in the tongue and presents as migratory, erythematous patches with serpiginous borders on the tongue. It has very similar histological features to psoriasis and is found at a much greater frequency in patients with psoriasis (Fig. 14.4). Annulus migrans is another potential finding in the mouth. It consists of annular or polycyclic, slightly raised, grey to white plaques on the dorsal tongue [4].

Differential Diagnosis

Psoriasis vulgaris needs to be differentiated from lichen simplex chronicus, lichen planus, pityriasis rubra pilaris, pityriasis rosea, secondary syphilis, tinea corporis, small and large plaque parapsoriasis, cutaneous T-cell lymphoma and cutaneous drug eruptions (such as acute generalized exanthematous pustulosis). On the scalp, it also needs to be distinguished from seborrheic dermatitis and tinea capitis.

The pustular forms need to be distinguished from bacterial, fungal and viral infections, drug eruptions, subcorneal pustular dermatosis and reactive arthritis [1]. The ocular manifestations need to be differentiated from idiopathic blepharitis, keratoconjunctivitis sicca and rosacea [5].

Biopsy

Histologically, plaque-type psoriasis will show confluent parakeratosis and hyperkeratosis, neutrophils in the stratum corneum (Munro microabscess) and spinous layer (spongiform pustules of Kogoj), regular acanthosis with clubbed rete ridges and dilated capillaries in the dermal papillae. The pustular forms of psoriasis will have similar histological features, but will also show more neutrophils in the stratum corneum forming obvious pustules and less acanthosis and hyperkeratosis [6].

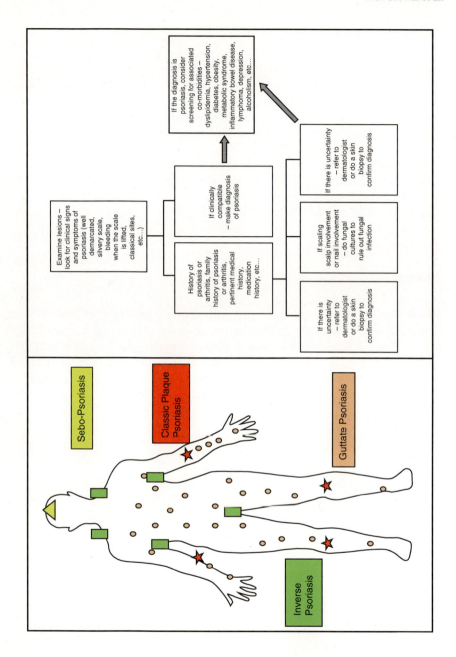

References

1. Bolognia JL, Jorizzo JL, Rapini RP. Dermatology. 2nd ed. Spain: Mosby Elsevier; 2008.
2. Mycrs WA, Gottleib AB, Mease P. Psoriasis and psoriatic arthritis: clinical features and disease mechanisms. Clin Dermatol. 2006;24:438–47.
3. Meier M, Sheth PB. Clinical spectrum and severity of psoriasis. Curr Probl Dermatol. 2009;38:1–20.
4. Wolff K, Goldsmith LA, Katz SI, Gilchrist BA, Paller AS, Leffel DJ. Fitzpatrick's dermatology in general medicine. 7th ed. New York: McGraw Hill Companies Inc.; 2008.
5. Psoriasis AR, Medscape medicine. 2009. http://emedicine.medscape.com/article/1197939-overview. Accessed 20 Mar 2010.
6. Rapini RP. Practical dermatopathology. Philadelphia: Elsevier Mosby; 2005.

Chapter 15
Inflammatory Bowel-Associated Spondyloarthropathy

Parbeer S. Grewal, Walter P. Maksymowych, and Alain Brassard

Inflammatory bowel disease is relatively common with a prevalence of 100–200/100,000 for Crohn's disease and 150–250/100,000 in ulcerative colitis. There is an equal sex distribution and a bimodal age distribution, with the greatest incidence in adolescence and young adults. Between 4 % and 11 % of patients with inflammatory bowel disease can develop spondyloarthropathy (SpA). Once again, males are more commonly affected than females, and patients have a higher prevalence of HLA-B27. In general, up to 36 % of patients with inflammatory bowel disease, with or without SpA, will develop extra-intestinal manifestations, many of which are mucocutaneous. These include erythema nodosum, pyoderma gangrenosum, pyoderma vegetans, vesiculopustular eruption of ulcerative colitis, cutaneous polyarteritis nodosa, metastatic Crohn's disease, Sweet's syndrome, linear IgA bullous dermatosis, psoriasis, perianal skin tags, and epidermolysis bullosa acquisita. Ocular manifestations include episcleritis and uveitis, retinal artery and vein occlusion, neuroretinitis, and ischemic optic neuropathy [1].

Erythema nodosum (EN) is a delayed hypersensitivity response to an as of yet unidentified antigen. It is clinically characterized by the acute eruption of tender, subcutaneous, erythematous nodules usually overlying the shins bilaterally. Rarely, it can localize to other surfaces of the body as well. Oftentimes there are also systemic symptoms, such as fever, chills, malaise, myalgias, and arthralgias. It can either accompany or precede the inflammatory bowel-associated SpA and usually

P.S. Grewal, M.D., FRCPC (✉)
Stratica Medical Centre for Dermatology, 10140-117 Street, Suite 200, Edmonton,
AB T5K1X3, Canada
e-mail: psgrewal@ualberta.ca

W.P. Maksymowych, M.D., FRCPC
Division of Rheumatology, Department of Medicine, University of Alberta,
8440-112 Street, Edmonton, AB T6G 2G3, Canada

A. Brassard, M.D., FRCPC
Division of Dermatology & Cutaneous Sciences, Department of Medicine, University of
Alberta, 2-125 Clinical Sciences Building, Edmonton, AB T6G 2G3, Canada

M. Matucci-Cerinic et al. (eds.), *Skin Manifestations in Rheumatic Disease*,
DOI 10.1007/978-1-4614-7849-2_15, © Springer Science+Business Media New York 2014

Fig. 15.1 Typical
presentation of erythema
nodosum with tender nodules
on the shins

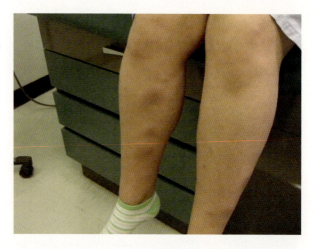

has a self-limited course, although recurrences can occur. The diagnosis is based on the clinical presentation and can be confirmed with an incisional wedge biopsy that includes the subcutaneous fat (Fig. 15.1) [2].

Pyoderma gangrenosum (PG) is a rare, inflammatory disorder thought to be due to abnormal immune reactivity and/or cross-reacting autoantibodies. Clinically, it can arise over a few days on any part of the skin or mucosa. It may present in one of four distinct forms: ulcerative, bullous, pustular, or vegetative. The ulcerative form presents as a large, painful, purulent, undermined ulceration. Bullous lesions present as painful, rapidly expanding superficial bullae that erode and ulcerate. Pustular lesions present as an acute, widespread eruption of painful pustules over any part of the body. This is the most characteristic presentation of PG in patients with inflammatory bowel disease. Vegetative lesions are rare and present as hypertrophic, mildly painful nodules, or abscesses. Patients can also have systemic symptoms of fever, chills, and malaise and internal organ involvement of the liver, kidney, and spleen. This is a diagnosis of exclusion on biopsy, and frequently other conditions, such as cutaneous infections, need to be ruled out [3] (Fig. 15.2a, b).

Pyostomatitis vegetans is thought to be a variant of pyoderma gangrenosum that occurs mainly in the oral or genital mucosa. It is characterized by an acute-onset, painful, pustular or erosive eruption alongside vegetating plaques. The vesiculopustular eruption of ulcerative colitis also presents very similarly with an acute eruption of vesicles and pustules on the skin that heal with residual hyperpigmentation.

Cutaneous polyarteritis nodosa is a medium vessel vasculitis that presents as painful, erythematous, purpuric, or ulcerated nodules on the lower extremities bilaterally.

Metastatic Crohn's is a non-caseating, granulomatous inflammatory disorder that appears clinically as erythematous or ulcerated nodules or plaques on the skin.

Sweet's syndrome, also known as acute febrile neutrophilic dermatosis, is characterized by fever, malaise, and an explosive eruption of dozens of erythematous, indurated, occasionally vesicular papules and plaques (Fig. 15.3).

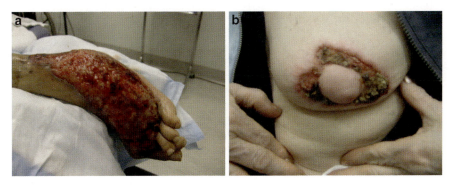

Fig. 15.2 (**a**, **b**): Two images of different patients with severe, necrotizing, ulcerating pyoderma gangrenosum

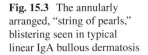

Fig. 15.3 The annularly arranged, "string of pearls," blistering seen in typical linear IgA bullous dermatosis

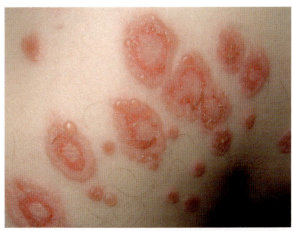

Linear IgA bullous dermatosis is an autoimmune blistering condition characterized by the eruption of multiple bullae in polycyclic or annular configurations.

Epidermolysis bullosa acquisita is an acquired autoimmune disorder of type VII collagen. Patients often complain of fragile skin that blisters at sites of friction or trauma and heals with residual scar formation and milia (tiny epidermoid inclusion cysts).

Psoriasis is a manifestation of inflammatory bowel-associated SpA that shares genetic features with both SpA and Crohn's disease as defined by genetic markers at the interleukin-23 locus.

Perianal skin tags, flesh-colored, well-defined, 1–10 mm, pedunculated papules, can also be found and are considered to be related to constant friction and trauma [1].

Differential Diagnosis

The differential diagnosis of erythema nodosum includes all other causes of panniculitis – morphea/scleroderma, alpha1-antitrypsin deficiency, pancreatic panniculitis, lupus panniculitis, lipodystrophic panniculitis, cold panniculitis, lipo-dermatosclerosis, and malignancy-related panniculitis. One also needs to rule out vasculitis, such as erythema induratum, nodular vasculitis, and polyarteritis nodosa [4]. The differential diagnosis for pyoderma gangrenosum, pyostomatitis vegetans, vesiculopustular eruption of ulcerative colitis, and metastatic Crohn's disease includes bacterial, viral, or fungal infections, vasculitis, neutrophilic disorders (Sweet's syndrome, Behcet's disease, bowel-associated arthritis dermatosis), drug eruptions, malignancy, and dermatitis artefacta. Polyarteritis nodosa also needs to be differentiated from other forms of vasculitis, panniculitis, drug eruptions, and infections. Perianal skin tags can often be confused with hemorrhoids and condylomata acuminata. Finally, epidermolysis bullosa acquisita needs to be differentiated from other autoimmune blistering conditions (such as pemphigus vulgaris, bullous pemphigoid, porphyria cutanea tarda, bullous lupus erythematosus), drug eruptions, and infections [5].

Biopsy

Histologically, erythema nodosum is a prototypical septal panniculitis of lympho-cytes, histiocytes, neutrophils, and/or eosinophils. Occasionally, multinucleate giant cells and fibrosis can be seen as well. Pyoderma gangrenosum, pyostomatitis vege-tans, and vesiculopustular eruption of ulcerative colitis can all appear as a bullous, pustular, necrotic, or ulcerative lesion with a predominant neutrophilic infiltrate. Pseudoepitheliomatous hyperplasia of the ulcer edge can also be seen. Metastatic Crohn's disease is often seen under the microscope as non-caseating, granuloma-tous inflammation with a predominance of histiocytes and lymphocytes. Polyarteritis nodosa has the prototypical leukocytoclastic vasculitis of small- and medium-sized blood vessels with intimal proliferation and/or thrombus. Sweet's syndrome shows a diffuse dermal neutrophilic infiltrate with prominent dermal edema and no evi-dence of true vasculitis. Psoriasis appears as regular acanthosis of the rete ridges with neutrophils on the stratum corneum and overlying hyperkeratosis or parakera-tosis. Perianal skin tags are papillomatous and acanthotic with dilated blood vessels. Epidermolysis bullosa acquisita is characterized by a subepidermal blister with lim-ited cellular infiltrate that will stain IgG and complement linearly along the dermal-epidermal junction on direct immunofluorescence [6].

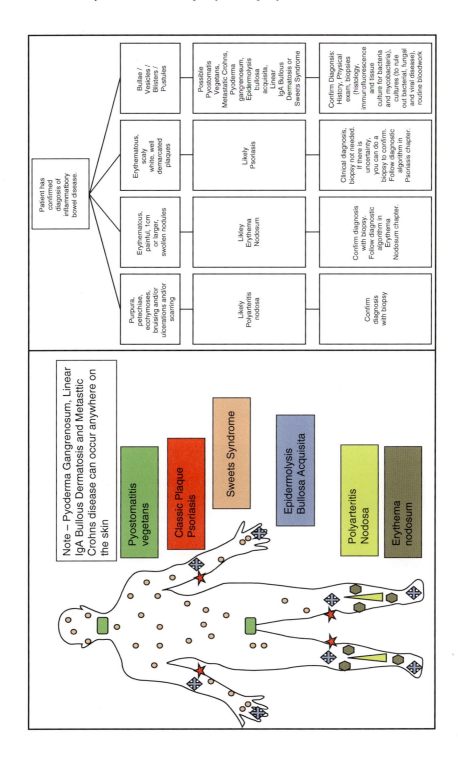

Patient has confirmed diagosis of inflammatbory bowel disease.

Purpura, petechiae, ecchymoses, bruising and/or ulcerations and/or scarring

Erythematous, painful, 1cm or larger, swollen nodules

Erythematous, scaly white, well demarcated plaques

Bullae / Vesicles / Blisters / Pustules

Likely Polyarteritis nodosa

Likley Erythema Nodosum

Likley Psoriasis

Possible Pyostomatis Vegetans, Metasttatic Crohns, Pyoderma gangrenosum, Epidermolysis bullosa acquisita, Linear IgA Bullous Dermatosis or Sweets Syndrome

Confirm diagnosis with biopsy

Confirm diagnosis with biopsy. Follow diagnostic algorithm in Erythema Nodosum chapter.

Clinical diagnosis, biopsy not needed. If there is uncertainty, you can do a biopsy to confirm. Follow diagnostic algorithm in Psoriasis chapter.

Confirm Diagonsis: History, Physical exam, biopsies (histology, immunofluorescence and tissue culture for bacteria and mycobacteria), cultures (to rule out bacterial, fungal and viral disease), routine bloodwork

Note – Pyoderma Gangrenosum, Linear IgA Bullous Dermatosis and Metasttic Crohns disease can occur anywhere on the skin

Pyostomatitis vegetans

Classic Plaque Psoriasis

Sweets Syndrome

Epidermolysis Bullosa Acquisita

Polyarteritis Nodosa

Erythema nodosum

References

1. Lichenstein GR. The clinician's guide to inflammatory bowel disease. Thorofare: Slack Incorporated; 2003. p. 1–9, 77–112
2. Requena L, Yus ES. Erythema nodosum. Dermatol Clin. 2008;26(4):435–8.
3. Ruocco E, Sangiuliano S, Gravina AG, Miranda A, Nicoletti G. Pyoderma gangrenosum: an updated review. J Eur Acad Dermatol Venereol. 2009;23(9):1008–17.
4. Bolognia JL, Jorizzo JL, Rapini RP. Dermatology. 2nd ed. Spain: Elsevier Mosby; 2008.
5. Wolff K, Goldsmith LA, Katz SI, Gilchrist BA, Paller AS, Leffel DJ. Fitzpatrick's dermatology in general medicine. 7th ed. New York: McGraw Hill Companies Inc.; 2008.
6. Rapini RP. Practical dermatopathology. Philadelphia: Elsevier Mosby; 2005.

Chapter 16
Nodules in Rheumatoid Arthritis

Beth S. Ruben and M. Kari Connolly

Definition

The most common nodules in rheumatoid arthritis (RA) are rheumatoid nodules (RN). Approximately 1 in 4 patients with long-standing rheumatoid arthritis will have classic rheumatoid nodules over the extensor surfaces of joints such as the elbow, Achilles tendon, fingers, and pressure points [1], (Fig. 16.1). RN are part of the RA classification criterion and associated with seropositive disease [2]. They tend to be large, starting at a few millimeters but grow to several centimeters. They are often non-tender, firm, flesh-colored subcutaneous masses that may or may not be bound down to the underlying periosteum. In classic cases, a biopsy is not necessary for diagnosis. In atypical cases, however, a biopsy can be helpful. Rheumatoid nodules can occur in other tissues such as the eye, larynx, lung, and nervous system. Methotrexate therapy is associated with rheumatoid nodulosis with rapid onset of multiple smaller lesions over the hands. Less commonly, smaller papules and plaques, occasionally linear, with smooth, umbilicated, or crusted surfaces occur symmetrically over the joints or extensor surfaces in patients with RA or systemic lupus erythematosus (SLE) and on biopsy show palisaded neutrophilic and granulomatous dermatitis (PNGD) [3] (Fig. 16.2).

B.S. Ruben, M.D. (✉)
Departments of Dermatology and Pathology, Dermatopathology Service,
University of California, 1701 Divisadero Street, #280, San Francisco, CA 94115, USA
e-mail: beth.ruben@ucsf.edu

M.K. Connolly, M.D.
Departments of Dermatology and Internal Medicine, University of California,
533 Parnassus Ave, Rm. U332, UCSF Box 0517, San Francisco, CA 94143-0517, USA
e-mail: connolly@derm.ucsf.edu

M. Matucci-Cerinic et al. (eds.), *Skin Manifestations in Rheumatic Disease*,
DOI 10.1007/978-1-4614-7849-2_16, © Springer Science+Business Media New York 2014

Fig. 16.1 Multiple
rheumatoid nodules in a
patient with advanced
rheumatoid arthritis and
destructive arthropathy
of the hands

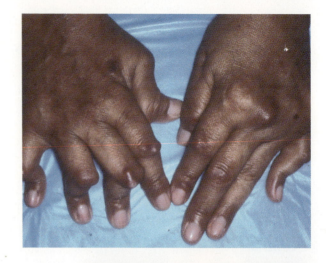

Fig. 16.2 Nodules and
plaques of palisaded
neutrophilic
and granulomatous dermatitis
in a somewhat linear
configuration on the extensor
forearm of a patient with
rheumatoid arthritis

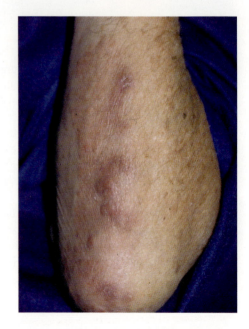

Differential Diagnosis

The differential diagnosis for rheumatoid nodules (RN) is broad [4, 5]. Acute rheumatic fever (ARF) is accompanied by subcutaneous nodules in 1 % of cases. ARF is
associated with group A streptococcal pharyngitis. The location of the nodules over
the olecranon and other joints is similar to rheumatoid nodules. Distinguishing features include that ARF nodules occur early in disease (first 1–3 weeks), tend to be

smaller in size, and resolve spontaneously. There are individuals who develop rheumatoid nodules in the absence of rheumatoid arthritis (RA); these are referred to as "benign nodules." Typically these occur in children on the scalp or posterior neck. Subcutaneous granuloma annulare is another entity that tends to occur in children or young adults and can present as subcutaneous nodules over joints. These have been referred as "pseudorheumatoid nodules." Calcinosis cutis forms whitish, rock hard subcutaneous nodules over joints and is more common in scleroderma and dermatomyositis than RA. The Gottron's papules of dermatomyositis occur over joints, but are violaceous and smaller than rheumatoid nodules. Tophi can mimic RN, but obviously occur in the setting of gout. Characteristic X-ray changes can be helpful to sort out the latter two entities. Multicentric reticulohistiocytosis occurs in middle-aged women, affects the skin and mucous membranes, and is associated with an erosive polyarthritis and increased risk of internal malignancy. There are multiple yellow-red papules that have a characteristic histology. A variety of xanthomas can occur as nodules over joints. They have a yellow-orange hue and are associated with abnormal lipids. Rheumatoid papules are distinctive because of their reddish-brown color, scale, and occurrence on the lower extremities. Approximately 10 % of SLE patients will have classic rheumatoid nodules that are clinically and histologically indistinguishable from nodules in an RA patient. Panniculitis typically affects larger areas of fat, is more amorphous than discrete nodules, and does not occur over joints. Similarly, medium vessel vasculitis such as polyarteritis nodosa typically occurs away from joints and may ulcerate, which RN do not. Infections tend to be more rapidly growing, tender, and may be associated with overlying erythema and suppurative ulceration. Urticaria is transient, and urticarial vasculitis is entirely macular without papules or nodules, so are easily distinguishable from RN.

Histologic Features

Rheumatoid nodules when well developed display a palisaded granulomatous pattern involving the deep dermis and/or subcutis, with a nodular infiltrate of histiocytes surrounding a homogeneous and eosinophilic zone containing altered collagen and typically fibrin centrally [6–8] (Fig. 16.3). Vasculitis may be evident in early lesions and fibrosis in late lesions. Deep granuloma annulare may present a similar pattern, but generally contains mucin in the centers of palisaded foci.

Palisaded neutrophilic and granulomatous dermatitis may present with a spectrum of histologic findings, depending on the age of the lesion [3, 6, 8]. Very early lesions display a pattern similar to urticaria, with a sparse infiltrate of neutrophils, eosinophils, and lymphocytes. Other lesions may contain leukocytoclastic vasculitic foci early in their evolution, with typical perivascular neutrophilic infiltrates with leukocytoclasis, and fibrin deposition within and surrounding vascular walls. Often, there is involvement of the deep dermis, and altered collagen may be present. Well-developed lesions also feature a palisaded to interstitial granulomatous pattern, but contain neutrophils and neutrophilic nuclear dust centrally as well as histiocytes at the periphery of such foci (Fig. 16.4). The infiltrate may form bands

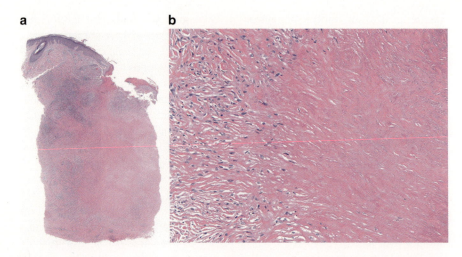

Fig. 16.3 Rheumatoid nodule: (**a**) large palisaded granulomata with an eosinophilic central zone at low magnification (40x); (**b**) palisaded histiocytes, and eosinophilic center, which contains fibrin and fibrosis typically, at higher magnification (200x)

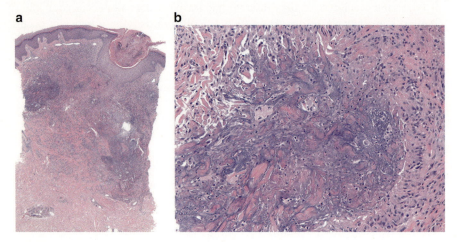

Fig. 16.4 Palisaded neutrophilic and granulomatous dermatitis: (**a**) a palisaded suppurative and granulomatous pattern at low magnification (40x); (**b**) neutrophils and altered basophilic and eosinophilic collagen at the centers of palisaded foci, with a rim of histiocytes at higher magnification (200x)

within the dermis and be "bottom-heavy," centered on the lower dermis. There is also altered basophilic degenerated collagenous material associated with the granulomas. Eosinophils may be present. Some histiocytes may have enlarged nuclei and mitotic figures may be present. The pattern is analogous to a so-called Churg-Strauss granuloma. In later lesions, fibrosis may supervene, with a palisaded infiltrate of histiocytes remaining, but a sparse neutrophilic component.

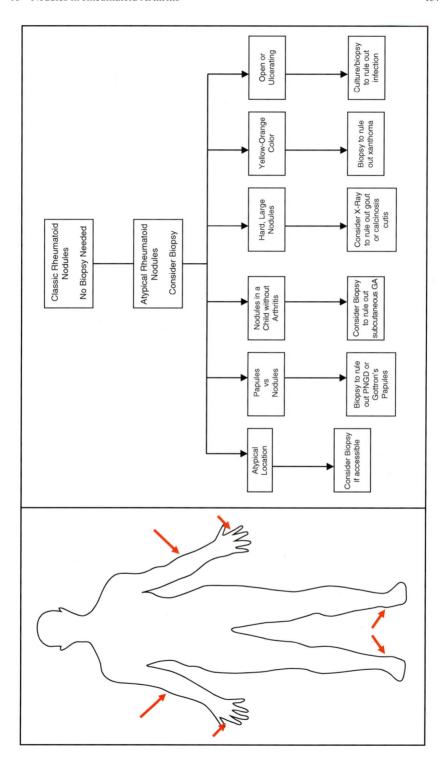

References

1. Harris ED, Firestein GS. Clinical features of rheumatoid arthritis. In: Firestein GS et al., editors. Kelley's textbook of rheumatology. 8th ed. Philadelphia: Saunders Elsevier; 2009. p. 1087–118.
2. Tehlirian CV, Bathon JM. Rheumatoid arthritis A. clinical and laboratory manifestations. In: Klippel JH et al., editors. Primer on the rheumatic diseases. 13th ed. New York: Springer Science; 2008. p. 114–21.
3. Chu P, Connolly MK, LeBoit PE. The histopathologic spectrum of palisaded neutrophilic and granulomatous dermatitis in patients with collagen vascular disease. Arch Dermatol. 1994; 130(10):1278–83.
4. García-Patos V. Rheumatoid nodule. Semin Cutan Med Surg. 2007;26(2):100–7.
5. Rencic A, Nousari CH. Other rheumatologic diseases. In: Bolognia JL et al., editors. Dermatology. 2nd ed. Philadelphia: Mosby Elsevier; 2008. p. 597–610.
6. Sangueza OP, Caudell MD, Mengesha YM, Davis LS, Barnes CJ, Griffin JE, Fleischer AB, Jorizzo JL. Palisaded neutrophilic granulomatous dermatitis in rheumatoid arthritis. J Am Acad Dermatol. 2002;47(2):251–7.
7. Collaris EJ, van Marion AM, Frank J, Poblete-Gutiérrez P. Cutaneous granulomas in rheumatoid arthritis. Int J Dermatol. 2007;46 Suppl 3:33–5.
8. Weedon D. Weedon's skin pathology. 3rd ed. London: Churchill Livingstone; 2009. p. 183–4.

Chapter 17
Genital Involvement as a Result of Reactive Arthritis

Richard M. Keating

Definition

Circinate balanitis (also termed balanitis circinata) is a characteristic reactive arthritis (ReA) skin lesion found at the meatus and on the glans penis, less often on the shaft, in patients who suffer from reactive arthritis (ReA).

Reactive arthritis (ReA) is an inflammatory arthritis that arises after certain types of gastrointestinal or genitourinary infections. It belongs to the group of inflammatory arthritides known as the spondyloarthropathies (SpAs). The classic syndrome, formerly known as Reiter's syndrome, is a triad of symptoms, including the urethra, conjunctiva, and synovium; however, the majority of patients do not present with this classic triad [1, 2]. Recently, there has been a welcomed effort to remove the term Reiter's syndrome from the literature in view of Reiter's Nazi party affiliation [3]. ReA may be thought of as an arthritis which develops soon after or during an infection elsewhere in the body, but in which the microorganisms cannot be recovered from the joint [4].

The lesion of circinate balanitis begins as an area of erythema that progresses to ulcerative papules and pustules on the corona and about the meatus of the penis. Circinate balanitis may take on a serpiginous appearance as the separate lesions coalesce on the glans penis. The lesions may appear moist and erosive on the uncircumcised penis and dry, hyperkeratotic, and crustier on the circumcised penis with a psoriasis-form appearance (Figs. 17.1 and 17.2).

Women too may demonstrate genital lesions as a manifestation of ReA in the form of circinate vulvitis and ulcerative vulvitis. Although ulcerative vulvitis is far less common than circinate balanitis, the lesions are themselves similar in

R.M. Keating, M.D. (✉)
Section of Rheumatology, Department of Medicine, The University of Chicago,
5841 S. Maryland Avenue, MC 0930, Chicago, IL 60637, USA
e-mail: rkeating@medicine.bsd.uchicago.edu

M. Matucci-Cerinic et al. (eds.), *Skin Manifestations in Rheumatic Disease*,   139
DOI 10.1007/978-1-4614-7849-2_17, © Springer Science+Business Media New York 2014

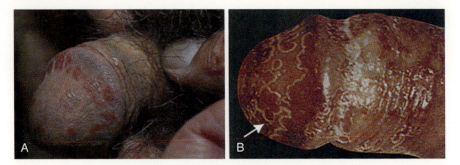

Fig. 17.1 Reactive arthritis – comparison of psoriasis (**a**) and reactive arthritis syndrome (B, bala-nitis circinata) involving the glans penis. Note the highly characteristic coalescence of lesions in this case of reactive arthritis (formerly called Reiter's syndrome) forming a wavy pattern *(arrow)* (Reprinted from Habif TP. Clinical Dermatology, 4th edition. Edinburgh, UK: Mosby; 2003. With permission from Elsevier)

Fig. 17.2 Reactive arthritis – classic serpiginous pattern of circinate balanitis (Reprinted from Wu IB, Schwartz RA. Reiter's syndrome: The classic triad and more. J Am Acad Dermatol 2008; 59:113–121. With permission from Elsevier)

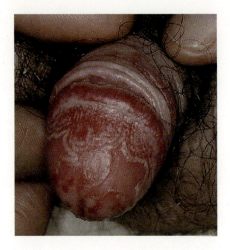

appearance with red, crusted plaques on the vulva and perineum. There may be papules on the vulva, labia minora, and vestibule as well as scattered, demarcated, shallow erosions over the entire genital area.

Differential Diagnosis

Recognizing the genital lesions of ReA is made easier by performing a thorough examination looking for other dermatologic manifestations of ReA. In addition to circinate balanitis, the affected patient may demonstrate keratoderma blennorrhagi-cum (see chapter "Skin Manifestations of Neonatal Lupus Erythematosus"), nail changes, and painless oral lesions.

In addition to the cutaneous lesion, the penis may demonstrate a bland urethritis – often mistakenly thought to be an STD discharge – that develops after the initial inciting infection, whether the inciting infection was an STD or enteric infection. Urethritis and cervicitis may occur in women, while prostatitis may occur in men.

Biopsy

Histopathologic findings of the early cutaneous lesions are essentially the same as in psoriasis. Early lesions balanitis circinata feature a spongiform pustule in the upper dermis. Later lesions demonstrate cornification and thickening overlying the pustule.

This thickening is the genesis for the clinical appearance of thickened excrescences. One eventually sees acanthosis and hyperkeratosis and a resemblance to psoriasis.

Diagnostic Flow Chart

The diagnosis of circinate balanitis and other genital lesions in ReA is made by obtaining a complete medical history and thoroughly examining the patient. The constellation of symptoms that confirm the clinical diagnosis of ReA may not occur contemporaneously, and the clinician must take a very careful history. No laboratory test confirms a diagnosis of ReA. HLA-B27 testing is neither diagnostic nor confirmatory although its presence does portend a possibly more aggressive form of the disease. The erythrocyte sedimentation rate (ESR) is often elevated as is the C-reactive protein (CRP). Leukocytosis and an anemia of chronic inflammation may be seen. The rheumatoid factor (RF) and antinuclear antibody (ANA) are both absent.

If early in the disease course, one might be able to culture Chlamydia from the urine or an enteric pathogen from the stool. HIV and syphilis testing should always be considered. Imaging studies of affected joints, at least in the early phase of symptoms, usually add little useful clinical information. Imaging of the sacroiliac (SI) joints may provide evidence for an unrecognized seronegative spondyloarthropathy if sacroiliitis is identified.

See Also

Chapter 8 – Skin Lesions as a Result of Spondyloarthritides
Chapter 9 – Mucosal Lesions as a Result of Spondyloarthritides
Chapter 10 – Psoriatic Arthritis: Nails and Papules

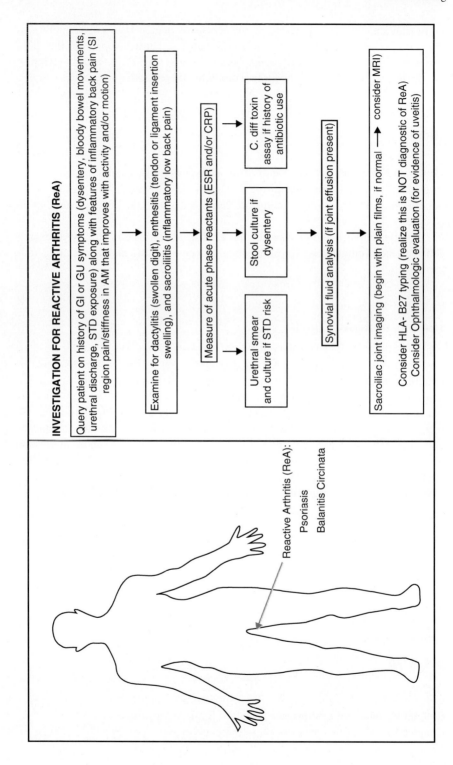

INVESTIGATION FOR REACTIVE ARTHRITIS (ReA)

Query patient on history of GI or GU symptoms (dysentery, bloody bowel movements, urethral discharge, STD exposure) along with features of inflammatory back pain (SI region pain/stiffness in AM that improves with activity and/or motion)

Examine for dactylitis (swollen digit), enthesitis (tendon or ligament insertion swelling), and sacroiliitis (inflammatory low back pain)

Measure of acute phase reactants (ESR and/or CRP)

Urethral smear and culture if STD risk

Stool culture if dysentery

C. diff toxin assay if history of antibiotic use

Synovial fluid analysis (if joint effusion present)

Sacroiliac joint imaging (begin with plain films, if normal → consider MRI)

Consider HLA- B27 typing (realize this is NOT diagnostic of ReA)
Consider Ophthalmologic evaluation (for evidence of uveitis)

Reactive Arthritis (ReA):

Psoriasis

Balanitis Circinata

References

1. Parker CT, Thomas D. Reiter's syndrome and reactive arthritis. J Am Osteopath. 2000;100(2): 101–4.
2. Carter JD, Hudson AP. Reactive arthritis: clinical aspects and medical management. Rheum Dis Clin North Am. 2009;35(1):21.
3. Panush RS, Wallace DJ, Dorff RE, Engleman EP. Retraction of the suggestion to use the term "Reiter's syndrome" sixty-five years later: the legacy of Reiter, a war criminal, should not be eponymic honor but rather condemnation. Arthritis Rheum. 2007;56:693.
4. Wu IB, Schwartz RA. Reiter's syndrome: the classic triad and more. J Am Acad Dermatol. 2008;59:113.

Chapter 18
Keratoderma Blennorrhagica as a Result of Reactive Arthritis

Richard M. Keating

Definition

Keratoderma blennorrhagica or keratoderma blennorrhagica (KD) is a characteristic reactive arthritis (ReA) skin lesion found on the palms and/or soles.

Reactive arthritis (ReA) is an inflammatory arthritis that arises after certain types of gastrointestinal or genitourinary infections. It belongs to the group of inflammatory arthritides known as the spondyloarthropathies (SpAs). The classic syndrome, formerly known as Reiter's syndrome, is a triad of symptoms, including the urethra, conjunctiva, and synovium; however, the majority of patients do not present with this classic triad [1]. Recently, there has been a welcomed effort to remove the term Reiter's syndrome from the literature in view of Reiter's Nazi Party affiliation [2]. ReA may be thought of as an arthritis which develops soon after or during an infection elsewhere in the body, but in which the microorganisms cannot be recovered from the joint.

This exanthem of KD initially begins as a clear vesicle on an erythematosus base that progresses to macules and/or waxy papules that progress and develop into a hyperkeratotic, scaly lesion that very much resembles pustular psoriasis. Individual lesions coalesce into larger areas of thick, keratotic scales. The lesions may remain small and appear as discrete, erythematosus, hyperkeratotic papules or coalesce into quite large plaques which resemble a more generalized hyperkeratosis. These lesions can be found on the scrotum, toes, plantar aspect of the feet, palms, trunk, and scalp. Coloration is that of yellow to brown. Often, there is an accompanying superficial painless ulceration on an erythematosus base seen on the buccal mucosa, palate, and tongue in ReA (Fig. 18.1). Nail dystrophy (thickening and ridging) may also be seen although pitting is unusual (Fig. 18.2) [3].

R.M. Keating, M.D. (✉)
Section of Rheumatology, Department of Medicine, The University of Chicago, 5841 S. Maryland Avenue, MC 0930, Chicago 60637, IL, USA
e-mail: rkeating@medicine.bsd.uchicago.edu

M. Matucci-Cerinic et al. (eds.), *Skin Manifestations in Rheumatic Disease*,
DOI 10.1007/978-1-4614-7849-2_18, © Springer Science+Business Media New York 2014

Fig. 18.1 Reactive arthritis – erosions on tongue (Reprinted from Wu IB, Schwartz RA. Reiter's syndrome: The classic triad and more. J Am Acad Dermatol 2008;59:113–121. With permission from Elsevier)

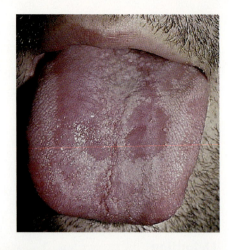

Fig. 18.2 Nail changes include nail dystrophy, subungual debris, and periungual pustules. (Reprinted from Wu IB, Schwartz RA. Reiter's syndrome: The classic triad and more. J Am Acad Dermatol 2008;59:113–121. With permission from Elsevier)

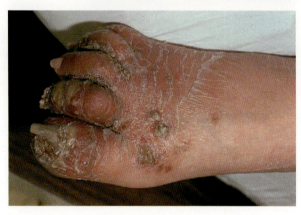

KD accompanies ReA and is one of its cardinal clinical manifestations, although the vast majority of patients with ReA never demonstrate cutaneous features and are never seen by a dermatologist. It is estimated that KD occurs in about 10 % of ReA patients.

Differential Diagnosis

The differential diagnosis for keratoderma blennorrhagica in the genital area includes Bowen's disease, candidiasis, Paget's disease, contact dermatitis, squamous cell carcinoma, erosive lichen planus, lichen sclerosus, fixed drug eruption, and, of course, psoriasis.

The differential diagnosis for lesions found on the palms and soles includes psoriasis as well as hyperkeratosis of the palms/soles, pustular eruption of the palms/soles, scabies, and dermatophytosis. Oral lesions of ReA may resemble aphthous ulcers, geographic tongue, lichen planus, candidiasis, and autoimmune bullous diseases.

Biopsy

KD lesions show spongiform macropustules in the upper epidermis, intraepidermal microabscesses, marked papillomatosis, and acanthosis. Older lesions show corni- fied and thickened layers and acanthosis. The histologic findings in KD are indistin- guishable from psoriasis (as are the clinical features). Subungual hyperkeratosis, found in KD, may also be indistinguishable from psoriasis.

Histopathologic findings of the early cutaneous lesions are essentially the same as in psoriasis. Early lesions of keratoderma blennorrhagicum feature a spongiform pustule in the upper dermis. Later lesions of keratoderma blennorrhagicum usually do not contain spongiform pustules but reveal the nonspecific findings of acantho- sis, hyperkeratosis, and parakeratosis.

Diagnostic Flow Chart

The diagnosis of KD and other dermatologic lesions in ReA is made by obtaining a complete medical history and thoroughly examining the patient. The constellation of symptoms that confirm the clinical diagnosis of ReA may not occur contempora- neously and the clinician must take a very careful history. No laboratory test con- firms a diagnosis of ReA. HLA-B27 testing is neither diagnostic nor confirmatory, although its presence does portend a possibly more aggressive form of the disease. The erythrocyte sedimentation rate (ESR) is often elevated as is the C-reactive pro- tein (CRP). Leukocytosis and an anemia of chronic inflammation may be seen. The rheumatoid factor (RF) and antinuclear antibody (ANA) are both absent. If early in the disease course, one might be able to culture Chlamydia from the urine or an enteric pathogen from the stool. HIV and syphilis testing should always be consid- ered. Imaging studies of affected joints, at least in the early phase of symptoms, usually add little useful clinical information.

The history of illness preceding the appearance of the lesion is the key to making the correct diagnosis. ReA is a systemic inflammatory disease with mucocutaneous and articular manifestations. An enteric or genitourinary infection triggers a response in a genetically predisposed patient that results in the arthritis, dermatitis, and sometimes ophthalmic manifestations. ReA is one of the four diseases included under the larger category of seronegative spondyloarthropathy (SNSA). The SNSAs include ankylosing spondylitis, inflammatory bowel disease associated arthritis, psoriatic arthritis, and ReA.

Common features to the SNSAs include an inflammatory oligoarthritis of the peripheral joints, an inflammatory arthritis of the spine (especially the sacroiliac joints), and enthesitis (inflammation where tendons, ligaments, or fascia attach to the bone). HLA-B27 presence is found at variable rates in the four forms of SNSA with over 90 % of ankylosing spondylitis patients positive, but far less so in ReA. ReA was previously catalogued as having a subcategory called Reiter's syndrome.

Reiter's syndrome included the triad of arthritis, dermatitis, and conjunctivitis. As Hans Reiter was a Nazi physician who took part in war crimes, the eponym has been recently abandoned and the larger category of ReA (which may not include the classic triad of eye, skin, and joint symptoms but only one or two organ systems involved) has been employed.

The clinician must carefully evaluate the patient for any signs or symptoms that would suggest an underlying ReA or an SNSA. The patient should be questioned about enthesitis (inflammation where tendons, ligaments, or fascia attach to the bone), dactylitis (swelling along the entire length of a toe or finger), nail changes (thickening and onychodystrophy – raising the possibility of psoriatic arthritis), inflammatory arthritis (pain along with joint effusions, especially of the lower extremities – usually oligoarticular and asymmetric), inflammatory back pain (sacroiliitis seen on plain films, pain lessening with activity), urethritis or cervicitis (in women), aphthous ulcerations (either oral or in genital mucosa), conjunctivitis, and uveitis [4].

The laboratory findings in ReA may include a number of nonspecific findings to include an anemia of chronic inflammation, polyclonal gammopathy, and increased acute-phase reactants (CRP, ESR). There is no serologic test specific for ReA or the SNSAs (hence the name "seronegative"). Although ReA is often triggered by an enteric or GU infection, by the time the patient presents with an inflammatory arthritis or exanthem, the organism is no longer easily cultured from the stool or mucosa. There is little utility to testing for the presence of the HLA-B27 antigen as the sensitivity and specificity for diagnosing ReA or SNSA are poorly established.

See Also

Chapter 8 – Skin Lesions as a Result of Spondyloarthritides
Chapter 9 – Mucosal Lesions as a Result of Spondyloarthritides
Chapter 10 – Psoriatic Arthritis: Nails and Papules

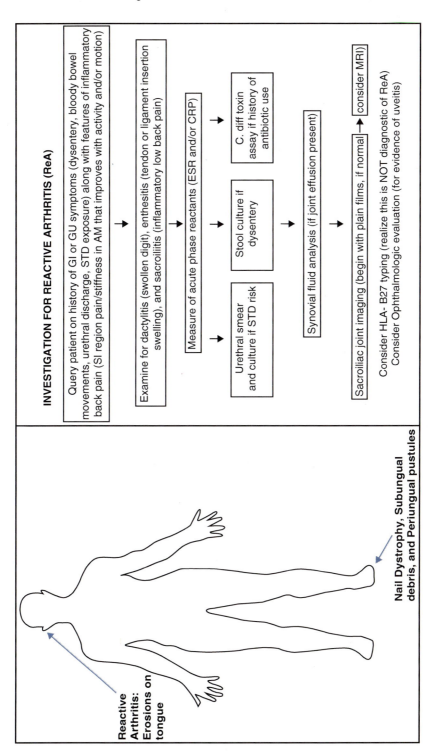

INVESTIGATION FOR REACTIVE ARTHRITIS (ReA)

Query patient on history of GI or GU symptoms (dysentery, bloody bowel movements, urethral discharge, STD exposure) along with features of inflammatory back pain (SI region pain/stiffness in AM that improves with activity and/or motion)

Examine for dactylitis (swollen digit), enthesitis (tendon or ligament insertion swelling), and sacroiliitis (inflammatory low back pain)

Measure of acute phase reactants (ESR and/or CRP)

Urethral smear and culture if STD risk

Stool culture if dysentery

C. diff toxin assay if history of antibiotic use

Synovial fluid analysis (if joint effusion present)

Sacroiliac joint imaging (begin with plain films, if normal → consider MRI)

Consider HLA- B27 typing (realize this is NOT diagnostic of ReA)
Consider Ophthalmologic evaluation (for evidence of uveitis)

Reactive Arthritis: Erosions on tongue

Nail Dystrophy, Subungual debris, and Periungual pustules

References

1. Parker CT, Thomas D. Reiter's syndrome and reactive arthritis. J Am Osteopath. 2000;100(2): 101–4.
2. Panush RS, Wallace DJ, Dorff RE, Engleman EP. Retraction of the suggestion to use the term "Reiter's syndrome" sixty-five years later: the legacy of Reiter, a war criminal, should not be eponymic honor but rather condemnation. Arthritis Rheum. 2007;56:693–4.
3. Wu IB, Schwartz RA. Reiter's syndrome: the classic triad and more. J Am Acad Dermatol. 2008;59:113–21.
4. Carter JD, Hudson AP. Reactive arthritis: clinical aspects and medical management. Rheum Dis Clin North Am. 2009;35(1):21–44.

Chapter 19
Parvovirus B19 Infection

Stanley J. Naides

Definition

Parvovirus B19 is a single-stranded, non-enveloped DNA virus of the family *Parvoviridae*, genus *Erythrovirus*. B19 causes asymptomatic infections; a flu-like illness; erythema infectiosum (fifth disease); hydrops fetalis and fetal loss; acute and chronic rheumatoid-like polyarthritis; chronic or recurrent bone marrow suppression in immunocompromised individuals; pancytopenia or isolated anemia, thrombocytopenia, and leukopenia; and, less commonly, hepatitis, fulminant liver failure, peripheral neuropathy, encephalopathy, and myocarditis or cardiomyopathy. Reports suggest that B19 may also be associated with vasculitis, including giant cell arteritis. B19 has tissue tropism for a broad array of tissues reflected by its clinical manifestations, but the virus productively replicates only in erythroid precursors. Classic erythema infectiosum is characterized by "slapped cheek" rash (Fig. 19.1). A macular or maculopapular eruption on the face and torso begins 7–18 days following infection. The rash spreads to the extremities, resolving in a centrifugal fashion. The rash is often mottled, lacy, reticulated, or fishnet-like in appearance. Rash may recur with exercise, sun exposure, or hot shower for weeks to months. Uncommon presentations include urticaria, a vesiculopustular rash, purpura with or without thrombocytopenia, Henoch-Schönlein purpura, and a "gloves and socks" acral erythema with or without papules [1–5].

S.J. Naides, M.D. (✉)
Immunology R&D, Quest Diagnostics Nichols Institute, 33608 Ortega Highway,
San Juan Capistrano, CA 92675, USA
e-mail: stanley.j.naides@questdiagnostics.com

M. Matucci-Cerinic et al. (eds.), *Skin Manifestations in Rheumatic Disease*, 151
DOI 10.1007/978-1-4614-7849-2_19, © Springer Science+Business Media New York 2014

Fig. 19.1 Classic "slapped" cheek rash of erythema infectiosum (fifth disease) on face and torso (Reprinted from Schneider AP, Naides SJ. Human Parvovirus Infection. Am J Family Physician. 39:165, 1989. With permission from American Academy of Family Physicians)

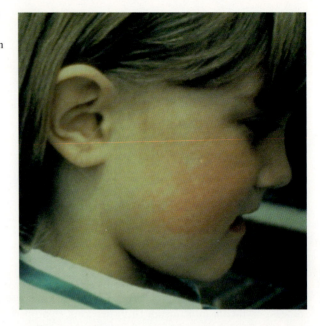

Differential Diagnosis

Bright-red "slapped" cheeks are highly suggestive of B19 infection. Macular or maculopapular rash is nonspecific and may be seen in a number of viral infections and drug eruptions. A history of exposure to B19 via a family contact or during a known outbreak is a helpful clue. Individuals with occupations that allow exposure to small children, e.g., school teachers or pediatric nurses, are at risk. Outbreaks typically occur in the winter and early spring, but outbreaks at other times of the year occur as do sporadic cases. A history of sudden-onset, symmetric, small joint polyarthralgia or polyarthritis should suggest the possibility of B19 infection. Rubella infection can present in the exact same manner with similar rash and poly-arthritis in a college age teen or young adult but is less common than B19 infection. Failure to confirm a recent B19 infection by the presence of serum anti-B19 IgM antibody should prompt consideration of testing for serum anti-rubella IgM antibody. Purpura may resemble many causes of purpura due to coagulopathy. Petechiae may resemble many causes of petechiae due to thrombocytopenia. Henoch-Schönlein purpura is suggested by the localization of purpura to the abdomen, buttocks, and lower extremities in the setting of arthritis, gastrointestinal symptoms, and/or hematuria following an antecedent respiratory illness; multiple triggers are known including B19 infection [1–4]. The differential diagnosis of the vesiculopus-tular eruption includes herpes simplex, varicella zoster, and vaccinia virus infection.

Fig. 19.2 (**a**) Arm showing finely papular eruption on an erythematous base with petechiae, evolving to (**b**) small, tense pustules and pseudopustules approaching confluence on an erythematous and slightly purpuric base (inset). Pustules and pseudopustules appear hemorrhagic 2 days later (Reprinted from Naides et al. Human parvovirus B19-induced vesiculopustular skin eruption. Amer J Med. 1988;84:968–972. With permission from Elsevier)

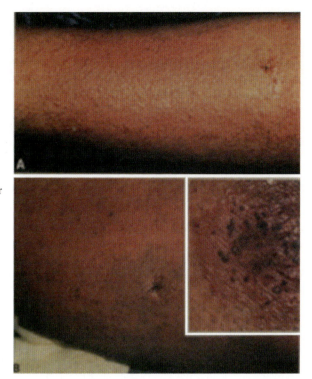

(Smallpox is also in the differential but not a routine consideration given its eradication from world populations.) "Gloves and socks" acral erythema is seen in B19.

Biopsy

Histological changes are not considered diagnostic. The putative receptor for B19, globoside, is present in the plasma membrane of endothelial cells. B19 may induce apoptosis in target cells nonpermissive for B19 replication through expression of its nonstructural protein, NS1, a helicase capable of damaging host cell genomic DNA. Electron microscopy may show B19 in lesional endothelial cells [6]. Catastrophic skin vascular endothelial cell injury has been described in B19 infection in which in situ reverse transcription and hybridization showed B19 RNA transcripts [3]. Vesiculopustular lesions show ballooning degeneration of keratinocytes with a mixed inflammatory cell infiltrate that may contain numerous eosinophils. Local edema, dilated vessels, and erythrocyte extravasation suggest local capillary leak. A lymphohistiocytic infiltrate with markedly abnormal atypical cells showing enlarged, hyperchromic nuclei may be present (Figs. 19.2 and 19.3) [7].

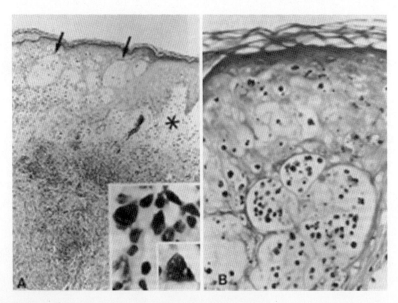

Fig. 19.3 Histology of biopsy site shown in Fig. 19.2. (**a**) *Arrows* show epidermal necrosis with vesicle formation. *Asterisk* shows prominent subepidermal edema. *Dermis* shows erythrocyte extravasation and lymphohistiocytic infiltrates including (large inset) atypical lymphohistiocytic cells and (small insert) binucleated giant cells. (**b**) *Pustule* showing ballooning degeneration and a multiloculated vesicle with neutrophilic infiltrate (Reprinted from Naides et al. Human parvovirus B19-induced vesiculopustular skin eruption. Amer J Med. 1988;84:968–972. With permission from Elsevier)

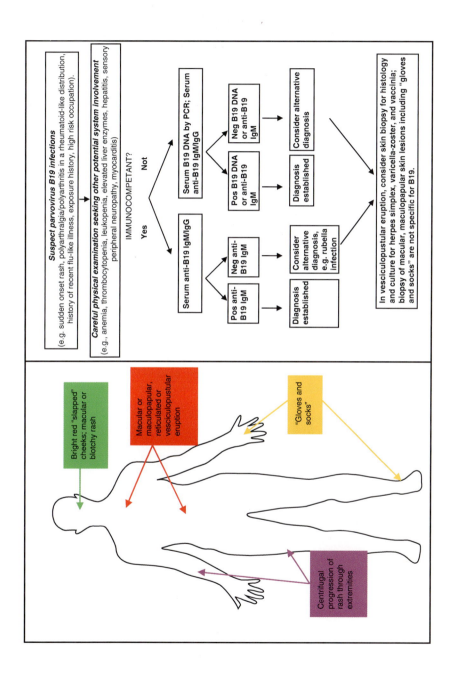

Suspect parvovirus B19 infections
(e.g. sudden onset rash, polyarthralgia/polyarthritis in a rheumatoid-like distribution, history of recent flu-like illness, exposure history, high risk occupation).

Careful physical examination seeking other potential system involvement
(e.g., anemia, thrombocytopenia, leukopenia, elevated liver enzymes, hepatitis, sensory peripheral neuropathy, myocarditis)

IMMUNOCOMPETANT?

Yes

Not

Serum anti-B19 IgM/IgG

Pos anti-B19 IgM

Neg anti-B19 IgM

Diagnosis established

Consider alternative diagnosis, e.g. rubella infection

Serum B19 DNA by PCR; Serum anti-B19 IgM/IgG

Pos B19 DNA or anti-B19 IgM

Neg B19 DNA or anti-B19 IgM

Diagnosis established

Consider alternative diagnosis

In vesiculopustular eruption, consider skin biopsy for histology and culture for herpes simplex, varicella-zoster, and vaccinia; biopsy of macular, maculopapular skin lesions including "gloves and socks" are not specific for B19.

Bright red "slapped" cheeks; macular or blotchy rash

Macular or maculopapular, reticulated or vesciculopustular eruption

"Gloves and socks"

Centrifugal progression of rash through extremities

References

1. Aractingi S, et al. Immunohistochemical and virological study of skin in the papular-purpuric gloves and socks syndrome. Br J Dermatol. 1996;135:599.
2. Cioc AM, et al. Parvovirus B19 associated adult Henoch Schönlein purpura. J Cutan Pathol. 2002;29:602.
3. Dyrsen ME, et al. Parvovirus B19-associated catastrophic endothelialitis with a Degos-like presentation. J Cutan Pathol. 2008;35 Suppl 1:20.
4. Hsieh MY, Huang PH. The juvenile variant of papular-purpuric gloves and socks syndrome and its association with viral infections. Br J Dermatol. 2004;151:201.
5. Naides SJ, et al. Human parvovirus B19-induced vesiculopustular skin eruption. Am J Med. 1988;84:968.
6. Takahashi M, et al. Human parvovirus B19 infection: immunohistochemical and electron microscopic studies of skin lesions. J Cutan Pathol. 1995;22:168.
7. Santonja C. Immunohistochemical detection of parvovirus B19 in "gloves and socks" papular purpuric syndrome: direct evidence for viral endothelial involvement. Report of three cases and review of the literature. Am J Dermatopathol. 2011;33:790.

Chapter 20
Rheumatic Fever

Fernanda Falcini

Definition

Acute rheumatic fever (ARF) is a nonsuppurative complication of sore throat by highly virulent group A streptococcus (GAS) strains with large hyaluronate capsules and M protein molecules containing epitopes cross-reactive with host tissues. It affects multiple organs of the body: heart, skin, joints, and nervous system. Cardiac involvement is the most serious manifestation accounting for the major clinical and public health effects due to the long-term damage to heart valves. ARF is rare in young children before full maturation of the immune system and peaks between 5 and 15 years. Males and females are equally affected except for chorea that is prevalent in girls. Host factors are important in the pathogenesis of disease, and a genetic susceptibility has been suggested. Its incidence is as high as 100–200/100,000 per year in Eastern Europe, Middle East, Asia, and Australia, while in America and Western Europe, it ranges from 0.5 to 3/100,000. The major clinical manifestations are as follows: (1) Arthritis (80 % of cases) is migratory, painful at rest, and exacerbated by movement, promptly responsive to aspirin, with no sequelae (Fig. 20.1). (2) Carditis (50 %) is the major cause of morbidity and mortality. The myocardium, endocardium, and pericardium are affected (Fig. 20.2); endocarditis is the main manifestation with mitral regurgitation and less commonly aortic insufficiency. (3) Erythema marginatum (5 %) is a macular, non-pruritic rash with serpiginous erythematosus spots located on the trunk and rarely on the face, commonly associated with arthritis or carditis (Figs. 20.3 and 20.4). Subcutaneous nodules are rare and located on the extensor surface of joints as knees, elbows, ankles, and knuckles, not painful, movable, and resembling benign rheumatoid nodules

F. Falcini, M.D. (✉)
Internal Medicine, Rheumatology Section, University of Florence,
Viale Pieraccini 18, Florence 50139, Italy
e-mail: falcini@unifi.it

M. Matucci-Cerinic et al. (eds.), *Skin Manifestations in Rheumatic Disease*,
DOI 10.1007/978-1-4614-7849-2_20, © Springer Science+Business Media New York 2014

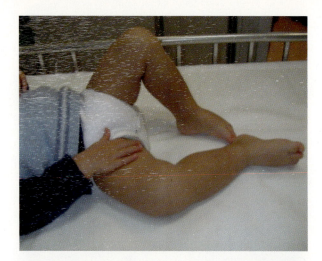

Fig. 20.1 Migrant, painful arthritis in a 6-year-old boy with ARF

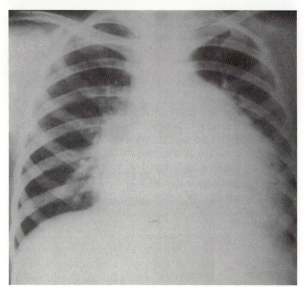

Fig. 20.2 Chest radiograph of an 8-year-old patient with acute carditis and pericardial effusion

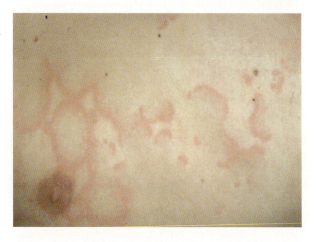

Fig. 20.3 Typical erythema marginatum in an 11-year-old girl with ARF. In this patient, erythema was also present on the face

Fig. 20.4 Subcutaneous nodules over the wrist in a 12-year-old boy with ARF. This boy developed mitral insufficiency

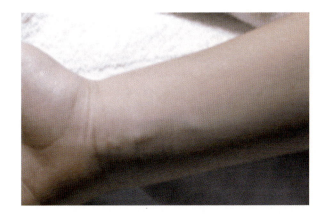

Fig. 20.5 Subcutaneous nodules on the extensor aspect of elbow in a 12-year-old boy with ARF. This boy developed pericarditis

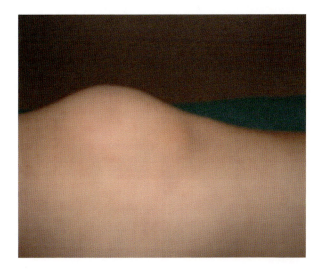

(Fig. 20.5). Sydenham's chorea, related to inflammation of the basal ganglia and caudate nucleus of the CNS, is a late complication characterized by involuntary, purposeless, symmetric, and uncoordinated movements of the extremities that disappear at sleep. According to the revised Jones' criteria, the diagnosis of ARF requires 2 major criteria or 1 major and 2 minor (fever, arthralgia, elevated acute phase reactants, or prolonged PR interval) with supporting evidence of antecedent GAS infection. This latter consists of positive throat culture or rapid test, or elevated or rising streptococcal antibody test. If arthritis is the major criteria, arthralgia may not be a minor criterion [1–5].

Differential Diagnosis

The most common conditions that may be differentiated by ARF include other rheumatic diseases with arthritis (septic arthritis, juvenile idiopathic arthritis, systemic lupus erythematosus, connective tissue diseases, post-streptococcal reactive arthritis, and all post-infectious arthritis). Chorea may be differentiated by other diseases with choreic movements: systemic lupus erythematosus, primary antiphospholipid syndrome, and neurological diseases.

Biopsy

No biopsy is required to diagnose ARF.

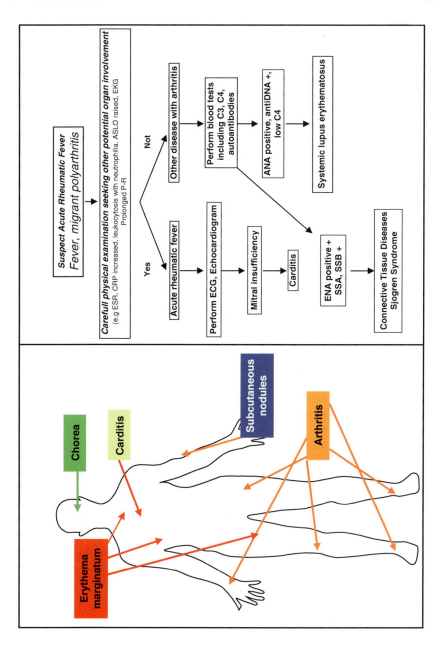

References

1. Bryant PA, et al. Some of the people, some of the time: susceptibility to acute rheumatic fever. Circulation. 2009;119:742–53.
2. Ferrieri P and for the Jones Criteria Working Group: Proceedings of the Jones Criteria Working Group, Circulation. 2002;106:2521–23.
3. Tani LY. Rheumatic fever in children younger than5 years: is the presentation different? Pediatrics. 2003;112:1065–8.
4. Gerber MA, et al. Prevention of rheumatic fever and diagnosis and treatment of acute Streptococcal pharyngitis. Circulation. 2009;119:1541–51.
5. Stollerman GH. Rheumatic fever in the 21st century. CID. 2001;33:806–14.

Part IV
Connective Tissue Diseases

Chapter 21
Skin Manifestations of Localized Scleroderma (LS)

Nicolas Hunzelmann, Gerd Horneff, and Thomas Krieg

Definition

Localized scleroderma (LS) encompasses a spectrum of sclerotic disorders of the skin, which, depending on the subtype and localization, may also affect nearby structures including fat tissue, muscles, joints, and bones. Involvement of internal organs (e.g., heart, lungs, kidneys, or gastrointestinal tract) is absent in localized scleroderma. The exceptions are (i) involvement of the brain (including the eye), which may complicate linear scleroderma of the head, and (ii) the occurrence of arthritis, which has particularly been observed in affected children.

The incidence of LS is reported at around 27 per 1 million inhabitants occurring more frequently in women than in men, at a ratio of 2.6–6 to 1 [1]. Recently, a classification has been suggested largely based on the classification described by Peterson et al. [2]. It incorporates both the extent of involvement and the depth of the fibrosis. According to this classification, localized scleroderma is divided into four basic types: limited, generalized, linear, and deep (Table 21.1). Some add a mixed group to this classification. This simple classification system has the advantage of

N. Hunzelmann, M.D.
Department of Dermatology, University Cologne, Kerpener Str. 62, Köln, Cologne 50937, Germany
e-mail: nico.hunzelmann@uni-koeln.de

G. Horneff, M.D.
Department of Pediatrics, Asklepios Clinic Sankt Augustin, Arnold-Janssen-Str. 29, Sankt Augustin 53757, Germany
e-mail: g.horneff@asklepios.com

T. Krieg, M.D. (✉)
Department of Dermatology and Venerology, University Hospital of Cologne, Kerpener Str. 62, Köln, Cologne 50937, Germany
e-mail: thomas.krieg@uni-koeln.de

M. Matucci-Cerinic et al. (eds.), *Skin Manifestations in Rheumatic Disease*, DOI 10.1007/978-1-4614-7849-2_21, © Springer Science+Business Media New York 2014

Table 21.1 Classification of localized scleroderma

Limited type
Morphea (plaque type)
Guttate morphea
Atrophoderma of Pasini and Pierini
Generalized type
Generalized localized scleroderma (3 or more anatomic sites)
Disabling pansclerotic morphea
Eosinophilic fasciitis
Linear type
Linear localized scleroderma (usually with involvement of the extremities)
Linear localized scleroderma, "en coup de sabre" type
Progressive facial hemiatrophy (synonym: Parry Romberg syndrome)
Deep type

reflecting the major prognostic and therapeutic aspects of localized scleroderma. For instance, in the limited type, LS resolves within about 2.5 years in around 50 % of patients [2, 3]. In generalized, linear, and deep types, the average duration of disease is longer, at about 5.5 years with secondary changes such as hyper- or depigmentation, contractures, and atrophy generally persisting. The frequencies of the subtypes vary depending on age. The linear type is more prevalent in children [4]. In pediatric patients it may also be observed that several disease types may occur simultaneously or over time, e.g., linear LS combined with limited LS.

Limited Type of Localized Scleroderma

The most common form of the limited type of LS is the plaque type (morphea). The plaque type is characterized by lesions measuring more than 1 cm in diameter affecting one or two areas of the integument. Characteristic sites of predilection are the trunk – especially the submammary region – and the area between the hip and inguinal regions. The often oval-shaped lesions have an erythematous appearance in the early phases, later hardening increasingly in the center and taking on a whitish or ivory color. Active lesions are characterized by a violet halo surrounding the fibrotic part well known as the "lilac ring." Fibrosis may be accompanied by the loss of skin appendages and alopecia. Often sclerotic lesions soften over time and even become atrophic, hypo-, or hyperpigmented.

The guttate type of limited scleroderma (morphea guttata) is characterized by multiple yellowish-whitish, small sclerotic lesions that have a glistening surface (<1 cm with a "lilac ring" in clinically active disease) and are located predominantly on the trunk. These lesions may at first simply present as erythematous maculae. Atrophoderma of Pasini and Pierini is possibly an early abortive type of guttate scleroderma. The clinical presentation of this variety, which frequently manifests during childhood, is characterized by symmetrical lesions on the trunk that measure

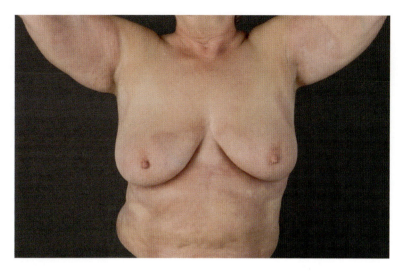

Fig. 21.1 Patient with a generalized form of LS. Please note the involvement of axillary, mammary, and abdominal regions

less than 1 cm in diameter. Loss of connective tissue can result in wedge-shaped depressions below the level of the skin. Histology corresponds to late atrophic phases of localized scleroderma.

Generalized Type of LS

The generalized type of LS is diagnosed if three or more anatomic sites are affected. The most commonly affected sites are the trunk, thighs, and lumbosacral region. The plaques are often distributed symmetrically and can coalesce into larger lesions representing different stages of the disease (Fig. 21.1).

A rare, severe variant of the generalized type of localized scleroderma is "disabling pansclerotic morphea." This variant, sometimes in combination with the linear type, leads to extensive skin involvement with only a limited tendency to regression. In these patients contractures and impaired wound healing develop, leading in some patients to ulceration.

Eosinophilic fasciitis (Shulman's syndrome) is by some experts considered to belong to the disease group of LS and in our opinion belongs to the generalized type.

Linear Type of LS

Linear localized scleroderma is characterized by longitudinally arranged linear, band-like, or systematic lesions often following Blaschko's lines [5]. In mild cases

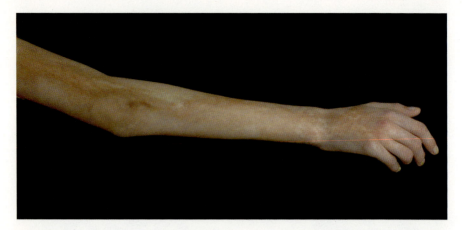

Fig. 21.2 Patient with linear scleroderma affecting the arm leading to atrophy and movement restriction

the lesions may heal with hyperpigmentation as the only residuum. However, in many patients the linear type is characterized by the formation of tough, sclerotic bands that sometimes cross joints and may restrict movement. Linear scleroderma can be accompanied by atrophy of the underlying muscle or bone at affected sites (Fig. 21.2). Antinuclear antibodies, usually of low titer and without further specificity, have been reported in up to 50 % of patients with the linear form of LS. The best known type is the "en coup de sabre" form, where the sclerotic tissue passes over the frontoparietal region, usually paramedian from the eyebrows into the hair-bearing scalp resulting in scarring alopecia (Fig. 21.3). Involvement of the underlying central nervous system (CNS), as detectable by MRI, is quite common. Clinically relevant associated neurological changes as, e.g., epilepsy and headache are, however, less frequent. More on the facial involvement of localized SSc is found in Chapter xxx.

Linear localized scleroderma is also related to progressive facial hemiatrophy (synonym: hemiatrophia faciei or Parry Romberg syndrome). Progressive facial hemiatrophy is characterized by primary atrophic transformation of the affected subcutaneous tissue, muscle, and bone. Skin fibrosis is rare. Onset is often during childhood or adolescence with involvement of subcutaneous tissue in the head region. Later on, the disease increasingly affects the underlying muscles, bone, and the tongue finally leading to severe facial asymmetry. Simultaneous occurrence of linear localized scleroderma of the "en coup de sabre" type and progressive facial hemiatrophy is quite frequent (up to 40 % of cases). In the classification proposed by the authors, the "en coup de sabre" type is thus listed under the linear types, although with exclusive involvement of extracutaneous structures, it may also be classified as a "deep type" of localized scleroderma. Involvement of the central nervous system is not uncommon. Antinuclear autoantibodies are found, usually in low titers, in up to 60 % and rheumatoid factors are described in up to 30 % of these patients. More on this facial lesion is found in Chapter xx.

Fig. 21.3 Patient with the "coup de sabre" variant of linear scleroderma. Please note the scarring alopecia

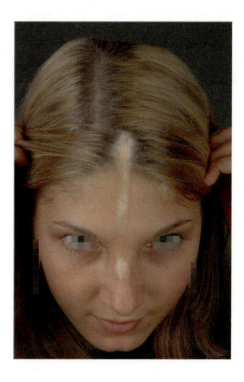

Deep Type of LS

The deep type of LS is very rare (<5 % of patients). Here, fibrosis mainly affects the deeper layers of the connective tissue, i.e., fat tissue, fascia, and underlying muscle. Lesions are typically arranged symmetrically on the extremities. The deep type of LS (deep morphea) can begin during childhood and may manifest without noticeable prior inflammation.

Differential Diagnosis

In long-standing LS, acrodermatitis chronica atrophicans, lipodystrophy, and lichen sclerosus should be excluded, and with lower leg involvement, necrobiosis lipoidica and pretibial myxedema should be considered.

In generalized localized scleroderma, the differential diagnoses include systemic scleroderma, pseudoscleroderma, scleroderma adultorum (Buschke's disease), scleromyxedema, sclerodermiform graft versus host disease, and nephrogenic systemic fibrosis.

Differential diagnoses in linear localized scleroderma – the "en coup de sabre" variant or progressive facial hemiatrophy – include panniculitis, progressive partial lipodystrophy, focal dermal hypoplasia, steroid atrophy, and lupus erythematosus profundus.

Biopsy

The characteristic plaque lesions are characterized by an inflammatory ring surrounding an area of sclerosis. Accordingly, in the inflammatory area, typical findings include dense perivascular and periadnexal inflammatory infiltrates in the reticular dermis which may extend into the subcutis (see Fig. 21.4). Lymphocytes predominate and plasma cells, histiocytes, and eosinophilic granulocytes may be present. The dermal connective tissue often contains thickened collagen fiber bundles with a superficial parallel arrangement as well as edema in the upper dermis. In the late phase, the dermis shows a cell poor fibrosis accompanied by a marked reduction of skin adnexa (Fig. 21.5).

On histological grounds systemic sclerosis and localized scleroderma cannot be differentiated. This holds also true for late stages of eosinophilic fasciitis. A clue may be the involvement of the fascia, underlining the importance of the depth of biopsy when eosinophilic fasciitis is considered.

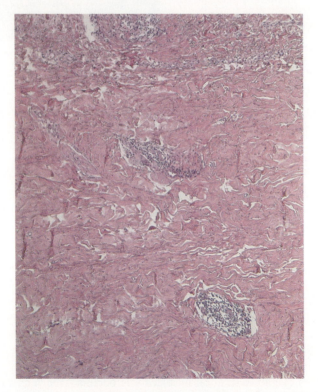

Fig. 21.4 Inflammatory stage of scleroderma. Please note the perivascular lymphoplasma cellular infiltrate

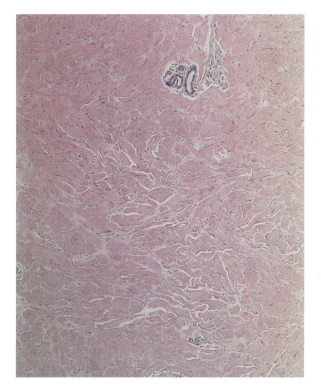

Fig. 21.5 Fibrotic stage of scleroderma. Please note the cell poor fibrosis and entrapment of eccrine glands by compacted bands of collagen

Diagnostics

Biopsy in a patient with characteristic clinical presentation will not be necessary, but may be needed to confirm or rule out differential diagnoses of LS as, e.g., necrobiosis lipoidica, acrodermatitis, eosinophilic fasciitis, and nephrogenic systemic fibrosis.

In linear localized scleroderma of the "en coup de sabre" type and in progressive facial hemiatrophy, patients who have neurological symptoms and suspected CNS involvement should undergo a cranial MRI.

See Also

Nephrogenic systemic fibrosis, Eosinophilic fasciitis, Scleroderma, Amyloidosis.

Identify other topics in the book where the lesion or the disease is also mentioned and described.

DIAGNOSTIC FLOW CHART

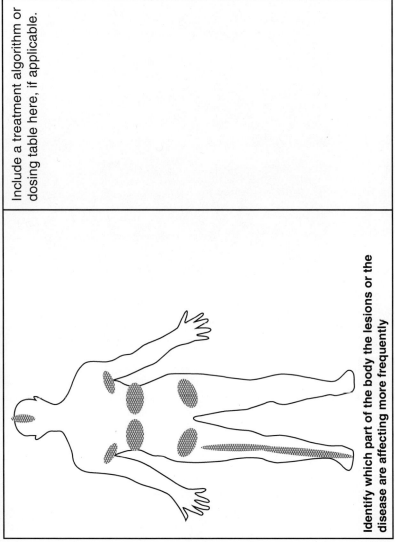

Include a treatment algorithm or dosing table here, if applicable.

Identify which part of the body the lesions or the disease are affecting more frequently

References

1. Silman A, Jannini S, Symmons D, Bacon P. An epidemiological study of scleroderma in the West Midlands. Br J Rheumatol. 1988;27:286–90.
2. Peterson LS, Nelson AM, Su WP. Classification of morphea. Mayo Clin Proc. 1995;70: 1068–76.
3. Christianson H, Dorsey C, O'Leary P, Kierland R. Localized scleroderma: a clinical study of two hundred thirty-five cases. Arch Dermatol. 1956;74:629–39.
4. Zulian F, Vallongo C, Woo P, et al. Localized scleroderma in childhood is not just a skin disease. Arthritis Rheum. 2005;52:2873–81.
5. Weibel L, Harper JI. Linear morphoea follows Blaschko's lines. Br J Dermatol. 2008;159: 175–81.

Suggested Reading

Bodemer C, Belon M, Hamel-Teillac D, Amoric JC, Fraitag S, Prieur AM, De Prost Y. Scleroderma in children: a retrospective study of 70 cases. Ann Dermatol Venerol. 1999;126:691–4.
Jablonska S. Facial hemiatrophy and it's relation to localized scleroderma. In: Jablonska S, editor. Scleroderma and pseudoscleroderma. Warsaw: PZWL; 1975. p. 537–48.
Kencka D, Blaszczyk M, Jablonska S. Atrophoderma Pasini-Pierini is a primary atrophic abortive morphea. Dermatology. 1995;190:203–6.
Kreuter A, Krieg T, Worm M, Wenzel J, Gambichler T, Kuhn A, Aberer E, Scharffetter-Kochanek K, Hunzelmann N. Diagnosis and therapy of circumscribed scleroderma. J Dtsch Dermatol Ges. 2009;7 Suppl 6:S1–14.
Sommer A, Gambichler T, Bacharach-Buhles M, von Rothenburg T, Altmeyer P, Kreuter A. Clinical and serological characteristics of progressive facial hemiatrophy: a case series of 12 patients. J Am Acad Dermatol. 2006;54:227–33.

Chapter 22
Localized Scleroderma of the Face

Francesco Zulian, Sabina Trainito, and Anna Belloni-Fortina

Localized scleroderma, also known as morphea, is a condition characterized by sclerosis of the skin and subcutaneous tissue, due to increased collagen content which can be either confined to the superficial layers of the dermis or extended to the deep dermis, fascia, and muscle. Localized scleroderma can be classified into five subtypes: circumscribed (plaque) morphea, linear scleroderma, generalized morphea, pansclerotic morphea, and a mixed subtype where a combination of two or more of the previous subtypes is present [1].

Conversely from adulthood, where systemic sclerosis is far more frequent, localized scleroderma is the predominant form of scleroderma in children, and the linear one is the most frequent subtype [2].

Linear scleroderma is characterized by streaks of skin induration affecting the limbs, the trunk, or the face, which can extend through the dermis to the muscle and bone and leading to significant functional limitations and aesthetical deformities. In the clinical practice, we can distinguish two types of linear scleroderma of the face (LSF). En coup de sabre (ECDS) scleroderma, so called because it resembles the stroke of a sword, affects the paramedial frontal area of the face and/or the scalp,

F. Zulian, M.D. (✉)
Pediatric Rheumatology Unit, Department of Pediatrics- Rheumatology Section,
University of Padua, Via Giustiniani 3, Padua 35128, Italy
e-mail: zulian@pediatria.unipd.it

S. Trainito
Pediatric Rheumatology Unit, University of Padua, Padua, Italy

A. Belloni-Fortina, M.D.
Pediatric Dermatology – Internal Medicine, Azienda Ospedaliera – Università di Padova,
Via C. Battisti, 206, Padova 35128, Italy
e-mail: belloni@pediatria.unipd.it

M. Matucci-Cerinic et al. (eds.), *Skin Manifestations in Rheumatic Disease*,
DOI 10.1007/978-1-4614-7849-2_22, © Springer Science+Business Media New York 2014

Fig. 22.1 *En coup de sabre*
scleroderma in a 10-year-old
girl: frontal-parietal linear
lesion resembling the stroke
of a sword

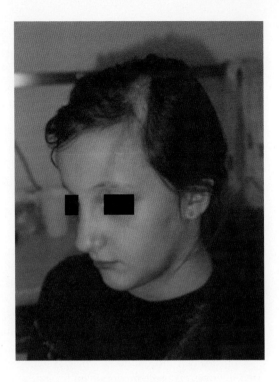

usually in association with scarring alopecia and skin discoloration (Fig. 22.1). Parry-Romberg syndrome (PRS), or progressive facial hemiatrophy, mainly affects subcutaneous tissue, muscle, and bone, often sparing the skin. The lesion, at onset, affects the muscles of the cheeks as well as the bone and tongue, progressively extending and leading to unilateral hypotrophy and undergrowth of the lower third of the face, with consequent severe cosmetic disfigurement (Fig. 22.2). While early, inflammatory lesions are usually surrounded by a violaceous border, late, chronic lesions appear sclerotic and/or atrophic [3, 4]. The significant overlap between these two conditions, the frequency of ocular and CNS complications [5, 6] and the prevalence of autoantibodies in both ECDS and PRS allow not to consider them as separate conditions but as part of the same disease spectrum [4, 7, 8].

Differential Diagnosis

LSF should be distinguished from other conditions affecting the dermis and subcutaneous tissue, such as partial progressive lipodystrophy, focal dermal hypoplasia, or atrophoderma after intramuscular injections of corticosteroids or vitamin K.

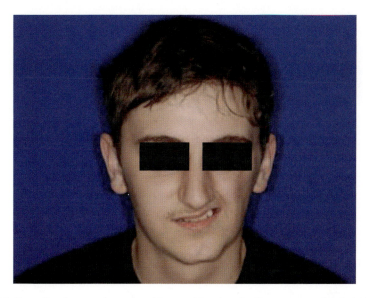

Fig. 22.2 Parry-Romberg syndrome in a 14-year-old patient, leading to progressive facial hemiatrophy of the left side of the face

The initial stage of LSF should be differentiated from annular erythema, erythema migrans, and sarcoidosis. The atrophic lesions of LSF should be distinguished from lichen sclerosus and atrophicus or other forms of panniculitis, especially the lupus-induced variety, called *lupus profundus*. The differential diagnosis of the latter with linear scleroderma as well as with deep morphea may be difficult. Even the biopsy is not always conclusive in this respect [9]. However, the circumscribed appearance of the lesions, presenting as sclerotic frontoparietal bands on one side of the face; the presence of serum autoantibodies; and the aggressive course, in most of the cases, are strongly suggestive of LSF [3].

Pathology

The skin biopsy is not mandatory to make the diagnosis of LSF; however, it could be advisable to confirm it in doubtful cases. When taking a specimen, the excision should be deep enough to include the subcutis, fat tissue, fascia, and muscle to exclude possible involvement of inner structures. Apart from the lack of intimal fibrosis due to microvascular damage, typical of systemic sclerosis (SSc), no reliable histological criteria of discernment between LSF and SSc are actually available. Despite the limitations of being invasive, skin biopsy should be performed

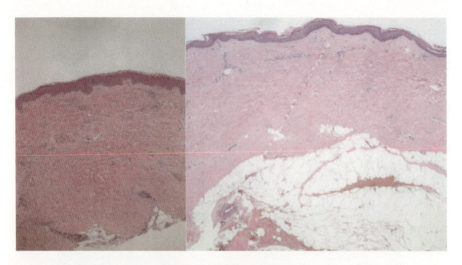

Fig. 22.3 Normal skin on the *left image* compared with morphea on the right. The latter is characterized by thickening of collagen bundles extending to the region of the subcutaneous fat, atrophy of the eccrine glands, and mononuclear cell infiltrates (*Hematoxylin and Eosin staining, original magnification 25x*)

mainly to confirm the diagnosis of LSF, to differentiate it from other fibrotic disorders, and to assess the depth of lesion. The early stage (inflammatory) is characterized by thickened collagen bundles with perivascular and periadnexal lymphoplasmacytic infiltrate in the reticular dermis, sometimes extended to the subcutis (Fig. 22.3). In the late stage (sclerotic), newly formed collagen replaces most of the subcutaneous fat, with resulting displacement of the eccrine glands higher in the dermis [10, 11].

Diagnostic Flowchart

The diagnosis of LSF is mainly clinical (Fig. 22.4). Despite the lack of specific serologic parameters, blood tests are considered the first step to confirm the diagnosis. Hypergammaglobulinemia and eosinophilia are quite common in children with LSF, while ANA positivity, regarded by many authors as an epiphenomenon, is nonetheless detectable in up to 50% of the patients [3].

Pivotal is the role of the biopsy, especially for differential diagnosis and assessment of therapeutic effectiveness. When the diagnosis of LSF is made, the involvement of both eye and CNS should be excluded by an ophthalmological examination and CNS imaging (cerebral MRI and/or CT scan), respectively.

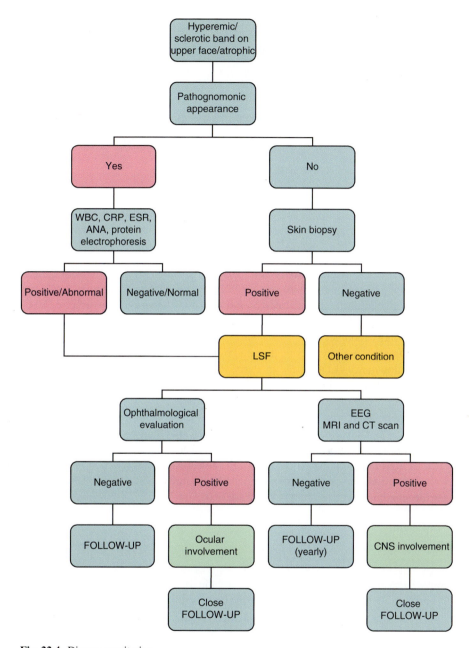

Fig. 22.4 Disease monitoring

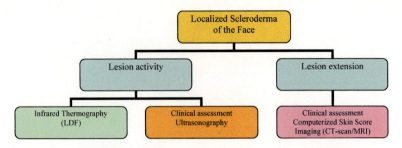

Fig. 22.5 Treatment approach of localized scleroderma of the face

Disease Monitoring

The assessment of lesion activity and extension is crucial to guide both the therapeutic approach and the follow-up (Fig. 22.5). Both lesion activity and extension can be evaluated through clinical scores (LoSSI) [12] and ultrasonography (USG) 20 MHz probes [13]. Unfortunately, both tools are operator dependent, and therefore not totally reliable.

Inflammatory activity may be detected by infrared thermography [14] or by laser Doppler flowmetry (LDF) [15]. In Parry-Romberg syndrome, thermography may sometimes give false-positive results on silent, atrophic lesions, so a correlation with a careful clinical examination is always needed.

Lesion extension can be also assessed by objective techniques, such as CT scan and MRI, which are also essential for the surgical planning. Despite their high reliability and reproducibility, these techniques present some limitations in children, such as high radiation exposure (CT scan), need for general sedation or prolonged immobilization, and costs. A computerized skin score (CSS) was recently proposed for the standardized assessment of disease extension [16].

Treatment

Since there are not validated guidelines, yet, the management and treatment of LSF is challenging (Fig. 22.6). Table 22.1 summarizes the drugs most frequently used in LSF with their dosage. While for circumscribed isolated lesions, a local treatment with topical agents and phototherapy has been suggested [17]; for linear active lesions, a more aggressive systemic therapy is recommended, given the progressive nature of the disease [1, 18, 19].

Methotrexate represents the most common and widely used drug during the recent years. It has been used successfully in children and adults with LSc [17, 18]. A recent randomized double-blind placebo-controlled trial comparing a 12-month

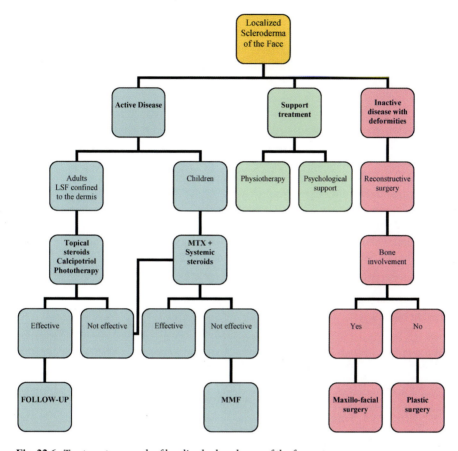

Fig. 22.6 Treatment approach of localized scleroderma of the face

Table 22.1 Treatments most frequently used in localized scleroderma of the face

Drug	Dose
Topical corticosteroids (moderately or highly potent)	Once daily for 3 months
Topical calcipotriol (0.005 %)	Once daily for 3 months
UVA1 phototherapy	20–80 J/cm^2 3–5/week, max 40 exposures
PUVA therapy	2–4/week, max 30 exposures
Methotrexate	12.5–25 mg/week in adults, 10–15 mg/m^2 once weekly in children, oral, sc, im
Systemic corticosteroids	Prednisone 0.5–1.0 mg/kg/day oral for 3 months, or 20–30 mg/kg IV methylprednisolone pulse therapy for 3 days monthly
Mycophenolate mofetil	600–1,200 mg/m^2 daily

course of oral methotrexate (15 mg/m^2) in combination with a 3-month course of oral prednisone (1 mg/kg/day, maximum dose 50 mg) with a 3-month course of oral prednisone only, at the same dosage, showed that methotrexate was effective and well tolerated in more than two-thirds of the patients with LSc [18]. A long-term follow-up study of the same patient cohort showed that prolonged remission off medication was achieved in patients treated for more than 24 months [20]. A relapse rate of 12.5 % was reported in a small group of patients treated for less than 24 months, whereas no relapses were noted in those treated longer.

In patients who are refractory to methotrexate and systemic corticosteroids, mycophenolate mofetil (MMF) may be considered [21]. In addition, physiotherapy is advised in order to prevent or relieve contractures and muscle atrophy. Given the disfiguring and evolutionary chronic course of the disease, a psychological support should be considered in order to help the patients and their families cope with the emotional impact of the disease [22]. Once the disease reaches a persistent inactive phase and when the child's growth is complete, surgical treatment may be planned, according to both functional and aesthetic needs [23].

References

1. Laxer RM, Zulian F. Localized scleroderma. Curr Opin Rheumatol. 2006;18:606.
2. Zulian F. Systemic sclerosis and localized scleroderma in childhood. Rheum Dis Clin North Am. 2008;34:239.
3. Zulian F. Juvenile localized scleroderma: clinical and epidemiological features in 750 children. An international study. Rheumatology (Oxford). 2006;45:614.
4. Tollefson MM, Witman PM. En coup de sabre morphea and Parry-Romberg syndrome: a retrospective review of 54 patients. J Am Acad Dermatol. 2007;56:257.
5. Zannin ME, et al. Ocular involvement in children with localised scleroderma: a multi-centre study. Br J Ophthalmol. 2007;91:131.
6. Zulian F, et al. Localized Scleroderma in childhood is not just a skin disease. Arthritis Rheum. 2005;52:2873.
7. Blaszczyk M, et al. Progressive facial hemiatrophy: central nervous system involvement and relationship with scleroderma en coup de sabre. J Rheumatol. 2003;30:1997.
8. Sommer A, et al. Clinical and serological characteristics of progressive facial hemiatrophy: a case series of 12 patients. J Am Acad Dermatol. 2006;54:227.
9. Jablonska S, Blaszczyk M. Scleroderma overlap syndromes. Adv Exp Med Biol. 1999;455:85.
10. Tuffanelli DL. Localized scleroderma. Semin Cutan Med Surg. 1998;17:27.
11. Vierra E, Cunningham BB. Morphea and localized scleroderma in children. Semin Cutan Med Surg. 1999;18:210.
12. Arkachaisri T, et al. The localized scleroderma skin severity index and physician global assessment of disease activity: a work in progress toward development of localized scleroderma outcome measures. J Rheumatol. 2009;36:2819.
13. Li SC, Liebling MS. The use of Doppler ultrasound to evaluate lesions of localized scleroderma. Curr Rheumatol Rep. 2009;11:205.
14. Martini G, et al. Juvenile-onset localized scleroderma activity detection by infrared thermography. Rheumatology (Oxford). 2002;41:1178.
15. Weibel L, et al. Laser Doppler flowmetry for assessing localized scleroderma in children. Arthritis Rheum. 2007;56:34.

16. Zulian F, et al. A new computerized method for the assessment of skin lesions in localized scleroderma. Rheumatology (Oxford). 2007;46:856.
17. Kreuter A, Altmeyer P, Gambichler T. Treatment of localized scleroderma depends on the clinical subtype. Br J Dermatol. 2007;156:1362.
18. Zulian F, et al. Methotrexate treatment in juvenile localized scleroderma. A randomized, double-blind, placebo-controlled trial. Arthritis Rheum. 2011;63:1998.
19. Li SC, et al. Development of consensus treatment plans for juvenile localized scleroderma: a roadmap toward comparative effectiveness studies in juvenile localized scleroderma. Arthritis Care Res. 2012;64:1175.
20. Zulian F, et al. A long-term follow-up study of methotrexate in juvenile localized scleroderma (morphea). J Am Acad Dermatol. 2012;67:1151.
21. Martini G, et al. Successful treatment of severe or methotrexate-resistant juvenile localized scleroderma with mycophenolate mofetil. Rheumatology (Oxford). 2009;48:1410.
22. Orzechowski NM, et al. Health-related quality of life in children and adolescents with juvenile localized scleroderma. Rheumatology (Oxford). 2009;48:670.
23. Palmero ML, et al. En coup de sabre scleroderma and Parry-Romberg syndrome in adolescents: surgical options and patient-related outcomes. J Rheumatol. 2010;37:2174.

Chapter 23
Skin Manifestations of Raynaud's Phenomenon

Noëlle S. Sherber and Fredrick M. Wigley

Definition

Raynaud's phenomenon describes an exaggerated response in the thermoregulatory vessels of the skin to cold exposure and/or emotional stress. Raynaud's phenomenon is characterized by episodic tissue ischemia, which most commonly involves the digits of the hands and feet (rarely also involving the ears, nose, face, tongue, or nipples).

When this clinically presents as cold skin with a mottled blue cyanotic appearance, this is indicative of reduced blood flow from vasoconstriction involving only the superficial thermoregulatory vessels (Fig. 23.1). If the vasoconstriction is more intense and involves the digital arteries, precapillary arterioles, and cutaneous thermoregulatory arteriovenous shunts, it can present with pallor of the skin (Fig. 23.2). This represents a true ischemic attack as the white appearance of the skin results from lack of perfusion to the skin and deeper tissue. An erythematous blush can then occur as a consequence of rebound perfusion (Fig. 23.3). These stages of cyanosis, pallor, and erythema can be seen concordantly.

During the ischemic phase, patients often experience numbness and paresthesias as a result of digital vessel vasospasm. True pain is a symptom of deprived tissue nutrition and is a warning symptom of potential impending tissue injury. Ischemic ulcerations can result from tissue injury (Fig. 23.4). An uncomplicated ischemic event is typically over in about 15 min.

N.S. Sherber, M.D. (✉)
Johns Hopkins Scleroderma Center, 5200 Eastern Avenue, Mason F. Lord Building,
Center Tower, Suite 4100, Baltimore, MD 21224, USA
e-mail: sherber@jhmi.edu

F.M. Wigley, M.D.
Division of Rheumatology, Johns Hopkins University School of Medicine, 5200 Eastern
Avenue, Mason F. Lord Building, Center Tower, Suite 4100, Baltimore, MD 21224, USA
e-mail: fwig@jhmi.edu

M. Matucci-Cerinic et al. (eds.), *Skin Manifestations in Rheumatic Disease*,
DOI 10.1007/978-1-4614-7849-2_23, © Springer Science+Business Media New York 2014

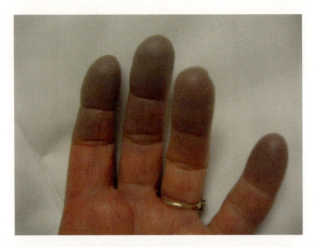

Fig. 23.1 Dusky cyanosis from vasoconstriction in Raynaud's phenomenon (Reprinted with from Wigley FM, Wung PK. Painful Digital Ulcers in a Scleroderma Patient with Raynaud's Phenomenon. In: Silver RM, Denton CP. (eds). Case Studies in Systemic Sclerosis. Springer-Verlag. London, UK; 2011: 95–105. With permission from Springer Science + Business Media)

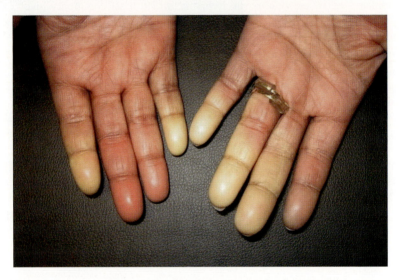

Fig. 23.2 Sharply demarcated pallor on several digits in the acute ischemic phase of Raynaud's phenomenon (Courtesy of Noëlle S. Sherber, Fredrick M. Wigley)

Differential Diagnosis

Raynaud's phenomenon (RP) may be an exaggerated normal response of the cutaneous thermoregulatory vessels and digital arteries to cold, stress, or trauma (primary Raynaud's phenomenon), or it can be associated with an underlying

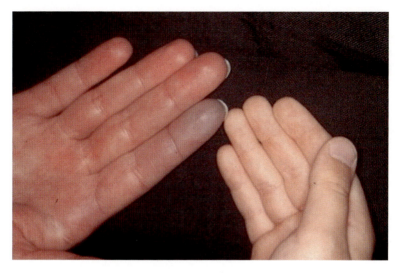

Fig. 23.3 Hyperemia in the blood flow recovery phase of Raynaud's phenomenon, with coexistent cyanosis of an adjacent digit, as compared to an unaffected hand (Courtesy of Noëlle S. Sherber, Fredrick M. Wigley)

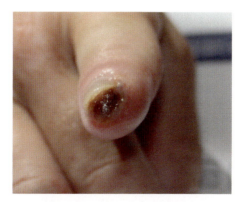

Fig. 23.4 Ischemic digital ulceration resulting from tissue injury in Raynaud's phenomenon (Reprinted with from Wigley FM, Wung PK. Painful Digital Ulcers in a Scleroderma Patient with Raynaud's Phenomenon. In: Silver RM, Denton CP. (eds). Case Studies in Systemic Sclerosis. Springer-Verlag. London, UK; 2011: 95–105. With permission from Springer Science + Business Media)

disease state, such as scleroderma (secondary Raynaud's phenomenon). Primary Raynaud's phenomenon is characterized by the absence of an underlying systemic disorder and is observed in approximately 3–5 % of individuals in the United States [1–3].

A frequent cause of secondary Raynaud's phenomenon is an underlying systemic rheumatic disease. The highest prevalence of RP among patients with a rheumatic disease is observed in systemic sclerosis (scleroderma) or in mixed connective tissue disease (MCTD), approaching 90 % or greater in most studies [4–7]. It is estimated that approximately 50 % of patients with undifferentiated connective tissue disease (UCTD) [8, 9], 21–44 % of patients with SLE [10, 11], up to 17 % of patients who have rheumatoid arthritis [12], and approximately 10 % of patients who have polymyositis demonstrate Raynaud's phenomenon as well.

Secondary Raynaud's can also be induced by trauma (hand-arm vibration syndrome), mechanical obstruction (thoracic outlet syndrome), pathologic serum proteins (cryoglobulinemia, cryofibrinogenemia), neurogenic stimuli (carpal tunnel syndrome), and exogenous vasoconstrictors (chemotherapeutic drugs).

Biopsy

There is no pathognomonic histology of Raynaud's, but, in disease states such as scleroderma, intimal hyperplasia of the digital vessels is characteristic.

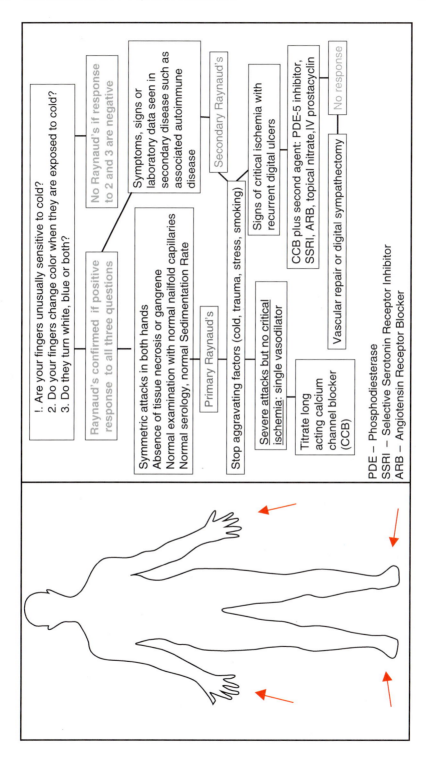

1. Are your fingers unusually sensitive to cold?
2. Do your fingers change color when they are exposed to cold?
3. Do they turn white, blue or both?

Raynaud's confirmed if positive response to all three questions

No Raynaud's if response to 2 and 3 are negative

Symptoms, signs or laboratory data seen in secondary disease such as associated autoimmune disease

Symmetric attacks in both hands
Absence of tissue necrosis or gangrene
Normal examination with normal nailfold capillaries
Normal serology, normal Sedimentation Rate

Primary Raynaud's

Secondary Raynaud's

Stop aggravating factors (cold, trauma, stress, smoking)

Severe attacks but no critical ischemia: single vasodilator

Signs of critical ischemia with recurrent digital ulcers

Titrate long acting calcium channel blocker (CCB)

CCB plus second agent: PDE-5 inhibitor, SSRI, ARB, topical nitrate, IV prostacyclin

No response

Vascular repair or digital sympathectomy

PDE – Phosphodiesterase
SSRI – Selective Serotonin Receptor Inhibitor
ARB – Angiotensin Receptor Blocker

References

1. Gelber AC, Wigley FM, Stallings RY, et al. Symptoms of Raynaud's phenomenon in an inner-city African-American community: prevalence and self-reported cardiovascular comorbidity. J Clin Epidemiol. 1999;52:441–6.
2. Block JA, Sequeira W. Raynaud's phenomenon. Lancet. 2001;357:2042–8.
3. Maricq HR, Carpentier PH, Weinrich MC, et al. Geographic variation in the prevalence of Raynaud's phenomenon: Charleston, SC, USA, vs Tarentaise, Savoie, France. J Rheumatol. 1993;20:70–6.
4. Sharp GC, Irvin WS, May CM, et al. Association of antibodies to ribonucleoprotein and Sm antigens with mixed connective-tissue disease, systematic lupus erythematosus and other rheumatic diseases. N Engl J Med. 1976;295:1149–4.
5. Tuffanelli DL, Winkelmann RK. Systemic scleroderma, a clinical study of 727 cases. Arch Dermatol. 1961;84:359–1.
6. Parker MD. Ribonucleoprotein antibodies: frequency and clinical significance in systemic lupus erythematosus, scleroderma, and mixed connective tissue disease. J Lab Clin Med. 1973;82:769–5.
7. Cohen ML, Dawkins B, Dawkins RL, et al. Clinical significance of antibodies to ribonucleo-protein. Ann Rheum Dis. 1979;38:74–8.
8. De Angelis R, Cerioni A, Del Medico P, et al. Raynaud's phenomenon in undifferentiated connective tissue disease (UCTD). Clin Rheumatol. 2005;24:145–51.
9. Mosca M, Neri R, Bencivelli W, et al. Undifferentiated connective tissue disease: analysis of 83 patients with a minimum followup of 5 years. J Rheumatol. 2002;29:2345–9.
10. Estes D, Christian CL. The natural history of systemic lupus erythematosus by prospective analysis. Medicine (Baltimore). 1971;50:85–95.
11. Hochberg MC, Boyd RE, Ahearn JM, et al. Systemic lupus erythematosus: a review of clinico-laboratory features and immunogenetic markers in 150 patients with emphasis on demographic subsets. Medicine (Baltimore). 1985;64:285–95.
12. Saraux A, Allain J, Guedes C, et al. Raynaud's phenomenon in rheumatoid arthritis. Br J Rheumatol. 1996;35:752–4.

Suggested Readings

Boin F, Wigley FM. Understanding, assessing and treating Raynaud's phenomenon. Curr Opin Rheumatol. 2005;17:752–60.

Flavahan NA. Regulation of vascular activity in scleroderma: new insights into Raynaud's phenomenon. Rheum Dis Clin North Am. 2008;34(1):81–7; vii.

Generini S, Seibold JR, Matucci-Cerinic M. Estrogens and neuropeptides in Raynaud's phenomenon. Rheum Dis Clin North Am. 2005; 31:177–86, x–xi.

Henness S, Wigley FM. Current drug therapy for scleroderma and secondary Raynaud's phenomenon. Curr Opin Rheumatol. 2007;19(6):611–8.

Herrick AL. Pathogenesis of Raynaud's phenomenon. Rheumatology. 2005;44:587–96.

Herrick AL. Therapy: a local approach to Raynaud phenomenon. Nat Rev Rheumatol. 2009;5:246–7.

Malenfant D, Catton M, Pope JE. The efficacy of complementary and alternative medicine in the treatment of Raynaud's phenomenon: a literature review and meta-analysis. Rheumatology (Oxford). 2009;48:791–5.

Steen V, Denton CP, Pope JE, Matucci-Cerinic M. Digital ulcers: overt vascular disease in scleroderma. Rheumatology (Oxford). 2009;48 Suppl 3:iii19–24.

Thompson AE, Pope JE. Calcium channel blockers for primary Raynaud's phenomenon: a meta-analysis. Rheumatology (Oxford). 2005;44:145–50.

Wigley FM. Raynaud's phenomenon. N Eng J Med. 2002;347:1001–8.

Chapter 24
Skin Manifestations of Systemic Sclerosis

Gabriele Valentini and Giovanna Cuomo

Systemic sclerosis (SSc) is a multisystem autoimmune rheumatic disease characterized by obliterative microvascular and proliferative small artery alterations, a distinct autoimmune response and deposition of collagen and other matrix constituents in the skin and target internal organs [1].

SSc presents with a number of skin manifestations (Table 24.1).

Telangiectasia and ulcerations/scars are addressed in other parts of the present book. This chapter is confined to the first three aspects.

Skin sclerosis represents the clinical hallmark of the disease. Actually, SSc is also referred to as *scleroderma* (i.e., hard skin) [1]. The extent of skin involvement has traditionally been divided into limited cutaneous and diffuse cutaneous disease, as the degree of skin involvement early in disease often predicts the longer-term prognosis of the patient [2] (Fig. 24.1). Diffuse disease includes involvement of the arms and legs proximal to the elbows and knees and may include the trunk. The limited cutaneous subset of scleroderma involves the arms/hands and/or legs/feet distal to the elbows and knees. The presence of face involvement does not differentiate the disease subtypes.

The indurative phase of skin involvement in SSc is usually preceded by an edematous phase in which the patient may complain about nonpitting edema causing swelling and puffiness of his/her fingers. In some patients, limbs and face are also involved. After months-years (the lag is shorter in patients with diffuse disease), definite skin sclerosis/indurations become apparent. The skin appears thickened, attached to the underlying subcutis, and sometimes shiny. The dermis is thickened by deposition of

G. Valentini, M.D. (✉)• G. Cuomo, M.D.
Department of Internal Medicine – Rheumatology Unit, Second University of Naples,
Via Pansini, 5, Naples, Italy 80130
e-mail: gabriele.valentini@unina2.it; giovanna.cuomo@unina2.it

M. Matucci-Cerinic et al. (eds.), *Skin Manifestations in Rheumatic Disease*,
DOI 10.1007/978-1-4614-7849-2_24, © Springer Science+Business Media New York 2014

Table 24.1 Cutaneous
manifestations of SSc

Skin sclerosis
Dispygmentation
Intradermal and subcutaneous calcinosis
Telangectasia
Ulcerations/scars

Fig. 24.1 Two main subsets:
limited cutaneous SSc and
diffuse cutaneous SSc

Skin sclerosis extent in the 2 main SSc subsets

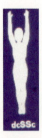 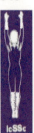

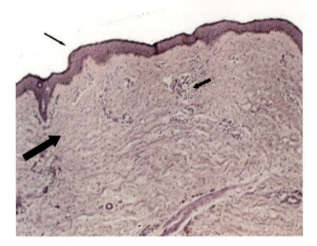

Fig. 24.2 Histopathology of scleroderma skin. E & E: 40× (original magnification). The epidermis is thinned (*small arrow*). The architecture of the dermis is replaced by collagen deposition with consequent rarefaction of skin appendages (*large arrow*). Small mononuclear perivascular infiltrates are detected (*medium arrow*)

collagen and other matrix constituents while the epidermis is thinned (Fig. 24.2). Loss of skin creases and destruction of hair follicles and sweat and sebaceous glands ensue. Skin sclerosis often reaches its maximal extent within 1–3 years from its onset. It involves the fingers and face in almost all patients and extends to the lower and upper limbs and trunk in some cases (Figs. 24.3 and 24.4) (see subsetting later).

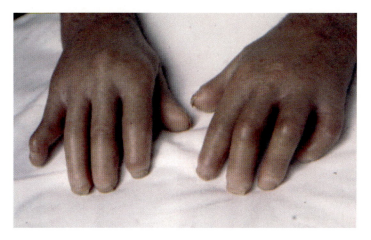

Fig. 24.3 Skin sclerosis of hands

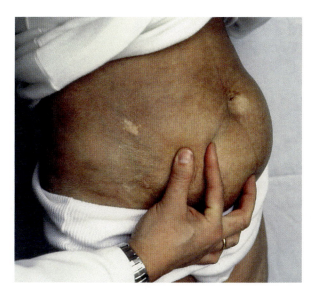

Fig. 24.4 Skin sclerosis (and hyperpigmentation) of trunk

The SSc patient in the sclerotic phase presents with typical features: the face becomes thickened and expression is difficult and the patient may seem expressionless (Fig. 24.5), the mouth opening is reduced (microstomy), the skin creases disappear, and hair loss and reduced sweating are apparent. A significant percentage (~20 %) of patients with diffuse cutaneous disease complain of pruritus as a result of mast cell activation and histamine release. It is most frequently in early disease and has recently been found to be significantly associated with the number of gastrointestinal

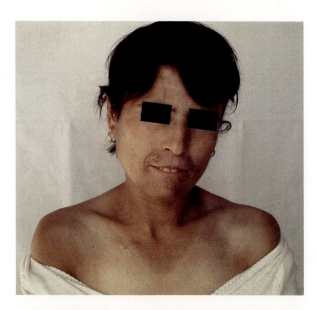

Fig. 24.5 The expressionless face of a patient with SSc

symptoms [3]. In addition, some patients, especially those with diffuse disease, have areas of skin **hyperpigmentation** and **hypopigmentation** (Fig. 24.6)**,** giving a "salt and pepper" appearance (Fig. 24.7). After some years, an atrophic stage ensues; the skin is tethered to the underlying tissue but is thinned. Again, the face has a typical feature characterized by lip retraction and radial furrowing around the mouth (Fig. 24.8). A few patients do not develop skin sclerosis (SSc sine scleroderma) [4].

Intradermal and subcutaneous calcinosis (Fig. 24.9) develops mainly, but not exclusively, in those with limited disease. Calcinosis occurs more frequently at the fingerpads and periarticular areas but can affect other districts. It consists of hydroxyapatite deposits which range from small to large lesions and can complicate with crystal-induced inflammation and/or skin ulceration with subsequent extrusion of white grains or toothpaste-like material.

Skin Involvement: Assessment

Skin involvement is commonly assessed by the modified Rodnan skin score (mRss). This is a measure of skin induration that the clinician evaluates by palpating and rating, from 0 (no thickening) to 3 (severe thickening), 17 body areas (Fig. 24.10)

Fig. 24.6 Diffuse
hyperpigmentation-
hypopigmentation of the
trunk and lower limbs

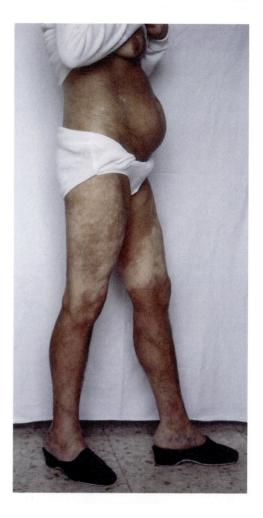

[5]. MRss is a validated measurement with defined reproducibility both in terms of intra- and interobserver variability. In early disease, it reflects the burden of skin disease and visceral involvement in patients with SSc. In long-standing disease, the skin becomes thinner and tethers to underlying tissues, losing the previous thickness and no longer correlating with visceral involvement (Fig. 24.11). Skin involvement has been assessed by other different methods. Among them, durometry [6] and ultrasonography [7] can have a role [8]).

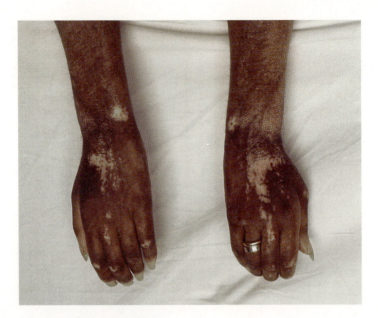

Fig. 24.7 Salt and pepper pattern

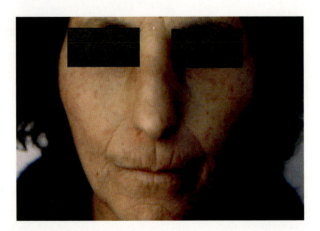

Fig. 24.8 Furrowing of the mouth

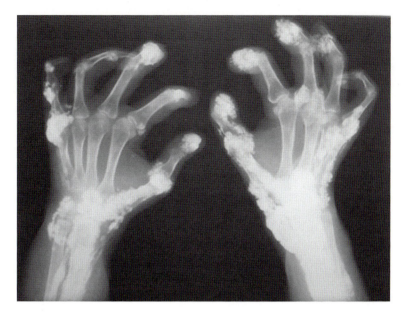

Fig. 24.9 Extensive subcutaneous calcinosis

Modified Rodnan skin score

	RIGHT	LEFT
Fingers	0 1 2 3	0 1 2 3
Hands	0 1 2 3	0 1 2 3
Forearms	0 1 2 3	0 1 2 3
Arms	0 1 2 3	0 1 2 3
Thighs	0 1 2 3	0 1 2 3
Legs	0 1 2 3	0 1 2 3
Feet	0 1 2 3	0 1 2 3

Face   0 1 2 3
Thorax   0 1 2 3
Abdomen 0 1 2 3

0=normal skin   **Total score**
1=slight thickening
2=moderate thickening
3= severe thickening

Fig. 24.10 Scheme for the evaluation of mRss

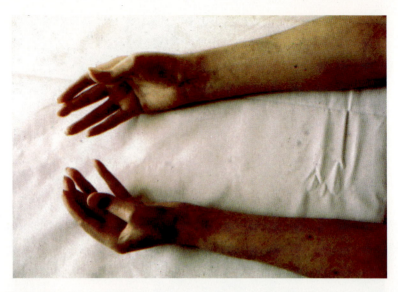

Fig. 24.11 Upper limbs of a patient with long-standing SSc. Note the tethering skin of hands

Table 24.2 Principal differential diagnosis

Conditions characterized by hardening of the skin	
Systemic Sclerosis	Toxic oil syndrome
Eosinophilic fasciitis	Eosinophilia-myalgia syndrome
Localized forms of scleroderma	GVH disease
Nephrogenic systemic fibrosis	Vinil chloryde disease
Scleredema of Buschke	Human adjuvant disease
Scleromyxedema	Diabetic sclerodactyly
Stiff skin syndrome	Drug – induced scleroderma like disease (eg bleomycin)

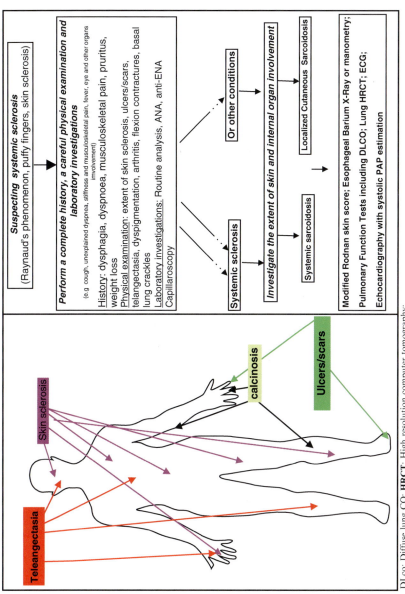

Suspecting systemic sclerosis
(Raynaud's phenomenon, puffy fingers, skin sclerosis)

Perform a complete history, a careful physical examination and laboratory investigations

(e.g cough, unexplained dyspnea, stiffness and musculoskeletal pain, fever, eye and other organs involvement)

History: dysphagia, dyspnoea, musculoskeletal pain, pruritus, weight loss
Physical examination: extent of skin sclerosis, ulcers/scars, telangiectasia, dyspigmentation, arthritis, flexion contractures, basal lung crackles
Laboratory investigations: Routine analysis, ANA, anti-ENA Capillaroscopy

Or other conditions

Systemic sclerosis

Investigate the extent of skin and internal organ involvement

Localized Cutaneous Sarcoidosis

Systemic sarcoidosis

Modified Rodnan skin score; Esophageal Barium X-Ray or manometry;
Pulmonary Function Tests including DLCO; Lung HRCT; ECG;
Echocardiography with systolic PAP estimation

Skin sclerosis

calcinosis

Ulcers/scars

Teleangectasia

DLco: Diffuse lung CO; **HRCT**: High resolution computer tomography;

References

1. Wigley FM. Scleroderma (Systemic Sclerosis). In: Goldman L, Ausiello D, editors. Cecil Medicine. 23rd ed. Philadelphia: Saunders- Elsevier; 2008. p. 2032–41.
2. LeRoy EC, Black C, Fleishmajer R, Jablonska S, Krieg T, Medsger Jr TA, Rowell N, Wollheim F. Scleroderma (systemic sclerosis): classification, subsets and pathogenesis. J Rheumatol. 1988;15:202–5.
3. Razykov I, Thombs BD, Hudson M, Bassel M, Baron M. Prevalence and clinical correlates of pruritus in patients with systemic sclerosis. Arthritis Rheum. 2009;61:1765–70.
4. Poormoghin H, Lucas M, Fertig N, Medsger Jr TA. Systemic Sclerosis sine scleroderma. Arthritis Rheum. 2000;43:444–51.
5. Clements PJ, Lachenbruch P, Seibold JR. Inter- and intraobserver variability of total skin thickness score (modified Ronan TSS) in systemic sclerosis. J Rheumatol. 1995;22:1281–5.
6. Aghassi D, Monoson T, Braverman I. Reproducible measurement to quantify skin involvement in scleroderma. Arch Dermatol. 1995;131:1160–6.
7. Scheja A, Akesson A. Comparison of high frequency (20 MHz) ultrasound and palpation for the assessment of skin involvement in systemic sclerosis (scleroderma). Clin Exp Rheumatol. 1997;15:283–8.
8. Valentini G, Matucci Cerinic M. Disease-specific quality indicators, guidelines and outcome measures in scleroderma. Clin Exp Rheumatol. 2007;25 Suppl 47:S159–62.

Chapter 25
Skin Manifestations of Neonatal Lupus Erythematosus

Ivan Foeldvari and Kristian Reich

Definition

The specific skin lesions occur in 2–10 % of children after delivery in anti-SSA/Ro- or anti-SSB/La-positive mothers. They are a consequence of the transplacental transfer of the antibodies. The lesions are similar to those seen in adult subacute cutaneous lupus erythematosus – scaly erythematous inflammatory lesions with a predominant annular or plaque-type appearance. The most common manifestation sites are the UV-exposed areas such as face and scalp, but lesions can also be disseminated. Skin lesions may be present at birth, but more often occur within the first weeks of life.

History and Clinical Picture

The clinical picture is that of plaques or annular erythemato-squamous lesions occurring congenitally but more often days to weeks after birth, sometimes after UV exposure [1]. They are usually transient, disappearing within weeks. Predilection sites are the scalp, the face, and the extremities (Fig. 25.1). Some children develop periorbital erythema leading to a masklike appearance [2].

I. Foeldvari, M.D.
Hamburger Zentrum für Kinder- und Jugendrheumatologie, Dehnhaide 120,
Hamburg 22081, Germany
e-mail: sprechstunde@kinderrheumatologie.de

K. Reich, M.D. (✉)
Dermatologikum Hamburg, Stephansplatz 5, Hamburg 20354, Germany
e-mail: reich@dermatologikum.de

M. Matucci-Cerinic et al. (eds.), *Skin Manifestations in Rheumatic Disease*,
DOI 10.1007/978-1-4614-7849-2_25, © Springer Science+Business Media New York 2014

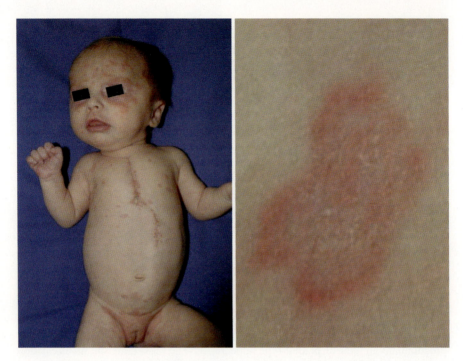

Fig. 25.1 Periorbital and inguinal distribution pattern of skin lesions of neonatal SCLE in a 2-month-old female baby (*left*). Single efflorescences appear as annular erythematous and scaly plaques (*right*). The sternal scar results from the implantation of a cardiac pacemaker for atrioventricular block grade III. (Reprinted from Heimann, S., M. Hertl, et al. (2009). "Scaling erythemas in an infant." J Dtsch Dermatol Ges 7(12):1087–1089. With permission from John Wiley & Sons, Inc.)

A positive history of connective tissue disease of the mother or positive serology for anti-Ro antibodies in the mother and child is supportive of the diagnosis [3, 4].

In unclear cases, a skin biopsy may be performed. Children with cutaneous involvement only have an excellent prognosis. The most life-threatening manifestation is a grade III atrioventricular block, which is not transient and may require pacemaker placement. Other manifestations are lymphopenia, thrombocytopenia, and a disturbance of liver function with elevated liver enzymes and hyperbilirubinemia.

Differential Diagnosis

- Erythema toxicum neonatorum is a common benign rash with papules or pustules on erythematous skin of unknown origin.
- Childhood seborrheic eczema is an inflammatory scaly dermatitis primarily of the scalp, face, and neck believed to involve an exaggerated cutaneous immune response to the yeast Malassezia furfur.

- Childhood psoriasis rarely manifests within the first year of life with erythemato-squamous lesions that may resemble neonatal LE.
- In principle, drug eruptions can mimic clinical manifestation of neonatal LE, for example, those occurring after treatment with antibiotics or antiepileptics.
- Transient neonatal pustular melanosis is a rare congenital dermatosis with collarette scaling and hyperpigmentation usually associated with formation of vesicles and pustules.
- Early congenital syphilis is caused by vertical transmission of syphilis in 50–80 % of exposed neonates and is associated with characteristic skin changes including a bullous eruption or macular rash that typically involves the palms and soles.
- NOMID/CINCA – Neonatal-onset multisystem inflammatory disease or chronic infantile neurologic cutaneous articular syndrome – skin symptoms are usually urticaria-like without a predominant epidermal component.
- Congenital candidiasis is a rare condition in which intrauterine Candida infection becomes manifest at birth. The cutaneous form presents with an extensive skin rash; clinically, a macular erythema can be seen, evolving from a macular pustular phase and finally resulting in extensive desquamation. The most commonly involved areas are neck and face.

Biopsy

The characteristic histopathology resembles that of subacute cutaneous lupus erythematosus with a lymphocytic infiltration at the basement membrane and signs of keratinocyte apoptosis, a pattern that is usually described as vacuolar interphase dermatitis [5]. Investigation by immunofluorescence can show deposition of IgG and complement at the dermoepidermal junction, which can be reproduced in human skin grafts in nude mice exposed systematically to anti-Ro antibodies [6]. The chemotactic activity of activated complement may explain the sometimes observed predominant infiltration of neutrophils [7].

See Also

SLE, cutaneous LE, SCLE.

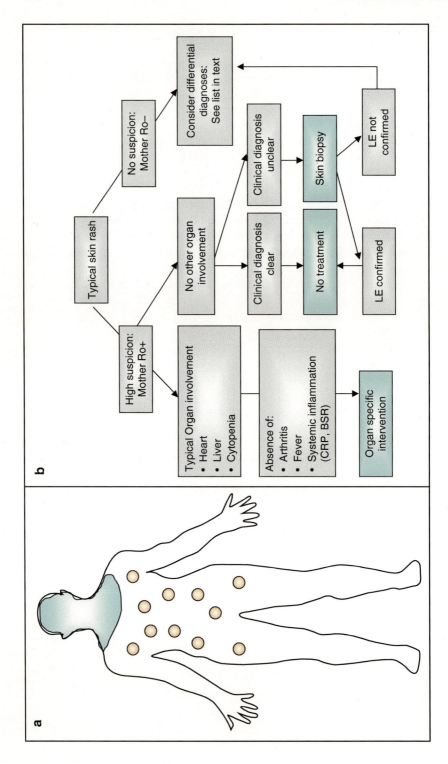

References

1. Renner R, Sticherling M. The different faces of cutaneous lupus erythematosus. G Ital Dermatol Venereol. 2009;144(2):135–47.
2. Lee LA. The clinical spectrum of neonatal lupus. Arch Dermatol Res. 2009;301(1):107–10.
3. Klauninger R, Skog A, et al. Serologic follow-up of children born to mothers with Ro/SSA autoantibodies. Lupus. 2009;18(9):792–8.
4. Buyon JP. Updates on lupus and pregnancy. Bull NYU Hosp Jt Dis. 2009;67(3):271–5.
5. Penate Y, Guillermo N, et al. Histopathologic characteristics of neonatal cutaneous lupus erythematosus: description of five cases and literature review. J Cutan Pathol. 2009;36(6):660–7.
6. Lee LA, Gaither KK, et al. Pattern of cutaneous immunoglobulin G deposition in subacute cutaneous lupus erythematosus is reproduced by infusing purified anti-Ro (SSA) autoantibodies into human skin-grafted mice. J Clin Invest. 1989;83(5):1556–62.
7. Satter EK, High WA. Non-bullous neutrophilic dermatosis within neonatal lupus erythematosus. J Cutan Pathol. 2007;34(12):958–60.

Chapter 26
Skin Manifestations and Sjögren's Syndrome

Chiara Baldini, Elisabetta Bernacchi, Rosaria Talarico,
and Stefano Bombardieri

Definition

Primary Sjögren's syndrome (pSS) is a systemic autoimmune disease characterized
by a focal lymphocytic infiltration of the exocrine glands potentially leading to
xerostomia and xerophthalmia. Although sicca symptoms are the hallmarks of the
disease, cutaneous manifestations are considered one of the most common extraglandular features of pSS, affecting up to half of the patients [1]. Cutaneous manifestations can be distinguished as _nonvascular lesions_ (NVL) (_xerosis (X), angular
cheilitis (AC), eyelid dermatitis (ED), and annular erythema (AE)_) and _vascular
lesions_ (VL) (_Raynaud's phenomenon_ (RP) and _vasculitis_). In addition, cutaneous
B-cell lymphoma has been reported, although rarely [1, 2]. Objective signs of xerosis are roughness, fine scaling, and loss of elasticity with subjective uncomfortable
symptoms of itchiness, burning, and a "pinprick-like" feeling [2, 3]. Decreased
activity of sebaceous and eccrine glands has been suggested as the pathogenetic
mechanism of pSS dry skin [2]. Recent immunohistochemical and functional studies have documented perturbed epidermal proliferation and differentiation and a
significant reduction ($p < 0.05$) of transepidermal water loss (TEWL) [3]. Angular
cheilitis is a well-known, frequent, and recurrent erythemato-squamous mucocutaneous lesion, often symmetrical, at the corners of the mouth [2, 4]. Eyelid dermatitis
is a lesion of the upper eyelid associated with xerosis, itching, and a foreign body

C. Baldini, M.D. • R. Talarico, M.D., Ph.D. • S. Bombardieri, M.D. (✉)
Department of Internal Medicine, Rheumatology Unit, University of Pisa,
Via Roma 67, 56126 Pisa, Italy
e-mail: chiara.baldini74@gmail.com; sara.talarico76@gmail.com;
s.bombardieri@int.med.unipi.it

E. Bernacchi, M.D.
Malattie Muscolo Scheletriche e Cutanee, Ospedale S. Chiara, Unità Operativa di
Reumatologia, AOUP, Via Roma 67, 56126 Pisa, Italy
e-mail: bettibernacchi@libero.it

M. Matucci-Cerinic et al. (eds.), _Skin Manifestations in Rheumatic Disease_,
DOI 10.1007/978-1-4614-7849-2_26, © Springer Science+Business Media New York 2014

sensation [2, 5]. *Annular erythema* is an annular erythema with central clearing and without atrophy, typical in Japanese SS, involving the face, the upper extremities, and the trunk, and correlated with anti-Ro/SSA and anti-La/SSB antibodies. The lesions are recurrent and not clearly related to sun exposure [6]. Among vascular lesions, palpable purpura (PP) of the lower extremities and buttocks is the most typical clinical sign of pSS vasculitis [7]. Urticaria-like lesions have also been described. Raynaud's phenomenon is detected in 20–45 % of pSS and is higher in the VL subgroup pSS patients [2].

Description and Differential Diagnosis

Xerosis. This is a common feature in pSS patients (32–67 %) significantly associated with SSA-SSB antibodies [1–3]. It is a nonspecific skin condition most commonly localized on the upper back, shoulders, and on the surface of the limbs (Figs. 26.1 and 26.2). Xerosis represents a "paraphysiological" condition in old-aged (>70 years) people [2]. Secondary xerosis is associated with various dermatological and systemic diseases or systemic and topical treatments (Table 26.1) [2]. Xerosis is enhanced in winter season and by repeated washing [2].

Angular Cheilitis. Synonyms: *perleche, commissural cheilitis*, and *angular stomatitis*. The term refers to inflammatory conditions that radiate from 1 or both angles of the mouth. Acute *angular cheilosis* is erythematous or erosive, stinging. Chronic cheilitis is erythemato-squamous and is often asymptomatic [4]. AC has some risk factors and may be present in various systemic conditions and dermatological diseases (Table 26.1) [4]. The most common etiology is infectious. In pSS, AC is related to xerostomia and to oral candidacies (more than 80 % pSS patients) [4].

Eyelid Dermatitis (Fig. 26.3). This can be found in various CTDs and particularly in the elderly. ED may be associated with continuous rubbing of the periorbital area due to ocular dryness and a foreign body sensation of xerophthalmia. ED is associated with xerosis in 86 % of pSS patients, typically involved the upper eyelid (types I and II ED), and ranged from slight erythema and infiltration to

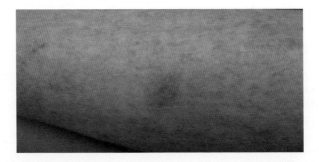

Fig. 26.1 Objective signs of xerosis (lower limbs)

Fig. 26.2 Objective signs of xerosis in SS female patients: roughness, fine scaling

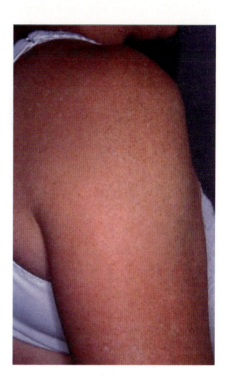

Table 26.1 Primary SS nonvascular skin lesions and their differential diagnosis

pSS skin lesions	Differential diagnosis
Skin xerosis	***Primary xerosis:*** "idiopathic xerosis," SS xerosis. ***Secondary xerosis:*** (a) *dermatological diseases* (atopic dermatitis, allergic and contact dermatitis, asteatotic and nummular eczema, autosomal dominant ichthyosis, stasis dermatitis), (b) *systemic therapy* (hypocholesterolemic drugs, aromatic retinoid, psoralens), (c) *topical treatments* (retinoid acid, benzyl benzoate (i.e. niacinamide)), (d) *systemic diseases* (hypothyroidism and autoimmune diseases such as lymphoma, leprosy, AIDS, anemia, sarcoidosis, liver and biliary disease, renal insufficiency, and diabetes mellitus), (e) *physiopathological conditions* (repeated washings, winter season), and (f) elderly skin xerosis
Angular cheilitis	***Risk factors:*** inadequate dentures, poor oral hygiene, excessive mouth washing and aggressive dental floss, age, abnormal skin folds at the corner of the mouth, licking, dry skin, and use of tobacco and alcohol. ***Infectious etiologies:*** Candida albicans, Staphylococcus aureus, and β-hemolytic streptococci. ***Noninfectious etiologies:*** (a) *systemic conditions* (iron deficiency anemia; riboflavin, foliate, and B12 deficiencies; diabetes mellitus; Crohn's disease; AIDS; Down's syndrome), (b) *dermatological conditions* (atopic and seborrheic dermatitis, contact allergy, perioral dermatitis, and orofacial granulomatosis)
Eyelid dermatitis	Allergic contact dermatitis, irritant dermatitis, atopic dermatitis, seborrheic dermatitis, urticaria (contact and systemic photo irritation), periocular rosacea, psoriasis, systemic lupus, dermatomyositis, infection (fungal/bacterial), secondary to conjunctivitis, or blepharitis
Annular erythema	**Cutaneous LE** (*LED*, *SCLE*, and *LET*), JKLS, REM, **Lyme disease** (*erythema chronicum migrans and linfocitoma benign cutis*), **rheumatic fever** (*erythema marginatum*), **specific paraneoplastic dermatitis** (*erythema gyratum repens*), and **hypersensitivity annular erythema** (*infectious, malignancy; liver diseases; autoimmune thyroiditis*)

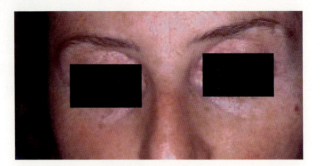

Fig. 26.3 Slight erythema of the upper eyelid in the same patients (Fig. 26.2)

lichenification and/or brown hyperpigmentation. Moreover, eyelid involvement is frequent in ophthalmological lesions. *Atopic dermatitis (AD)* is the most common cause of chronic eyelid involvement and patients should be questioned for a personal and family history of asthma, atopy, or eczema; in atopy, it is characteristic of the Dennie-Morgan infraorbital fold of the lower eyelid. In *allergic contact dermatitis (ACD)* or *irritant contact dermatitis (ICD)*, occupational history, domestic interest, and hobbies are important aspects of diagnosis; moreover, in ACD present in the face and neck, patch-testing positivity improves after allergen removal. *Contact urticaria ED* is rare and usually includes other symptoms such as rhinitis, edema, gastrointestinal disturbance, and angioedema; a diagnostic feature is the expression of dermatitis after exposure or contact (30–60 min/4–6 h) to an allergen. In *ocular rosacea*, *ED* is characterized by eyelid margin telangiectasia rather than by periorbital papules, meibomian inflammation, recurrent chalazia, and the typical facial involvement. In seborrhea ED, the eyelids show greasy-appearing scales, crusting, and erythema. Moreover, the typical nasolabial fold scaling is present. In *psoriasis ED*, the lid and eyelid present erythematous scaling plaques and in more severe forms edema of the lower lids and ectropion.

Annular Erythema. This is rare in Caucasians. Three types of *AE* are described [1]: type I, isolated donut ring erythema with an elevated border [2]; type II, SCLE-like polycyclic erythema [3]; and type III or papular-like erythema [6]. The common characteristic is the presence of infiltrated, indurated, non-scaling lesions with central clearing without discromia or atrophy not clearly related to sunlight exposure [1]. *AE* shares many clinical, histological, and immunological features with cutaneous LE and related LE skin disorders such as Jessner-Kanof lymphocytic infiltrate (JKLI) and reticular erythematous mucinosis (REM). Histopathological findings, rather than clinical findings (see biopsy below), are useful for the differential diagnosis, in particular with respect to *subacute* cutaneous lupus erythematosus (*SCLE*) which is considered the corresponding Caucasian form of AE [1, 6]. In *SCLE*, polycyclic scaling not infiltrating the margins, achromia, and a subacute course are distinctive features [6]. Moreover, a strong association with sun exposure has been detected. Discoid lupus erythematosus *(LED)* can be distinguished due to the

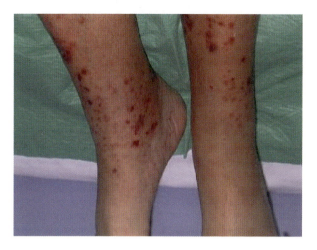

Fig. 26.4 Skin vasculitis (lower limbs)

presence of hyperkeratosis and scleral atrophy. Lupus tumidus *(LET)* is characterized by an intermittent course, high photosensitivity, and edematous lesions [7]. Annular lesions and specific features of the underlying disease should be detected in Lyme disease (erythema chronicum migrans), rheumatic fever (erythema marginatum), and paraneoplastic dermatitis (erythema ageratum reopens). Finally, an annular erythema can be present in various pathological conditions such as a nonspecific hypersensitivity manifestation (Table 26.1) [6].

Vascular Lesions

Vasculitic lesions in pSS are mainly related to a leukocytoclastic vasculitis (LCV) of the small and medium dermal vessels [2, 8–10]. LCV is an immune complex-mediated process and is related to a B-cell-driven autoimmune response [2, 8–10]. SS-LCV is associated with anti-Ro/SSA, anti-La/SSB, and RF positivity and hypergammaglobulinemia [2, 8–10]. Positive cryoglobulins and decreased levels of complement factors are considered negative prognostic markers. Moreover, the presence of LCV during pSS course may be associated to lymphoma [2, 8–10].

Palpable purpura is the most common type (84 %) of *LCV* in pSS patients, consisting of widespread, symmetrical, and asymptomatic erythematous purple papules that do not blanch when pressure is applied (Fig. 26.4). It is located on the extremities and sometimes on shoulders [2]. *PP* may represent a nonspecific sign of other systemic or cutaneous LCV (hypersensitivity vasculitis) (Table 26.2). In systemic lupus erythematosus (SLE) and rheumatoid arthritis (RA), other types of vasculitic lesions are usually present (palmar and digital pulp ischemic lesions and depressed punctuated scares on fingertips) [2]. Henoch-Schonlein purpura affects young boys and is characterized by gastrointestinal involvement, prodromic upper respiratory tract infection, and

Table 26.2 Primary SS vascular lesions and their differential diagnosis

pSS vasculitis	Differential diagnosis
Palpable purpura	**Cutaneous leukocytoclastic vasculitis (hypersensitivity vasculitis and allergic vasculitis),** *idiopathic, exercise induced, and drugs (almost every class, chemicals, food, vitamins, nutritional supplement, tumor necrosis factor-alpha),* **infections** *(all virus, bacteria, fungi, parasites),* **malignancy** (hematologic malignancies, *myelodisplastic syndrome, lymphoma, carcinomas),* **leukocytoclastic vasculitis** *(autoimmune disorders, CTD, CM, hypocomplementemic vasculitis, S-H purpura, Kaposi sarcoma,; malignancy, hepatitis B–C infection, endocarditis, ANCA-associated vasculitis, Behcet's disease*
	Lymphocytic vasculitis *(rickettsial-viral infections), drugs, CTD (Behcet's disease and Degos' disease)*
Urticarial vasculitis	**Idiopathic, MC, CTD, monoclonal gammopathy, leukocytoclastic vasculitis (other), and drugs:** *infliximab, formaldehyde, paroxetina, and others*

immunoglobulin IgA deposition within the affected vessels. Pauci-immune vasculitis is characterized by the presence of ANCA autoantibodies, DIF negativity, and specific clinical features related to the systemic vasculitic process [10].

Urticarial vasculitis *(UV)* is the second most frequent type of VL in pSS, but it is uncommon relative to *PP*. UV lasts longer than 24 h, burns rather than itches, and heals with hyperpigmentation. The hypocomplementemic form (UHV) is characterized by circulating anti-C1q antibodies and is more often associated with pSS and other CTDs. Also, UV represents a nonspecific lesion and could be associated to other cutaneous and systemic VLC conditions (Table 26.2) [2].

The morphology of the lesions is a direct reflection of the size and extent of the vessels (small-medium) affected and is nonspecific. Petechiae, not palpable purpura, bullous lesions, erythematous maculopapules, livedo reticularis other than PP, and UV can be present. Isolated cases of nodular and livedoid vasculitis have also been described [2].

Biopsy

Skin Xerosis (X), Angular Cheilitis (AC), and Eyelid Dermatitis (ED). The diagnosis of dry skin is clinical, and skin biopsy is usually not performed. Similar considerations can be made for AC and ED [1, 2].

Generally, histological examination of xerotic skin shows common aspecific features (slight epidermal hyperorthokeratosis and dermal elastosis) which may be associated to other characteristic features of the various dermatological conditions, eventually associated to xerosis [1, 2].

Annular Erythema. Histopathological examination shows an interface dermatitis with absent or scarcely epidermal changes (light atrophy, parakeratosis) and perivascular lymphocytic infiltrate with a mixture of neutrophils or plasma cells in the middle-deep dermis. *AE* is characterized by lack of hydropic degeneration of keratinocyte's basal layer specific of chronic, subacute, and acute cutaneous LE. Moreover, in *AE* the hyperkeratosis and follicular plugging of LED and the mucinosis of LET are absent [6].

Vasculitis (Palpable Purpura and Urticarial Vasculitis). Vasculitis in pSS is an LVC immune complex-mediated and directed immunofluorescence (DIF)-positive process involving small and medium vessels. A mononuclear pattern, DIF negative, of the inflammatory vessel infiltrate can also be detected. The LCV pattern is characterized by an inflammatory and mostly fragmented neutrophilic infiltrate. LV lesions typically display fibrinoid necrosis, lumen occlusion, and extravasations of red blood cells. The mononuclear inflammatory vascular disease is characterized by a lymphocytic inflammatory infiltrate with invasion of the blood vessel walls. Fibrinoid necrosis is present, but less prominent than the neutrophilic inflammatory infiltrate [10]. The optimal time for LV skin biopsy is <48 h from the appearance of the lesion; 24 h after biopsy, it may show lymphocytic-mononuclear infiltrate. In addition, DIF positivity is inversely related to the age of the vasculitic lesion biopsied. Despite the evidence of these two forms of vasculitis, their clinical expression is very similar, so that one cannot predict the histopathology pattern of vascular insult in examining the skin. Nonetheless, LCV is statistically associated with antinuclear antibodies, high titres of anti-Ro/SSA and anti-La/SSB antibodies, hypergammaglobulinemia, RF, and hypocomplementemia [2, 10]. The histology of UV shows a sparse neutrophilic infiltrate with focal small vessel vasculitis and frequent presence of eosinophils; the fibrinoid change or necrosis is less common in urticarial vasculitis lesions than in the fully developed lesions of palpable purpura [2, 10].

See Also

Raynaud phenomenon, Systemic sclerosis; Cryoglobulinemia, Systemic vasculitis

Treatment:

Skin lesions	Treatment
Xerosis	Urea-based cream/ Emollient body cream and wash/ topical products containing glycerol /dexpanthenol ointment
Eyelid dermatitis	Base–emollient cream/ Topical steroids Low corticosteroids
Angular cheilitis	Base-emollient cream/ Fluconazole-azoles systemic and topical ointment
Annular erythema	Topical steroids; tacrolimus ointment 0,1 %
Skin vasculitis	Low-medium corticosteroids + hydroxychloroquine

The diagnosis of pSS should be made according to the AECG criteria 2002 (see the AECG revised rules)

Acknowledgment We thank Laura Maria Fatuzzo for her valuable contribution in reviewing the text.

References

1. Soy M, Piskin S. Coetaneous findings in patients with primary Sjogren's syndrome. Clin Rheum. 2007;26:1350–2.
2. Bernacchi E, Amato L, Parodi A, Cottoni F, Rubegni P, De Pità O, Papini M, Rebora A, Bombardieri S, Fabbri P. Sjögren's syndrome: a retrospective review of the cutaneous features of 93 patients by the Italian Group of Immunodermatology. Clin Exp Rheumatol. 2004; 22(1):55–62.
3. Bernacchi E, Bianchi B, Amato L, Giorgini S, Fabbri P, Tavoni A, Bombardieri S. Xerosis in primary Sjögren syndrome: immunohistochemical and functional investigations. J Dermatol Sci. 2005;39(1):53–5.
4. Gonsalves WC, Chi AC, Neville BW. Common oral lesions: part I. Superficial mucosal lesions. Am Fam Physician. 2007;75(4):501–7.
5. Zug KA, Palay DA, Rock B. Dermatologic diagnosis and treatment of itchy red eyelids. Surv Ophthalmol. 1996;40(4):293–306.
6. Katayama I, Kotobuki Y, Kiyohara E, Murota H. Annular erythema associated with Sjögren's syndrome: review of the literature on the management and clinical analysis of skin lesions. Mod Rheumatol. 2010;20(2):123–9.
7. Kuhn A, Bein D, Bonsmann G. The 100th anniversary of lupus erythematosus tumidus. Autoimmun Rev. 2009;8(6):441–8.
8. Ramos-Casals M, Anaya JM, García-Carrasco M, Rosas J, Bové A, Claver G, Diaz LA, Herrero C, Font J. Cutaneous vasculitis in primary Sjögren syndrome: classification and clinical significance of 52 patients. Medicine (Baltimore). 2004;83(2):96–106.
9. Kluger N, Francès C. Cutaneous vasculitis and their differential diagnoses. Clin Exp Rheumatol. 2009;27(1 Suppl 52):S124–38.
10. Carlson JA. The histological assessment of cutaneous vasculitis. Histopathology. 2010;56(1): 3–23.

Chapter 27
Skin Manifestations of Systemic Lupus Erythematosus

Martin Aringer and Annegret Kuhn

Systemic lupus erythematosus (SLE) is a prototypical autoimmune disease. Organ manifestations caused by autoantibodies and immune complexes can affect essentially all organ systems. Like other organ manifestations, skin manifestations in SLE can be strikingly heterogeneous. Indeed, the 11 SLE classification criteria of the American College for Rheumatology (ACR), which comprise four different skin and mucosal manifestations, underline this fact [1, 2].

Apparently, the nature of the specific autoantibody and the properties of the immune complexes determine pathology. For example, immune complexes from autoantibodies against double-stranded DNA (dsDNA) and chromatin deposit in the glomeruli, thereby leading to severe, proliferative immune complex nephritis, while antibodies to phospholipids, present in membranes of thrombocytes and endothelial cells, induce thrombotic events and foetal loss. Cutaneous manifestations of the disease probably are likewise caused by autoantibodies and immune complexes, independent of the question of whether skin lesions are the primary sign of the disease, as in cutaneous LE (CLE), or part of a disease spectrum, as in SLE. In fact, immune complex deposition and complement activation can be demonstrated in tissue samples of both CLE and SLE.

Several disease activity scores (SLEDAI, ECLAM, BILAG) have been established for SLE to determine the disease activity of individual patients. Although the disease activity scores include dermatological criteria, such as butterfly rash, generalised erythema and oral ulcer, they are not suitable for judging activity of CLE

M. Aringer, M.D. (✉)
Division of Rheumatology, Department of Medicine III, University Medical Centre Carl Gustav Carus at the Technical University of Dresden, Fetscherstrasse 74, 01037 Dresden, Germany
e-mail: martin.aringer@uniklinikum-dresden.de

A. Kuhn, M.D.
Department of Dermatology, University of Muenster, Von-Esmarch-Strasse 58, D-48149 Muenster, Germany
e-mail: kuhnan@uni-muenster.de

M. Matucci-Cerinic et al. (eds.), *Skin Manifestations in Rheumatic Disease*,
DOI 10.1007/978-1-4614-7849-2_27, © Springer Science+Business Media New York 2014

subtypes. For this reason, a modified scoring system (RCLASI=revised cutaneous lupus erythematosus disease area and severity index) has been developed for LE patients with skin lesions to determine activity and damage of the disease [3]. Some of the skin manifestations are specific for LE, and these will constitute the main focus of this overview; however, several non-specific findings are likewise too important to not be mentioned. We will therefore start with photosensitivity, an important aspect of the disease, and proceed to inflammatory skin lesions, beginning with those specific for SLE.

Photosensitivity

Definition

Sensitivity to UV light is fairly common in SLE and not only limited to skin eruptions but also associated with SLE flares afflicting internal organs. Therefore, avoidance of UV light and consistent skin protection are of major importance [4].

Photosensitivity in SLE may be difficult to judge from the patient's history. In contrast to other UV-induced skin changes, such as polymorphic light eruption (PLE), which develop rapidly after exposure, SLE skin changes commonly take several days up to weeks to start developing. Therefore, patients will often not link UV exposure to clinical worsening of their disease. Other patients may give a history of clear photosensitivity, but suffer from other UV-induced skin diseases, such as PLE. Therefore, standardised phototesting on non-exposed skin may help decide for or against UV sensitivity [5].

Differential Diagnosis

Ultraviolet light (UV) can induce a wide variety of skin changes. Simple sunburn is usually rather obvious, and phototoxic reactions as well as polymorphic light eruption (PLE) are a very rapid response, whereas SLE UV sensitivity leads to inflammatory changes days to a few weeks after the UV exposure. Mostly, the lesions evolving are fairly typical SLE lesions (see below). The likewise UV-sensitive rash of dermatomyositis has a somewhat different localisation in the face (above the butterfly area) and commonly a lilac hue.

Histology

Fully developed skin lesions after UV exposure will show specific cutaneous features of LE (see below). However, biopsies are also of interest, because they may lead to a better understanding of the pathophysiology of the disease. Days after UV exposure, late apoptotic cells accumulate in the skin of patients with LE in contrast to healthy controls [6]. Since there are no indications for increased cell death, this phenomenon may be due to deficient clearance of apoptotic cells.

Acute Cutaneous Lupus Erythematosus (ACLE)

Definition

ACLE lesions commonly occur concomitant with generalised disease activity and nearly always point to SLE rather than CLE. Like the other LE-specific lesions, ACLE develops predominantly in UV-exposed areas. The most common ACLE manifestation is the malar rash, but it can also involve dorsal fingers, sparing the knuckles, and can lead to a generalised rash. ACLE is a non-scarring subtype and does usually not lead to depigmentation (Fig. 27.1).

Malar erythema – the butterfly rash – is the prototypical SLE picture and, not surprisingly, constitutes one of the ACR classification criteria. This type of skin lesions develops in areas with thermoregulatory vessels, i.e. those that turn reddish upon overheating. Thus, the erythema prominently affects the nose and the cheeks, but leaves out the nasolabial folds. It commonly starts with small, symmetrical erythematous macules or papules that then become confluent. The erythematous area is usually palpably indurated. Sometimes, fine scales are found on the lesions [7].

Generalised ACLE often involves the UV-exposed aspects of toes and fingers, characteristically sparing the knuckles and thus resulting in a negative picture as compared to the Gottron papules of dermatomyositis. This subtype can also involve

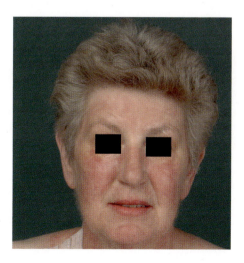

Fig. 27.1 Localised ACLE with discrete butterfly rash in a patient with SLE

large portions of the integument and occasionally mimic toxic epidermal necrolysis in its most acute forms. Even if less acute, the rash can be pruritic. In addition to the skin changes, ACLE is often accompanied by superficial mucosal ulcers, which constitute yet another ACR criterion. These ulcers typically afflict the hard palate, but may be found anywhere in the oral cavity as well as the nose.

Differential Diagnosis

Several relevant differential diagnoses have to be distinguished from malar rash. Acne rosacea is characterised by small pustules and telangiectasias. The rash of dermatomyositis is more oedematous and has a more violet hue, as well as a slightly different localisation pattern, with predominant involvement of the front and lids. Solar erythema can occasionally be misleading, but so can seborrheic eczema, tinea faciei, perioral dermatitis and erysipelas, in particular, and non-specific erythema, as in febrile patients [7].

Histology

Histologically, ACLE is often less impressive than in the clinical picture. Nevertheless, lymphocyte infiltrates around vessels and adnexes are found in both superficial and deep layers, as well as in the dermoepidermal junction, a picture called interface dermatitis, which is typical for all specific LE skin lesions. Likewise, immune complex and complement split product deposition can be shown.

Subacute Cutaneous Lupus Erythematosus (SCLE)

Definition

Skin lesions of patients with SCLE develop in sun-exposed areas, mostly of the face, the upper extremities and the trunk in a symmetrical fashion, where erythematosus macules or papules evolve into scaly lesions that appear either polycyclic (Fig. 27.2) or psoriasiform and heal with depigmentation, but not scarring [8]. SCLE lesions are not part of the ACR classification criteria, but are arguably covered by photosensitivity within these criteria.

SCLE constitutes an isolated cutaneous condition in more than half of the patients, whereas a smaller portion suffers from SLE. SCLE is associated with the HLA haplotype B8 DR3 and with autoantibodies to Ro/SSA and La/SSB. Lesions can be triggered by UV light and several drugs, among them terbinafine, thiazide diuretics and several calcium channel blockers.

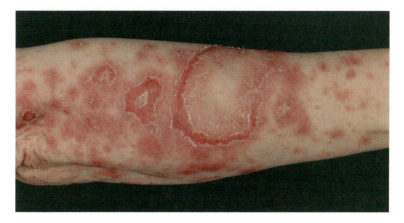

Fig. 27.2 Annular type of SCLE with multiple confluent lesions on the lower arm

Differential Diagnoses

The differential diagnoses of SCLE include tinea corporis, psoriasis, mycosis fungoides, erythema exsudativum multiforme/toxic epidermal necrolysis, erythema annulare centrifugum, erythema gyratum repens, drug eruption, nummular eczema and seborrhoeic eczema [7].

Histology

Histologically, SCLE is characterised by interphase dermatitis leading to keratinocyte necrosis and vacuolar degeneration at the dermoepidermal junction, as well as lymphocytic infiltrates and moderate hyperkeratosis.

Chronic Cutaneous Lupus Erythematosus (CCLE)

Definition

CCLE includes discoid LE (DLE) and lupus panniculitis or lupus erythematosus profundus (LEP). Chilblain lupus is the topic of a specific chapter of this book.

DLE consists of well-defined, coin-shaped erythematous plaques, on which adherent scales develop. Removal of the scale exposes follicle-sized keratotic spikes, the "carpet tack sign" [8]. This form of CCLE can lead to atrophy and scaring (Fig. 27.3). DLE lesions occur in approximately 15 % of patients with SLE, but more than 95 % of patients with DLE lesions suffer from CLE only.

LEP/lupus panniculitis is characterised by indurated nodules or plaques that will result in deep lipoatrophy. Commonly, LEP is associated with DLE lesions.

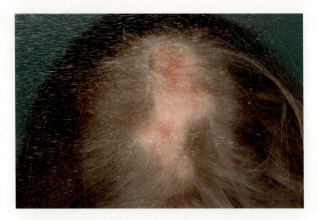

Fig. 27.3 In a patient with SLE, scarring alopecia due to DLE lesions with active erythematous plaques

Differential Diagnosis

There are several diagnoses that need to be distinguished from DLE, such as tinea faciei, actinic keratosis, lupus vulgaris, and sarcoidosis. LEP/lupus panniculitis needs to be differentiated from other forms of panniculitis, including subcutaneous sarcoidosis, panarteriitis nodosa, malignant lymphoma (in particular subcutaneous panniculitis-like T-cell lymphoma), morphea profunda and subcutaneous granuloma annulare [7].

Histology

Histologically, DLE lesions show the typical interface dermatitis and vacuolar degeneration of the dermoepithelial junction but also gross epidermal involvement with pronounced hyperkeratosis and follicular plugging (Fig. 27.4).

LEP is characterised by lobular lymphocytic panniculitis, which may be difficult to differentiate from other forms of panniculitis in the absence of DLE lesions.

Lupus Erythematosus Tumidus: Intermittent CLE

Definition

LE tumidus (LET) is the latest addition to the family of specific skin manifestations in CLE, which is rarely associated with SLE [9]. This subtype is a non-scarring skin manifestation consisting of succulent, swollen, almost urticaria-like plaques with

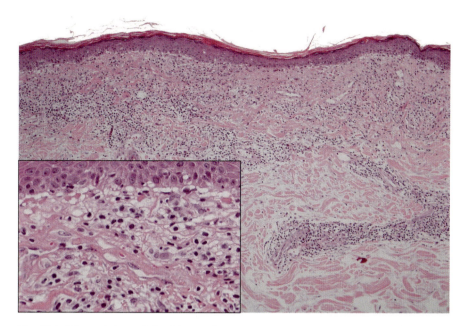

Fig. 27.4 Histopathology of discoid lupus erythematosus. Note the vacuolar degeneration of the dermoepidermal junction and the periadnexal lymphocytic infiltrate

smooth surface, i.e. no epidermal involvement, which distinguishes it from SCLE in the case of annular lesions. LET colour shades range from bright red to violacious. In sun-exposed areas, both single and multiple plaques can appear. In the latter case, these lesions can coalesce in their periphery and thus produce a gyrate configuration, while single lesions may flatten in the centre, but swell in the periphery [10].

In contrast to SCLE, LET is rarely associated with autoantibodies to Ro/SSA or with other defined autoantibodies. LET is extremely prone to photosensitivity and can commonly be reproduced by phototesting [11].

Differential Diagnosis

The differential diagnoses of LET include lymphocytic infiltration Jessner-Kanof/ erythema arciforme et palpabile, PLE, pseudolymphoma, B-cell lymphoma, plaque-like cutaneous mucinosis and light urticaria [7].

Histology

Histologically, LET lacks epidermal involvement and the vacuolar degeneration of the dermoepidermal junction seen in other CLE lesions. In addition, LET is characterised by lymphocytic infiltration and abundant mucin deposition between collagen bundles.

LE-Non-specific Skin Manifestations

Definition

In addition to the above-mentioned specific lesions, skin manifestations of SLE may include a wide variety of changes that are also found in the framework of other diseases. Many of these non-specific manifestations are vascular lesions, ranging from Raynaud's phenomenon and livedo patterns to overt leukocytoclastic or urticarial vasculitis.

Hair loss is fairly common in SLE. Discoid lesions of the scalp will lead to coin-shaped scarring alopecia, which may occasionally evolve to subtotal or total hair loss over time. In contrast, diffuse hair loss is common in active SLE, and non-scarring, reversible diffuse alopecia may result. Therefore, it may be highly relevant to distinguish scarring from non-scarring follicular changes.

Raynaud's phenomenon in SLE is fairly common, with degree and variability depending on the autoantibodies [12]. Most SLE patients have relatively mild episodes of Raynaud's phenomenon, which are commonly associated with overall SLE activity. In contrast, those with autoantibodies against U1RNP, which are otherwise associated with mixed connective tissue disease (MCTD), suffer from severe Raynaud's phenomenon, which is more stable over time. The latter patients are also prone to develop occlusive angiopathy, although fingertip ulcers are rare in SLE. Raynaud's phenomenon rarely needs provocation testing, being rather obvious in most cases. Capillary microscopy may add significant information.

Livedo reticularis is a typical, but harmless, condition. However, its reticular pattern is associated with antiphospholipid antibodies in SLE and may thus alert to the risk of severe vascular complications [12]. In contrast, the more flame-like livedo racemosa speaks to vasculitis itself. Other vasculitic lesions in SLE include palpable purpura, splinter haemorrhages and the urticarial form of vasculitis. All of these types can be associated with vasculitic internal organ involvement, albeit isolated skin vasculitis is more common. Histological analysis of livedo racemosa and other vasculitic lesions typically show the picture of leukocytoclastic vasculitis.

Conclusions

SLE, with its wide variety of skin and internal organ manifestations, will always remain a diagnostic and therapeutic challenge. Some of the skin manifestations are typical for the disease, but even those will need to be distinguished from other lesions. Other skin lesions, such as splinter haemorrhages, will provoke a search for both infectious (endocarditis) and other autoimmune manifestations, and histology may also prove inconclusive. Overtreatment, such as unwarranted cyclophosphamide therapy, may be as harmful as failure to recognise severe or disfiguring disease. Therefore, sufficient experience and an open, interdisciplinary approach will be essential to optimise care for SLE patients. Even under these circumstances, and despite all due caution, the disease will sometimes not adhere to any textbook, and all unexpected reactions should prompt rethinking and reinvestigation.

See Also

Chilblain Lupus Erythematosus by Min Ae Lee-Kirsch, Martin Aringer and Annegret Kuhn. Identify other topics in the book where the lesion or the disease is also mentioned and described.

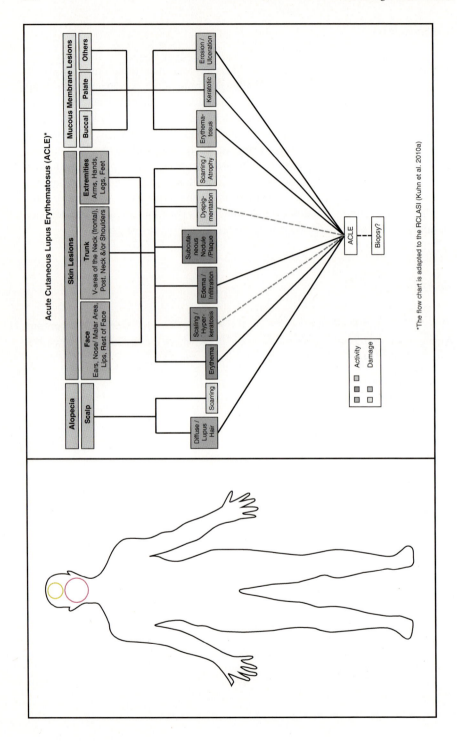

*The flow chart is adapted to the RCLASI (Kuhn et al. 2010a)

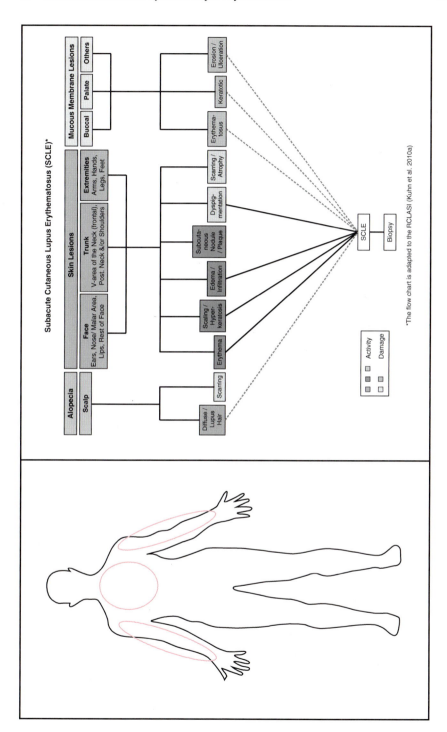

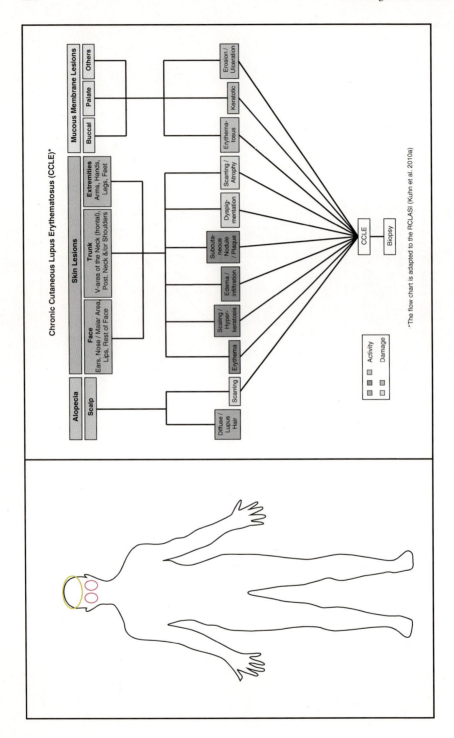

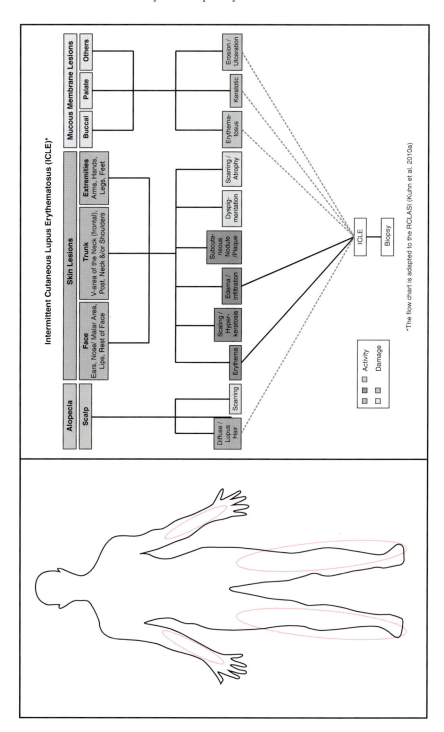

Acknowledgments We thank P. Wissel, J. Bückmann and Professor T. A. Luger, University Muenster, Germany, for providing the clinical figures and Professor D. Metze, University Muenster, Germany, for providing the histological figures.

References

1. Albrecht J, et al. Dermatology position paper on the revision of the 1982 ACR criteria for systemic lupus erythematosus. Lupus. 2004;13:839–49.
2. Tan EM, et al. The 1982 revised criteria for the classification of systemic lupus erythematosus. Arthritis Rheum. 1982;25:1271–7.
3. Kuhn A, et al. Revised cutaneous lupus erythematosus disease area and severity index (RCLASI): a modified outcome instrument for cutaneous lupus erythematosus. Br J Dermatol. 2010;163:83–92.
4. Kuhn A, et al. Photosensitivity, phototesting, and photoprotection in cutaneous lupus erythematosus. Lupus. 2010;19:1125–36.
5. Kuhn A, et al. Photosensitivity in lupus erythematosus. Autoimmunity. 2005;38:519–29.
6. Kuhn A, et al. Accumulation of apoptotic cells in the epidermis of patients with cutaneous lupus erythematosus after ultraviolet irradiation. Arthritis Rheum. 2006;54:939–50.
7. Kuhn A, et al. Leitlinien Kutaner Lupus Erythematodes (Entwicklungsstufe 1). In: Korting HC, Callies R, Reusch M, Schlaeger M, Sterry W, editors. Dermatologische Qualitätssicherung: Leitlinien und Empfehlungen. Berlin: ABW Wissenschaftsverlag GmbH; 2009. p. 214–57.
8. Kuhn A, et al. Clinical manifestations of cutaneous lupus erythematosus. In: Kuhn A, Lehmann P, Ruzicka T, editors. Cutaneous lupus erythematosus. Heidelberg: Springer; 2004. p. 59–92.
9. Kuhn A, et al. The 100th anniversary of lupus erythematosus tumidus. Autoimmun Rev. 2009;8:441–8.
10. Schmitt V, et al. Lupus erythematosus tumidus is a separate subtype of cutaneous lupus erythematosus. Br J Dermatol. 2010;162:64–73.
11. Kuhn A, et al. Phototesting in lupus erythematosus tumidus – review of 60 patients. Photochem Photobiol. 2001;73:532–6.
12. Kuhn A, et al. Differential diagnosis of dermatological peripheral cutaneous circulatory disorders. In: Müller-Ladner U, editor. Raynaud's phenomenon and peripheral ischemic syndromes. Bremen: Uni-Med Verlag; 2008. p. 53–71.

Chapter 28
Skin Manifestation in Dermatomyositis

László Czirják and Endre Kálmán

Definition

Dermatomyositis (DM) is a systemic autoimmune disorder with skin, muscle involvement, and other manifestations including polyarthritis, lung fibrosis, and, occasionally, a coexistent malignancy. Muscle symptoms include proximal limb weakness, myalgia, and tenderness [1–4]. Altogether in classic dermato-/polymyositis, cutaneous manifestation occurs in 30–40 % of the adult and 95 % of the juvenile cases. With regard to DM, it is unusual that cutaneous manifestation precedes the muscle disease, and even if this is the case, muscle symptoms usually appear within 6 weeks. Adult patients with a recent onset of DM have a coexistent malignant disease in 20–25 % of the cases. Conversely, 4–8.2 % of the patients with DM show exclusively skin symptoms and never develop muscle involvement.

Description

Skin symptoms usually include Gottron's papules appearing over the metacarpophalangeal, interphalangeal, elbow, and knee joints (Figs. 28.1 and 28.2). This particular violaceous erythema is symmetric. In its full-blown form, the papules show a slight central depression with a white, atrophic appearance. Further, dermatomyositis-related skin symptoms include periorbital violaceous (heliotrope)

L. Czirják, M.D., Ph.D. (✉)
Department of Rheumatology and Immunology, Clinical Center,
University of Pécs, Akác u. 1, Pécs, Hungary H-7632
e-mail: laszlo.czirjak@aok.pte.hu

E. Kálmán, M.D.
Department of Pathology, Clinical Center, University of Pécs, Pécs, Hungary

M. Matucci-Cerinic et al. (eds.), *Skin Manifestations in Rheumatic Disease*,
DOI 10.1007/978-1-4614-7849-2_28, © Springer Science+Business Media New York 2014

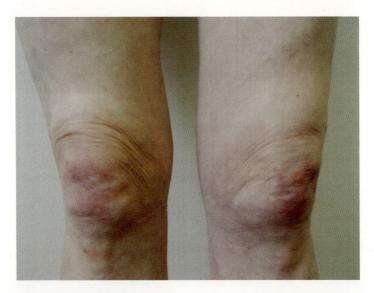

Fig. 28.1 Gottron's papule of the knee

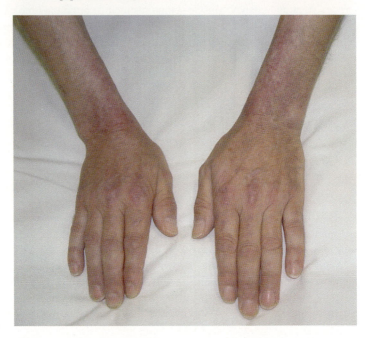

Fig. 28.2 Gottron's papules of the hands

rash overlying of the eyelids and periorbital tissue often accompanied by edema (Fig. 28.3). This particular confluent, macular violaceous erythema (diffuse flat purple-red skin) may also be present on the dorsal surface of the arms and fingers (over the extensor tendon sheaths); over the deltoids, posterior shoulders, and neck ("shawl sign"); V area of anterior neck and upper chest; and central aspect of the

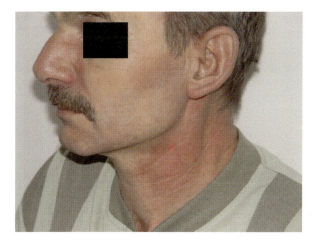

Fig. 28.3 Heliotrope rash and periorbital edema in a young patient with DM

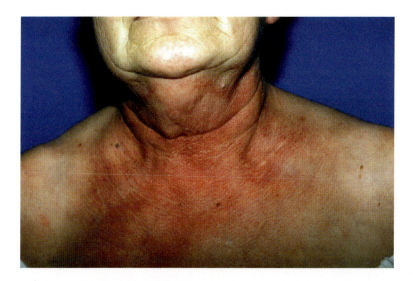

Fig. 28.4 V sign in DM (Courtesy of Katalin Dankó)

face (Fig. 28.4). The patches of violaceous erythema can become confluent over large areas of affected skin. The involvement of the face is typically present in the periocular region, and this particular heliotrope rash involving the eyelids (often most notable on the upper lids) and periorbital tissue is the most characteristic skin symptom of DM (Fig. 28.3). Periungual telangiectasia with or without skin dystrophy also belongs to the typical DM-related skin signs. Further secondary changes of DM include scale, follicular hyperkeratosis, pigmentary changes, subepidermal bullous change, and ulceration. Poikiloderma atrophicans vasculare (poikilodermatomyositis) that is a circumscribed violaceous erythema with associated telangiectasia, hypopigmentation, hyperpigmentation, and superficial atrophy may be present in certain parts of the body including the V area of anterior neck and upper chest, back, flanks, and buttocks. Occasionally, calcinosis cutis may also appear. Photosensitivity is an important clinical feature of DM.

The term amyopathic DM (ADM) (synonymous with "DM sine myositis") and furthermore a closely related form of DM, "hypomyopathic DM," (HDM) are characterized by the appearance of typical skin disease for at least 6 months without having any muscle weakness [5].

Cancer-associated DM is a subset that is probably much more prevalent in adults than it has previously been suspected, and the majority of patients develop skin symptoms characteristic of DM. Almost all children with DM also develop cutaneous manifestations usually before the diagnosis of myositis [1–4].

Differential Diagnosis

Skin symptoms should be differentiated from those seen in cutaneous manifestations of lupus. Exposure to UV light is a provoking factor in both cases. Pruritus is often an early event in DM that is typically missing in cutaneous lupus. The overall clinical presentation, and autoantibody findings (anti-double-stranded DNA in lupus), usually easily differentiates between these two connective tissue disorders. Skin involvement together with inflammatory disease is typical and characteristic for DM.

Skin biopsy may also help, but by itself does not clearly differentiate between DM and cutaneous manifestation of lupus; however, the lupus band test is negative in most of the cases [6]. Vascular deposits of C5b-9 are described in DM, but not in lupus.

Some other conditions with muscle symptoms should also be differentiated from DM. Infectious myopathies (HIV-1, coxsackie, adenovirus, echovirus, Epstein-Barr virus, hepatitis B virus) and drug-induced myopathies caused by a series of agents (antimalarial, lipid-lowering drugs/statins, and fibrates, colchicines, cyclosporine) as well as alcohol, cocaine, and heroin abuse should be considered in differential diagnosis. Furthermore, endocrine disorders (hypo- and hyperthyroidism, Cushing's disease) with myopathy also should be considered. There are a large number of myopathies (inclusion body myositis, muscular dystrophies, metabolic myopathies) that should also be carefully considered in differential diagnosis. All of these particular disorders can be differentiated from DM by the specific findings of muscle biopsy and the lack of the classic skin symptoms described above. Detection of myositis-specific autoantibodies is also useful. Patients with anti-Mi2 usually have DM.

The aim of the DM management after a careful confirmation of the diagnosis is to assess all disease manifestations and define the disease activity and the extent of irreversible damage. Then an individualized treatment plan can be developed. The first-line therapy for myositis is corticosteroids. If the response is not sufficient, corticosteroids are supplemented with immunosuppressive agents. Methotrexate and azathioprine are the most commonly used drugs [7]. Physical therapy to restore muscle strength is also important. In refractory cases, other agents including mycophenolate, cyclosporine, tacrolimus, cyclophosphamide, and intravenous gamma globulin may also be efficient.

Biopsy

Muscle histology includes infarcts, myocyte-specific MHC-I upregulation, perifascicular atrophy, endothelial cell swelling/necrosis, and vessel wall membrane attack complex (MAC) deposition.

Skin histology of DM is quite variable and often subtle (Figs. 28.5 and 28.6). It includes hyperkeratosis, epidermal basal cell vacuolar degeneration/apoptosis, and focally thinned epidermis. Increased dermal mucin deposition and a cell-poor interface dermatitis consisting of lymphocytes at the dermal-epidermal junction can also be present [8]. Vascular ectasia and fibrin deposition, C5b-9 (MAC) [9] deposition in both dermal vasculature and the dermoepidermal junction, and a perivascular lymphocytic infiltrate are also typical findings [1].

The predominant infiltrating cell is the CD4+ T lymphocyte, localized predominantly in the perivascular areas of the upper dermis. These particular lymphocytes usually belong to the activated/memory phenotype. A significantly increased number of both CD-40+ cells (including keratinocytes and mononuclear cells in the dermis) as well as infiltrating CD4+ CD-40L+ T lymphocytes are also found in skin biopsies from patients with DM. Activation of the CD-40/CD-40L system may

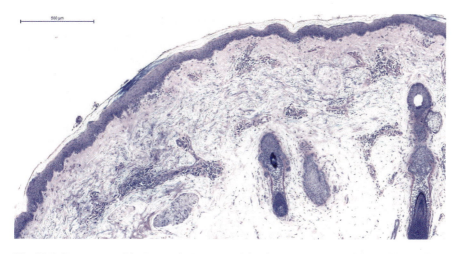

Fig. 28.5 Dermatomyositis. Lennert's Giemsa 4x. The changes are quite subtle. Mild superficial perivascular infiltrate of lymphocytes with some increase of metachromatic interstitial mucin is visible. Subtle lichenoid tissue reaction can be noticed

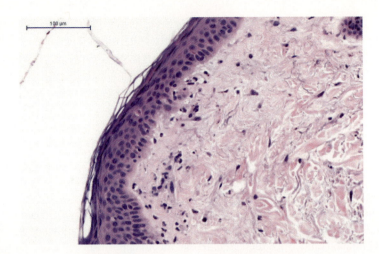

Fig. 28.6 Dermatomyositis. H&E 20x subtle lichenoid tissue reaction can be seen, mild vacuolar degeneration of the basal keratinocytes with few lymphocytes. An apoptotic keratinocyte is in the *upper part* of the epidermis

be involved in the upregulation of certain pro-inflammatory molecules, including IL-6, IL-15, IL-8, and MCP-1. The association between UVB exposure and TNF-α release is consistent with a model in which UV light triggers cytokine-mediated inflammation and keratinocyte apoptosis [1]. Type I IFNs (α and β) are thought to play an important role in the pathogenesis of DM as well [10].

See Also

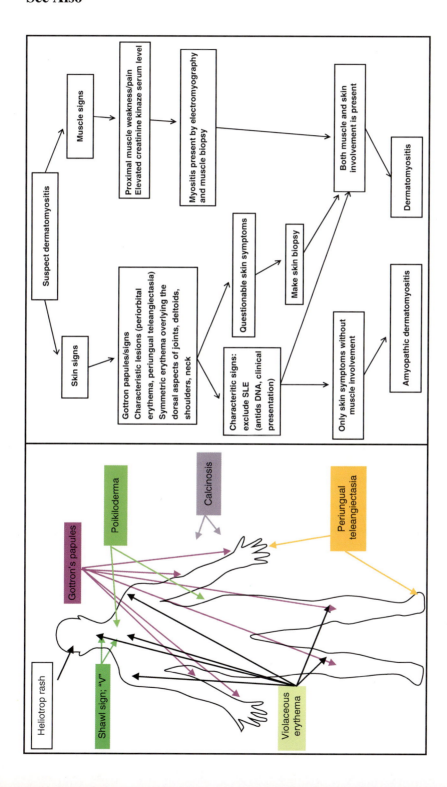

References

1. Sontheimer RD, Euwer RL, Costner MI. Dermatomyositis. In: Sontheimer RD, Provost TT, editors. Cutaneous manifestations of rheumatic diseases. Philadelphia: Lippincott Williams and Wilkins; 2004. p. 65–103.
2. Franks AG. Skin manifestations of internal disease. Med Clin North Am. 2009;93:1265.
3. Krathen MS, Fiorentino D, Werth VP. Dermatomyositis. Curr Dir Autoimmun. 2008;10:313.
4. Callen JP. Cutaneous manifestations of dermatomyositis and their management. Curr Rheumatol Rep. 2010;12:192.
5. Gerami P, Schope JM, McDonald L, Walling HW, Sontheimer RD. A systematic review of adult-onset clinically amyopathic dermatomyositis (dermatomyositis sine myositis): a missing link within the spectrum of the idiopathic inflammatory myopathies. J Am Acad Dermatol. 2006;54:597.
6. Vaughan Jones SA, Black MM. The value of direct immunofluorescence as a diagnostic aid in dermatomyositis: a study of 35 cases. Clin Exp Dermatol. 1997;22:77–81.
7. Miller FW. New approaches to the assessment and treatment of the idiopathic inflammatory myopathies. Ann Rheum Dis. 2012;71(Suppl II):i82–5.
8. Weedon D. Dermatomyositis. In: Weedon's skin pathology. Churchill Livingstone Elsevier; 2010. p. 64–66.
9. Magro CM, Crowson AN. The immunofluorescent profile of dermatomyositis: a comparative study with lupus erythematosus. J Cutan Pathol. 1997;24:543–52.
10. Greenberg SA. Dermatomyositis and type 1 interferons. Curr Rheumatol Rep. 2010;12:198.

Chapter 29
Stiff Skin Syndrome

Serena Guiducci, Mirko Manetti, Eloisa Romano, Silvia Bellando Randone, and Lidia Ibba Manneschi

Definition

Stiff skin syndrome (SSS) is clinically characterized by stone-hard skin (Fig. 29.1) bound firmly to the underlying tissues, leading to a secondary limitation of joint mobility, often associated mild overlying hypertrichosis, and postural and thoracic wall abnormalities. Notably lacking are visceral, bone, or muscular involvement; immunologic abnormalities; vascular disturbances; or mucopolysacchariduria [1]. First manifestations of SSS are usually observed between birth and early childhood [2] with rock-hard skin that is most prominent in areas with abundant fascia such as on the buttocks and thighs [3], and the disease progresses until the skin of the entire body becomes fibrotic with subsequent growth retardation and joint contractures. Extracutaneous features of SSS include contractures, especially of the large joints, often resulting in scoliosis, a tiptoe gait, and a narrow thorax in relation to the arm girdle. Skin fibrosis can also lead to decreased costovertebral joint mobility with restrictive changes of lung function [2]. The disease is slowly progressive and nonfatal.SSS was first described in 1968 in a boy with joint contractures and skin changes resembling scleroderma [2] and, in 1971, in four patients showing skin hardening and secondary limitation of joint mobility [4]. Jablonska et al. [5] further characterized this condition as a generalized, noninflammatory fascial disorder and proposed the name "congenital fascial dystrophy." Until now, about 40 SSS patients have been described in the literature, with few familial cases [4–7]. The pathogenesis of SSS remains unknown. Initially, an abnormal mucopolysaccharide metabolism limited to the skin, in absence of mucopolysacchariduria, has been suggested [4]. Cutaneous lesions in SSS were attributed to deposits of acid mucopolysaccharides

S. Guiducci, M.D., Ph.D. (✉) • M. Manetti, Ph.D. • E. Romano, Ph.D.
S.B. Randone, M.D., Ph.D. • L.I. Manneschi
Department of Biomedicine Section of Rheumatology, University of Florence,
Viale Pieraccini 18, Florence 50139, Italy
e-mail: s.guiducci@hotmail.com

M. Matucci-Cerinic et al. (eds.), *Skin Manifestations in Rheumatic Disease,*
DOI 10.1007/978-1-4614-7849-2_29, © Springer Science+Business Media New York 2014

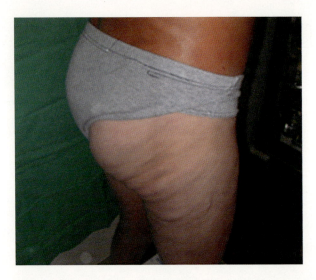

Fig. 29.1 The most relevant sign was the stone-hard skin induration of buttocks and thighs

localized within collagen fibers in the dermis and hypodermis [2, 4, 8–10]. Recently, the most relevant modifications were localized in the fascia, which was thickened by a hyalinized, collagenous tissue [5, 9]. In skin fibroblasts, collagen synthesis was upregulated as shown by increased activity of prolyl hydroxylase and lysyl hydroxylase [5].

Differential Diagnosis

SSS is a diagnosis of exclusion, with a distinctive clinical presentation without pathognomonic laboratory or pathological findings. The clinical differential diagnosis of stone-hard and thickened skin areas includes systemic sclerosis, overlap syndromes (e.g., sclerodermatomyosists), morphea, scleroderma, eosinophilic fasciitis, and scleromyxedema. The appearance of the disease in early childhood, the limitation of joint mobility, the proximal rather than a distal stiffness, and the absence of organ involvement are the main clinical findings that differentiate SSS from systemic sclerosis. Moreover, microvascular abnormalities, Raynaud's phenomenon, and autoantibodies were absent in SSS. Several features can help differentiate SSS from scleredema. In SSS, disease is centered on or around the pelvic and shoulder girdle, whereas scleredema is centered on the face, head, neck, and back. Joint restriction, although common in SSS, is rare in scleredema and is more often due to a "bulk" effect of the thick skin usually affecting the eyelids, neck, mouth, and shoulder. The skin stiffness in SSS is often well demarcated, uneven, or lumpy and may not involve an entire anatomic unit, while the stiffness in scleredema is more uniform, typically encompassing an entire involved anatomic unit. The abrupt onset often seen in scleredema is not a feature of SSS.

Sclerodermatomyositis presents with arthralgias, arthritis, sclerodermoid skin lesions, and joint restriction. Features that distinguish this entity from SSS are evidence of muscle involvement, autoantibodies, and vascular hyperreactivity. Localized scleroderma (morphea) tends to have a later onset as well as more localized and asymmetric indurations and alterations of the skin. Generalized morphea, a form of localized scleroderma, must also be distinguished from SSS. In deep morphea, there is typically a lymphocytic or lymphoplasmacytic infiltrate at the junction of the dermis and subcutis with abnormal, sclerotic collagen in the deep reticular dermis or subcutaneous septa, and fascial involvement is exceptional. In addition, many of the clinical features of SSS, such as the characteristic distribution involving the pelvic area and/or shoulder girdle and the often-present hypertrichosis, are typically not observed with generalized or localized morphea. Eosinophilic fasciitis classically presents with rapidly appearing tender swelling on the arms and legs evolving into brawny induration, often following exertion. Localized morphea-like skin changes and joint contractures may be present, and the induration is often more distal than proximal. Hematologic abnormalities including peripheral blood eosinophilia, hypergammaglobulinemia, and elevated erythrocyte sedimentation rate are often present. Histopathologic findings demonstrate thickened fascia with a cellular inflammatory infiltrate of lymphocytes and plasma cells, with or without eosinophils.

Biopsy

Several histologic patterns have been described in literature. Early reports described increased dermal mucin and large, bizarre fibroblasts that stained metachromatically with toluidine blue. Jablonska described underlying fascial thickening as "four times beyond normal" with "amianthoid-like" collagen fibers and bundles composed of incompletely organized microfibrils. Several subsequent reports confirmed a thickened fascia, but others reported normal fascia. In the SSS dermis (Fig. 29.2), Guiducci et al. [11] clearly showed an increase of fibrotic molecules (col1A2, fibronectin-1, and thrombospondin-1) and the presence of irregularly distributed collagen bundles, flattening of dermal papillae, and absence of sebaceous glands (Fig. 29.3); inflammatory mediators (IL-6, IL-1b, FGFR-3, and MCP-1) were downregulated in agreement with the absence of dermal inflammatory infiltrates (Fig. 29.4); no differences in pro-fibrotic cytokines (TGF-b, ET-1, and CTGF) were detected; and a loss of microvessels was clearly evident at the dermal–epidermal junction and in the papillary dermis, despite the overexpression of VEGF found in the dermis. In a previous work, circulating levels of pro-inflammatory cytokines (IL-6 and TNF-_ and TGF-b2) were found to be increased, whereas collagen production and DNA biosynthesis were normal [12]. In agreement with other authors [12], Guiducci et al. [11] did not report mucopolysaccharide deposits in the dermis. However, Geng et al. [13]

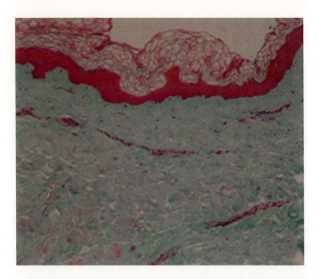

Fig. 29.2 Masson's trichrome staining of SSS skin. Mild fibrosis and dense, tightly packed, and irregularly distributed collagen bundles are evident in SSS dermis (original magnification x20)

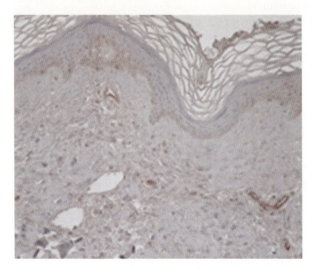

Fig. 29.3 Immunostaining for the panendothelial marker (vWF) in SSS skin (blue hematoxylin counterstaining, original magnification _20)

reported mild deposits of mucopolysaccharides between the collagen bundles throughout the dermis, hypothesizing that SSS could be a localized form of mucopolysaccharidosis.

Possibly, SSS exhibits a spectrum of histopathologic findings and different disease stages might also account for controversial results.

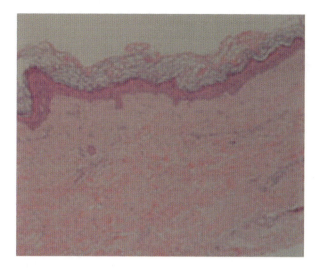

Fig. 29.4 H&E staining of SSS skin from the right femoral region (original magnification _20). No inflammatory infiltrates are present in SSS dermis

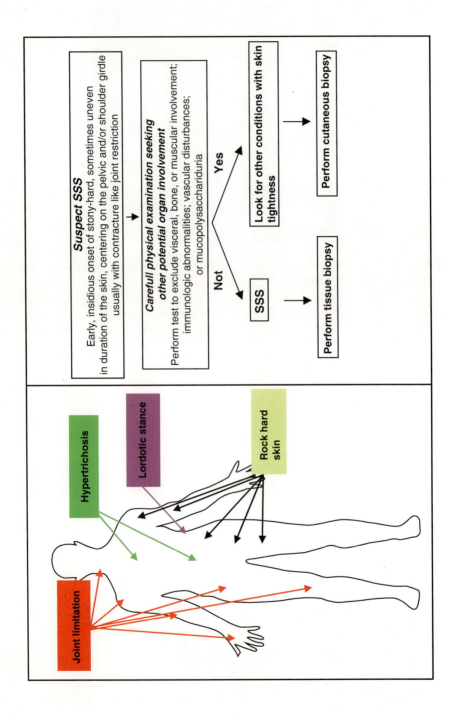

References

1. Jablonska S, Blaszczyk M. Scleroderma-like indurations involving fascias: an abortive form of congenital fascial dystrophy (stiff skin syndrome). Pediatr Dermatol. 2000;17(2):105–10.
2. Kikuchi I, Inoue S, Hamada K, Ando H. Stiff skin syndrome. Pediatr Dermatol. 1985;3: 48–53.
3. Jablonska S, Blaszczyk M. Scleroderma-like disorders. Semin Cutan Med Surg. 1998;17(1): 65–76.
4. Esterly NB, McKusick VA. Stiff skin syndrome. Pediatrics. 1971;47:360–9.
5. Jablonska S, Groniowski J, Krieg T, et al. Congenital fascial dystrophy—a noninflammatory disease of fascia: the stiff skin syndrome. Pediatr Dermatol. 1984;2(2):87–97.
6. Helm TN, Wirth PB, Helm KF. Congenital fascial dystrophy: the stiff skin syndrome. Cutis. 1997;60:153–4.
7. Liu T, McCalmont TH, Frieden IJ, Williams ML, Connolly MK, Gilliam AE. The stiff skin syndrome: case series, differential diagnosis of the stiff skin phenotype, and review of the literature. Arch Dermatol. 2008;144:1351–9.
8. Jablonska S, Schubert H, Kikuchi I. Congenital fascia dystrophy: stiff skin syndrome. A human counterpart of the tight skin mouse. J Am Acad Dermatol. 1989;21:943–50.
9. Bodemer C, Habib K, Teillac D, Munich A, De Prost Y. Un nouveau cas de stiff skin syndrome. Ann Dermatol Venereol. 1991;118:805–6.
10. Gilaberte Y, Saenz-de Santamaria MC, Garcia-Latasa FJ, Gonzalez-Mediero I, Zambrano A. Stiff skin syndrome: a case report and review of the literature. Dermatology. 1995;190: 148–51.
11. Guiducci S, Distler JH, Milia AF, Miniati I, Rogai V, Manetti M, Falcini F, Ibba-Manneschi L, Gay S, Distler O, Matucci-Cerinic M. Stiff skin syndrome: evidence for an inflammation-independent fibrosis? Rheumatology (Oxford). 2009 Jul;48(7):849–52.
12. Richard MA, Grob JJ, Philip N, et al. Physiopathogenic investigations in a case of familial stiff-skin syndrome. Dermatology. 1998;197:127–31.
13. Geng S, Lei X, Toyohara JP, Zhan P, Wang J, Tan S. Stiff skin syndrome. J Eur Acad Dermatol Venereol. 2006;20:729–32.

Chapter 30
Nephrogenic Systemic Fibrosis

Jonathan Kay and Rosalynn M. Nazarian

Definition

Nephrogenic systemic fibrosis (NSF) is a progressive fibrosing disorder that presents with brawny hyperpigmentation and tethering of the skin, predominantly on the extremities [1, 2] (Fig. 30.1). Characteristic cutaneous features include patterned plaques, "cobblestoning," and marked induration with a *peau d'orange* appearance (Fig. 30.2). Other cutaneous findings may include puckering or linear banding, superficial plaques, and dermal papules.

This condition has been observed almost exclusively among patients with compromised renal function following exposure to gadolinium-containing contrast agents during imaging procedures [3, 4]. The majority of patients with NSF develop skin changes within three months of receiving a gadolinium-containing contrast agent [5].

Description

Typically, both distal lower extremities are involved initially; skin changes usually progress proximally to involve both legs and thighs and both hands, forearms, and upper arms [2]. Although occurring infrequently, skin changes may be present over the chest and abdomen and on the back. Many patients with NSF also have slightly

J. Kay, M.D. (✉)
Rheumatology Division, Department of Medicine, University of Massachusetts School of Medicine, 119 Belmont Street, Worcester, MA 01605, USA
e-mail: jonathan.kay@umassmemorial.org

R.M. Nazarian, M.D.
Dermatopathology Unit, Department of Pathology, Massachusetts General Hospital and Harvard Medical School, 55 Fruit Street, WRN 831B, Boston, MA 02114, USA

M. Matucci-Cerinic et al. (eds.), *Skin Manifestations in Rheumatic Disease*, DOI 10.1007/978-1-4614-7849-2_30, © Springer Science+Business Media New York 2014

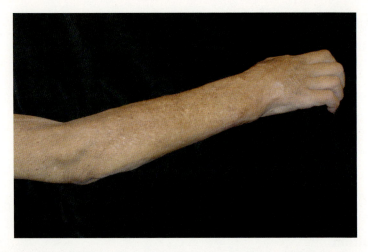

Fig. 30.1 Thickened, hardened skin with brawny hyperpigmentation and raised plaques on the arm of a patient with NSF. There are fixed flexion contractures of the elbow and fingers

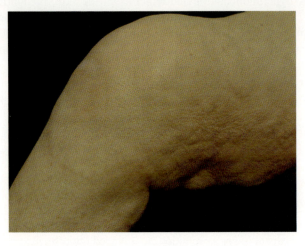

Fig. 30.2 "Cobblestoning" and marked induration of skin with a *peau d'orange* appearance on the thigh of a patient with NSF

raised, yellow plaques on the sclera of their eyes, medial and/or nasal to the iris, which often are accompanied by conjunctival injection (Fig. 30.3). However, the skin of the face is almost never affected.

As the skin around joints tightens, patients develop fixed flexion contractures that typically affect the knees, ankles, elbows, and fingers, resulting in a claw-like appearance to the hand [1, 2] (Fig. 30.4). These fixed deformities compromise physical function, often limiting the patient's ability to walk independently and to perform fine motor functions involving the hands.

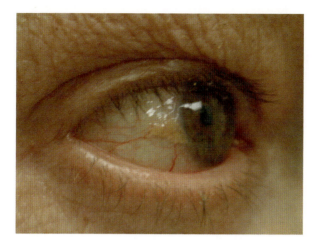

Fig. 30.3 A yellow scleral plaque on the eye of a patient with NSF

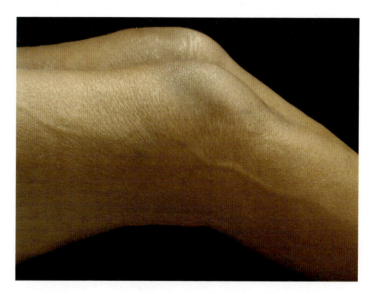

Fig. 30.4 Hardened and tethered skin around the knees of a patient with NSF causing fixed flexion contractures

Although initially recognized as a cutaneous disorder and named "nephrogenic fibrosing dermopathy" [6], extensive systemic involvement has been identified in patients with NSF, including fibrosis of lymph nodes, thyroid, esophagus, heart, lungs, liver, diaphragm, skeletal muscle, genitourinary tract, and dura mater [7, 8].

Differential Diagnosis

The vast majority of cases of NSF have occurred in patients with stage 5 chronic kidney disease (GFR <15 mL/min/1.73 m^2 or requiring dialysis). Thus, other conditions should be considered in the differential diagnosis, especially when a patient has lesser degrees of renal dysfunction [2]. The appearance of NSF skin changes on the lower extremities is very similar to that of lipodermatosclerosis occurring in the setting of chronic venous stasis. However, the indurated and dyspigmented lesions of lipodermatosclerosis typically are confined to the leg below the knee and are not accompanied by joint contractures.

Although the histological appearance of NSF may be indistinguishable from that of scleromyxedema, the numerous firm, minute papules of scleromyxedema occur on the face and neck, as well as on the hands, arms, and upper trunk. Patients with NSF lack the facial involvement and paraproteinemia typically associated with scleromyxedema. Unlike scleroderma, NSF does not involve the face and is not associated with Raynaud's phenomenon or circulating autoantibodies. The clinical appearance of NSF is similar to that of chronic graft-versus-host disease, but chronic graft-versus-host disease occurs in the setting of prior bone marrow transplantation and often involves the trunk.

Scleredema diabeticorum occurs in individuals with diabetes mellitus and presents with cutaneous induration on the shoulders and upper back. Morphea presents with a localized, linear area of cutaneous sclerosis and lacks the symmetrical distribution of scleroderma or NSF. Beta-2 microglobulin amyloidosis, which occurs exclusively in patients with stage 5 chronic kidney disease, and Dupuytren's contracture both manifest with subcutaneous thickening on the palms of the hands that results in fixed flexion contractures of the fingers which resemble the claw-like appearance of the hand in NSF; however, neither of these conditions is associated with the cutaneous changes that cause the finger joint contractures in NSF.

Biopsy

Histopathological findings in NSF include increased cellularity in the dermis comprised of spindle-shaped fibroblast-like cells with dual CD34- and procollagen I-positive immunohistochemical staining [2, 6] (Fig. 30.5a, b). In the vast majority of cases of NSF, the degree of cellularity exceeds 30 cells per high-power microscopic field [9]. Intervening collagen bundles are thickened, eosinophilic, and characteristically separated by adjacent clefts (Fig. 30.6). Elastic fibers are preserved and often elongated (Fig. 30.7). Variable histologic features include the presence of a mild chronic inflammatory infiltrate, calcification, osseous metaplasia, and osteoclast-like giant cells. Gadolinium has been detected and quantified in biopsies of skin and other tissues taken from patients with NSF [8, 10].

The histologic differential diagnosis of NSF includes scleromyxedema, which may be differentiated by the presence of "pools" of dermal mucin in the latter.

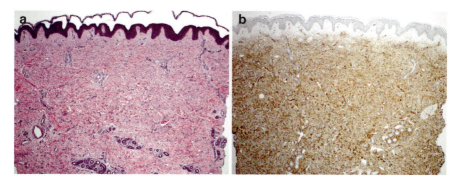

Fig. 30.5 (**a**): NSF is characterized by increased dermal cellularity (H&E, 40x; *left panel*). (**b**): Positive staining of dermal fibroblast-like cells for CD34 in NSF (CD34, 40x; *right panel*)

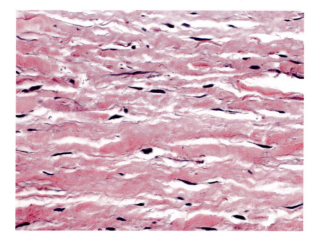

Fig. 30.6 Eosinophilic collagen bundles are thickened with adjacent clefts interspersed between spindle-shaped cells in the dermis (H&E, 400x)

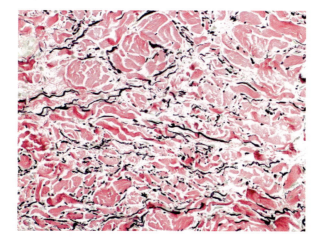

Fig. 30.7 Dermal elastic fibers are preserved and may be elongated (Verhoeff-van Gieson, 200x)

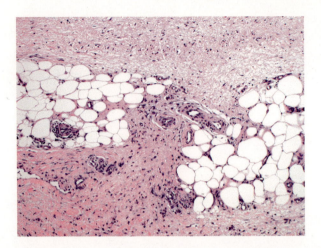

Fig. 30.8 NSF characteristically involves interlobular septae of subcutaneous fat (H&E, 100x)

Unlike scleredema, there is involvement of interlobular septae of the subcutaneous adipose tissue in NSF (Fig. 30.8). Thus, a deep skin punch biopsy and clinicopathologic correlation are essential to make the diagnosis of NSF [2].

See Also

Scleroderma, scleromyxedema

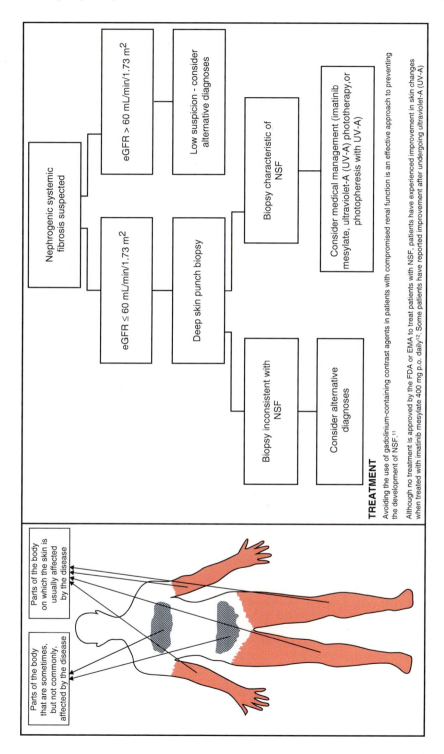

TREATMENT

Avoiding the use of gadolinium-containing contrast agents in patients with compromised renal function is an effective approach to preventing the development of NSF.[11]

Although no treatment is approved by the FDA or EMA to treat patients with NSF, patients have experienced improvement in skin changes when treated with imatinib mesylate 400 mg p.o. daily[12]. Some patients have reported improvement after undergoing ultraviolet-A (UV-A).

Nephrogenic systemic fibrosis suspected

eGFR ≤ 60 mL/min/1.73 m²

eGFR > 60 mL/min/1.73 m²

Low suspicion - consider alternative diagnoses

Deep skin punch biopsy

Biopsy characteristic of NSF

Biopsy inconsistent with NSF

Consider medical management (imatinib mesylate, ultraviolet-A (UV-A) phototherapy, or photopheresis with UV-A)

Consider alternative diagnoses

Parts of the body that are sometimes, but not commonly, affected by the disease

Parts of the body on which the skin is usually affected by the disease

References

1. Cowper SE, Robin HS, Steinberg SM, Su LD, Gupta S, LeBoit PE. Scleromyxoedema-like cutaneous diseases in renal-dialysis patients. Lancet. 2000;356:1000–1.
2. Girardi M, Kay J, Elston DM, LeBoit PE, Ali Abu-Alfa A, Cowper SE. Nephrogenic systemic fibrosis: clinicopathological definition and work-up recommendations. J Am Acad Dermatol. 2011;65:1095–1106.e7.
3. Grobner T. Gadolinium–a specific trigger for the development of nephrogenic fibrosing dermopathy and nephrogenic systemic fibrosis? Nephrol Dial Transplant. 2006;21:1104–8.
4. Todd DJ, Kagan A, Chibnik LB, Kay J. Cutaneous changes of nephrogenic systemic fibrosis: predictor of early mortality and association with gadolinium exposure. Arthritis Rheum. 2007;56:3433–41.
5. Abujudeh HH, Kaewlai R, Kagan A, Chibnik LB, Nazarian RM, High WA, Kay J. Nephrogenic systemic fibrosis after gadopentetate dimeglumine exposure: case series of 36 patients. Radiology. 2009;253:81–9.
6. Cowper SE, Su LD, Bhawan J, Robin HS, LeBoit PE. Nephrogenic fibrosing dermopathy. Am J Dermatopathol. 2001;23:383–93.
7. Koreishi AF, Nazarian RM, Saenz AJ, Klepeis VE, McDonald AG, Farris AB, Colvin RB, Duncan LM, Mandal RV, Kay J. Nephrogenic systemic fibrosis: a pathologic study of autopsy cases. Arch Pathol Lab Med. 2009;133:1943–8.
8. Kay J, Bazari H, Avery LL, Koreishi AF. Case records of the Massachusetts General Hospital. Case 6–2008. A 46-year-old woman with renal failure and stiffness of the joints and skin. N Engl J Med. 2008;358:827–38.
9. Nazarian RM, Mandal RV, Kagan A, Kay J, Duncan LM. Quantitative assessment of dermal cellularity in nephrogenic systemic fibrosis: a diagnostic aid. J Am Acad Dermatol. 2011;64:741–7.
10. High WA, Ayers RA, Cowper SE. Gadolinium is quantifiable within the tissue of patients with nephrogenic systemic fibrosis. J Am Acad Dermatol. 2007;56:710–2.
11. Wang Y, Narin O, Alkasab TK, Nazarian RM, Kaewlai R, Kay J, Abujudeh HH. Incidence of nephrogenic systemic fibrosis following adoption of a restrictive gadolinium policy. Radiology. 2011;260:105–11.
12. Kay J, High WA. Imatinib mesylate treatment of nephrogenic systemic fibrosis. Arthritis Rheum. 2008;58:2543–8.

Chapter 31
Graft-Versus-Host Disease (GvHD): Cutaneous Manifestations

Peter Häusermann and Alan Tyndall

Definition

Graft-versus-host disease (GvHD) is the major complication of allogeneic hematopoietic stem cell transplantation (HSCT). Over the last decades, this complex therapeutic procedure has become a worldwide important therapy for hematological malignancies, nonmalignant stem cell disorders, certain genetic diseases (e.g., immunodeficiencies), and even some solid tumors. More than 40 years of tremendous scientific work has concluded that GvHD is an acquired immune-mediated disease in the stem cell recipient that arises when donor-immunocompetent T cells respond to genetically defined proteins on host cells [1].

The most important recognized proteins are human leucocyte antigens (HLAs), which are highly polymorphic and are encoded by the major histocompatibility complex (MHC). Donor T cells react against class I HLA (A, B, and C, expressed on almost all nucleated cells of the body) and class II proteins (DR, DQ, and DP, mainly expressed on hematopoietic cells, e.g., B cells, dendritic cells, and monocytes) of the host. Frequency and severity of GvHD, that overall occurs in about 50 % of patients undergoing that procedure, are directly related to the degree of mismatch between HLA proteins [2, 3].

The pathophysiology of acute GvHD is well understood and initially involves activation of antigen-presenting cells (APCs) of the host by the underlying disease and the conditioning regimen. Subsequently, donor T cells proliferate and

P. Häusermann, M.D., FMH (✉)
Department of Dermatology, University Hospital Basel, Petersgraben 4,
4031 Basel, Switzerland
e-mail: phaeusermann@uhbs.ch

A. Tyndall, Ph.D., M.D.
Department of Rheumatology, Felix Platter Spital, University Hospital Basel,
Burgfelderstrasse 101, Basel, Switzerland
e-mail: alan.tyndall@fps-basel.ch

M. Matucci-Cerinic et al. (eds.), *Skin Manifestations in Rheumatic Disease*,
DOI 10.1007/978-1-4614-7849-2_31, © Springer Science+Business Media New York 2014

Fig. 31.1 Acute cutaneous GvHD: characteristic morbilliform/maculopapular exanthema involving most of the body in a patient 30 days after allogeneic HSCT

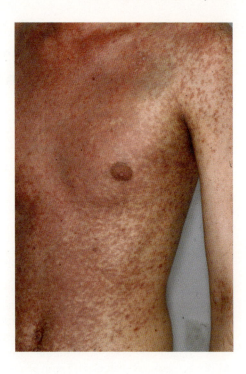

differentiate in response to activated APCs of the recipient that finally induces T-cell-mediated attack against host tissue. In contrast, the mechanisms underlying chronic GvHD are still obscure. Potentially many different cells are involved including T cells, B cells, macrophages, and regulatory cells. Furthermore, it is assumed that thymic injury related to conditioning, immunosuppression, and aGvHD may impair negative selection of T cells emigrating from the thymus [1, 2, 4].

Clinically, acute GvHD predominantly involves fast-proliferating organs such as skin, liver, and gastrointestinal tract. The hallmark cutaneous finding is a distinct maculopapular rash with follicular prominence (Fig. 31.1). Characteristically, acral sites such as head, hand, and feet are involved as well (Fig. 31.2). Severe manifestations include erosive lesions of mucous membranes and bullae formation reminiscent of drug-induced toxic epidermal necrolysis. In contrast, chronic GvHD can involve almost any organ and structures concurrently or consecutively. This disease complex often mimics systemic autoimmune diseases such as lupus erythematosus, Sjögren's syndrome, systemic sclerosis, or mixed connective tissue disease. Skin manifestations include a wide spectrum, e.g., ichthyosis-like changes, erythematosquamous and eczematous lesions, lichen planus-like features, as well as sclerotic and fibrosing changes of superficial or deep dermal structures (lichen sclerosus-like, morpheaform, eosinophilic fasciitis-like) (Figs. 31.3–31.5). Frequently, mucous membranes and adnexal structures (hair, nails, and eccrine, apocrine, and sebaceous glands) are affected as well (Fig. 31.6) [5, 6].

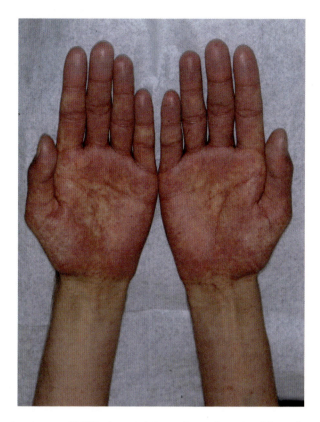

Fig. 31.2 Acute cutaneous GvHD: characteristic acral exanthema involving palms and soles in a patient 30 days after allogeneic HSCT

In the past, acute and chronic GvHD have been separated stringently by time point after allogeneic HSCT. Any manifestations of GvHD present at ≥100 days posttransplant were arbitrary defined as chronic GvHD. As a result of newer conditioning and immunosuppressive regimens and multiple interventions (e.g., donor lymphocyte infusions), the distinction between simple categories such as acute and chronic GvHD is blurred. For instance, acute GvHD can be precipitated ≥100 days posttransplant by donor T-cell infusions to treat relapse and discontinuation of immunosuppressive medications (which initially prevented or treated acute GvHD). As a consequence, categories of acute and chronic GvHD were recently redefined by the NIH consensus development project groups. Acute GvHD is thus divided into classic (symptoms ≤ 100 days) and persistent, recurrent, or late-onset (symptoms ≥ 100 days) disease. Chronic GvHD is today categorized as classical (no time limit of symptoms, no presence of acute GvHD features) or overlap syndrome (no time limit, presence of acute and chronic features of GvHD) [6, 7].

Fig. 31.3 Chronic cutaneous
GvHD: disseminated
erythemato-squamous
plaques and patches involving
most parts of the body in a
patient more than 2 years
after allogeneic HSCT.
Clinicopathological
correlation is consistent with
overlap syndrome

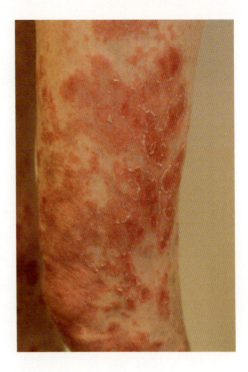

Differential Diagnosis

In the appropriate setting of allogeneic HSCT, the differential diagnosis of acute cutaneous GvHD includes morbilliform drug exanthema, chemotherapy-related toxic exanthema, morbilliform viral exanthema (especially CMV), but also engraftment syndrome, eruption of lymphocyte recovery, or bacterial infections such as secondary syphilis. Depending on the predominant type of skin lesions and mucous membrane involvement, chronic cutaneous GvHD can imitate psoriasis, atopic dermatitis, drug-induced exanthema, vitiligo, or lichen planus. Often, the distinction to systemic autoimmune disorders such as lupus erythematosus, Sjögren's syndrome, systemic sclerosis, or mixed connective tissue diseases can be challenging. Fibrosing disease is particularly reminiscent of lichen sclerosus, morphea, eosinophilic fasciitis (Shulman's syndrome), and systemic sclerosis (limited or diffuse). Unlike systemic sclerosis, cGVHD does not manifest small vessel disease such as Raynaud's phenomenon and nail typical fold capillaroscopy changes [5, 8].

Biopsy

Histologically, acute cutaneous GvHD is characterized by apoptosis of keratinocytes within the basal or lower spinosum layers of the epidermis, outer root sheath of the hair follicle, or acrosyringium (Fig. 31.7). Most often, a sparse lymphocytic

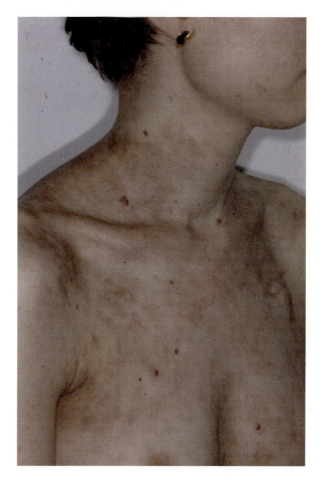

Fig. 31.4 Chronic lichenoid GvHD: characteristic livid and hyperpigmented patches in a patient 6 months after allogeneic HSCT

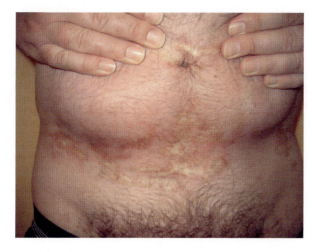

Fig. 31.5 Chronic sclerodermatous GvHD: characteristic sclerotic plaques in a patient more than 3 years after allogeneic HSCT

Fig. 31.6 Chronic cutaneous
GvHD involving the nails:
characteristic lichen
planus-like changes of nails
in a patient more than 2 years
after allogeneic HSCT

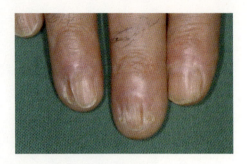

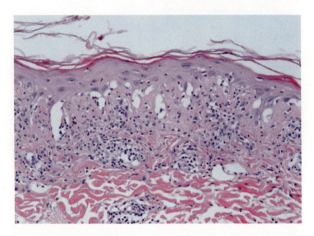

Fig. 31.7 Acute cutaneous GvHD: hallmark histological features of T-cell-mediated cytotoxic interface dermatitis with apoptosis, dyskeratosis, and satellite necrosis of epidermal keratinocytes

T-cell infiltrate can be found around superficial vessels and close to apoptotic keratinocytes. According to the severity of these inflammatory changes, acute GvHD was traditionally graded from grade I (only vacuolar changes) up to grade IV (subepidermal bullae). To date, no single histologic feature has been shown pathognomonic of acute cutaneous GvHD [9].

Chronic lichenoid GvHD of skin presents with a rather pronounced T-cell-mediated interface dermatitis characterized by either a lichenoid pattern of T lymphocytes (with or without lymphocyte-induced satellite necrosis) or primarily vacuolar changes of the basal layers devoid of relevant amounts of T cells. Acanthosis, compact orthohyperkeratosis, and hypergranulosis are classical epidermal findings in lichenoid type of chronic GvHD. Chronic fibrosing GvHD of skin demonstrates compactation and homogenization of collagenous matrix of papillary or reticular dermis and involves fascial septa of muscles in deep fibrosing disease (e.g., eosinophilic fasciitis-like lesions) (Fig. 31.8) [5, 9].

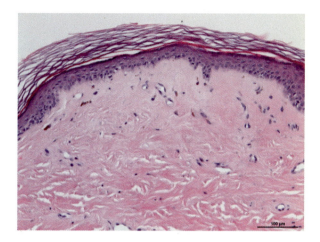

Fig. 31.8 Chronic cutaneous GvHD: increase and compactation of collagenous matrix and vessel rarification characteristic of chronic sclerodermatous GvHD

See Also

Lupus erythematosus, Systemic sclerosis, Morphea, Dermatomyositis, Mixed connective tissue disease, and Sjögren's syndrome

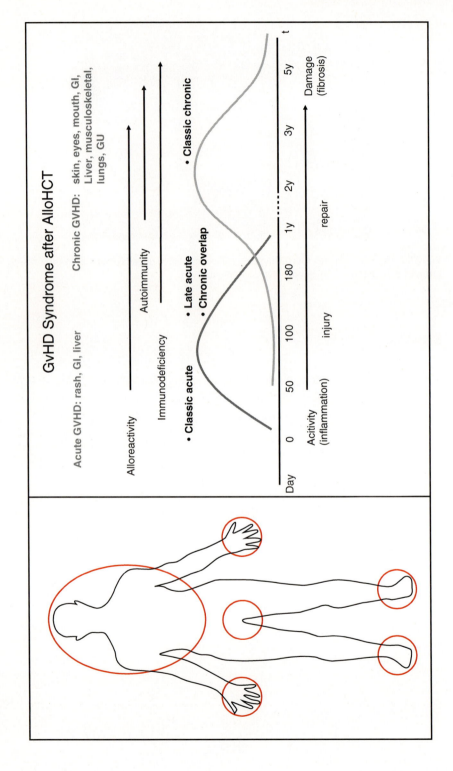

References

1. Copelan EA. Hematopoietic stem-cell transplantation. N Engl J Med. 2006;354:1813.
2. Ferrara JLM, et al. Graft-versus-host disease. Lancet. 2009;373:1550.
3. Shlomchik WD. Graft-versus-host disease. Nature Rev Immunol. 2007;7:340.
4. Wagner JL, Murphy GF. Pathology and pathogenesis of cutaneous graft-versus-host disease. In: Ferrara JLM, Cooke KR, Deeg HJ, editors. Graft-vs-host disease. 3rd ed. New York: Marcel Dekker; 2005. p. 229–57.
5. Häusermann P, et al. Cutaneous graft-versus-host disease: a guide for the dermatologist. Dermatology. 2008;216:287.
6. Filipovitch AH et al. 14. National Institutes of Health consensus development project on criteria for clinical trials in chronic graft-versus-host disease: I. Diagnosis and staging working group report, Biol Blood Marrow Transplant. 2005;11:945.
7. Schaffer JV. The changing face of graft-versus-host disease. Semin Cutan Med Surg. 2006;25:190.
8. Mays SR, et al. Approach to the morbilliform eruption in the hematopoietic transplant patient. Semin Cutan Med Surg. 2007;26:155.
9. Shulman HM, et al. Histopathologic diagnosis of chronic graft-versus-host disease: National Institutes of Health Consensus Development Project on Criteria for Clinical Trials in chronic Graft-versus-Host Disease: II. Pathology working Group Report. Biol Blood Marrow Transplant. 2006;12:31.

Chapter 32
Scleromyxoedema

Catherine H. Orteu and Christopher P. Denton

Introduction

Scleromyxoedema is a rare disorder of unknown etiology that is an important potential mimic of other sclerosing skin diseases and, in particular, of disorders within the scleroderma spectrum [1]. It is characterised by the presence of infiltrative and confluent skin induration with papule formation. The histopathological hallmark is an increase in mucin-rich extracellular matrix in the involved skin, although this may diminish with time and be replaced by fibrosis [2]. There has been historical confusion between this disorder and other forms of skin thickening associated with increased acid mucin deposition in the skin by histological examination. There are, however, distinct features that define scleromyxoedema. As proposed by Rongioletti, the term should be reserved for patients with a generalised papular and sclerodermoid eruption, cutaneous mucin deposition, fibroblast proliferation and fibrosis, a monoclonal gammopathy and no evidence of thyroid disease. In contrast with localised forms of papular mucinosis which have no associated systemic manifestations and run a benign course, it tends to run a progressive course with a poor outcome and in many cases leads to potentially life-threatening complications [3]. The most important manifestations relate to dysphagia, aspiration and difficulties with facial movement, eating, nutrition and eyelid closure. Some 150 cases have been described in the English literature although it is a well-recognised condition in specialist dermatology clinics and probably under-reported.

C.H. Orteu, B.Sc., M.D., FRCP
Department of Dermatology, Royal Free Hospital, NW3 2QG London, UK
e-mail: cate.orteu@nhs.net

C.P. Denton, Ph.D., FRCP (✉)
Centre for Rheumatology, Royal Free Hospital, NW3 2QG London, UK
e-mail: c.denton@medsch.ucl.ac.uk

M. Matucci-Cerinic et al. (eds.), *Skin Manifestations in Rheumatic Disease*,
DOI 10.1007/978-1-4614-7849-2_32, © Springer Science+Business Media New York 2014

Clinical Features

The average age of onset is 55 years. Males and females are affected equally. Patients develop multiple, firm, 1–3 mm dome-shaped, white- to skin-coloured, waxy, infiltrative papules and/or diffuse cutaneous sclerosis. Papules may be arranged linearly or give a cobblestone appearance. Acute stages may be erythematous and oedematous; later, fibrosis predominates. Pruritus is common. The face, postauricular areas, neck, extensor forearms and backs of the hands are typically involved [1–3] (see Fig. 32.1). Less commonly the trunk and legs are affected. Progressive thickening and hardening of the skin can cause contractures and limit function (see Fig. 32.2).

Extracutaneous manifestations are common. Over 80 % of cases have a serum paraprotein, usually IgG λ. Its level does not parallel disease activity. Gastrointestinal (oesophageal dysmotility) and neurological manifestations (epilepsy, aphasia, motor impairment, carpal tunnel syndrome, peripheral neuropathy, depression, memory loss, dementia and psychosis) are commonest. Exertional dyspnoea, restrictive or obstructive lung disease, upper airway involvement and more rarely pulmonary hypertension can occur. Proximal muscle weakness, inflammatory myopathy, inflammatory polyarthritis and other haematological disorders are documented [2, 3].

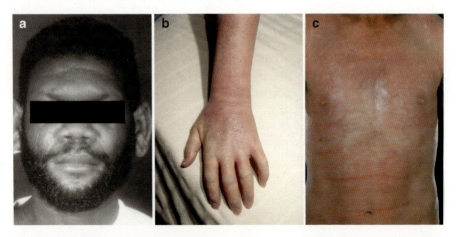

Fig. 32.1 Facial and hand features of scleromyxoedema. (**a**) Diffuse skin thickening of the face particularly involving the glabella and forehead, with multiple firm papules 1–3 mm on the ears (Reprinted from Lister RK, Jolles S, Whittaker S, et al. Scleromyxoedema: Response to high-dose intravenous immunoglobulin (hdIVIg). J Am Acad Dermatol 2000;43:403–8. With permission from Elsevier). (**b**) Sclerodermoid appearance of the hands. (**c**) Involvement of the trunk showing a significant inflammatory component

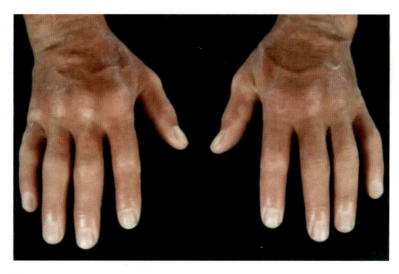

Fig. 32.2 Contractural changes and skin induration in advanced disease. Skin thickening with marked accentuation of skin folds

Differential Diagnosis

Scleroderma, scleroedema, nephrogenic systemic fibrosis, eosinophilic fasciitis and pretibial and generalised myxoedema are included in the differential diagnosis (see Table 32.1). The presence of waxy papules giving the skin a cobblestone appearance helps to distinguish scleromyxoedema from scleroedema and scleroderma. Raynaud's phenomenon, nailfold capillary abnormalities, telangiectases, calcinosis and positive antinuclear autoantibodies (ANA), often with defined specificity and nucleolar staining pattern by immunofluorescence, are typically present in systemic sclerosis but rare in scleromyxoedema (and the other differentials listed). Scleroedema occurs in children and adults and typically affects the upper back, neck and face. The skin induration is nonpitting and hard, and there is no sharp demarcation between the normal and affected skin. Diabetes (typically long-standing and insulin dependent), recent infection (particularly streptococcal) and IgG k paraproteinaemia are associated. Both scleroedema and scleromyxoedema may be associated with paraproteinaemia and with a plasma cell dyscrasia and less commonly with multiple myeloma [4]. NSF and eosinophilic fasciitis commonly involve the extremities and rarely the face. Normal renal function and absence of exposure to gadolinium-based contrast media exclude NSF. In eosinophilic fasciitis there is woody induration of the limbs, usually sparing the hands and feet. At sites of vessels, the overlying skin shows typical guttering. Marked peripheral eosinophilia commonly occurs. Normal thyroid function and absent thyroid autoantibodies exclude both generalised and pretibial myxoedema. A diagnostic skin biopsy, preferably a deep incisional ellipse, is essential. A diagnostic flow chart summarising the key clinical and investigational features that underpin the diagnosis of scleromyxoedema is shown in Fig. 32.3.

Table 32.1 Differential diagnosis of scleromyxoedema: comparative features of related skin diseases

	Scleromyxoedema	Scleroderma	Scleroedema	Nephrogenic systemic fibrosis	Eosinophilic fasciitis
Collagen	Thickened increased collagen clefting	Enlarged eosinophilic collagen bundles orientated parallel to skin surface. Loss of adnexal structures	Swollen collagen bundles look fenestrated	Thickened increased collagen	Thickened increased collagen
CD34+ fibrocytes	Yes, stellate	No	No	Yes	No
Mucin (mainly hyaluronic acid)	++++	+	++	+++	No
Depth of skin involvement	To mid-reticular dermis	Into subcutis fascia and muscle	Into subcutis (fat replaced by collagen)	Into panniculus	Fat and deep fascia
Inflammation	Perivascular upper dermis	Perivascular prominent	No	No/less obvious	Yes ± eosinophils
Site	Face hands forearms	Generalised	Back, sides neck, face	Extremities	Extremities
ANA	±ANA	ANA++ ENA++	No	No	ANA ± eosinophilia
Familial			Yes		
Other associations	Paraprotein IgG λ	Calcinosis, Raynaud's, abnormal nailfold capillaries	Diabetes, infection (especially streptococcal) Paraprotein IgG κ, IgA	Renal failure, gadolinium exposure	Morphoea, immune cytopenias, haematological malignancy

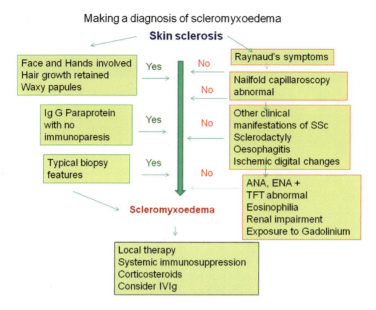

Fig. 32.3 Making a diagnosis of scleromyxoedema. Flow chart summarising key clinical and laboratory features of scleromyxoedema. Positive features are indicated in *green* and significant negative features in *red*

Biopsy Findings

Histological similarities between scleroedema, scleromyxoedema and nephrogenic systemic suggest that similar pathogenic mechanisms may be involved [5]. Typical histological features of scleromyxoedema are shown in Fig. 32.4. They include a diffuse deposition of mucin in the papillary and mid-reticular dermis. The deep dermis and subcutis are not involved. A mild perivascular inflammatory cell infiltrate may be present in the early stages. There is increased collagen deposition and a proliferation of irregularly arranged, stellate and bipolar fibroblasts. Later stages show more sclerosis and thickening of collagen bundles. Deposited mucin is mainly composed of hyaluronic acid and can be visualised with alcian blue or toluidine blue stains. The overlying epidermis may be normal or thinned. Elastic fibres may be fragmented and reduced in numbers. Underlying pathogenic mechanisms are poorly understood [1]. Patient serum has been shown to stimulate DNA synthesis and fibroblast proliferation in vitro, but the serum factor was not paraprotein. Patient serum has also been documented to increase hyaluronic acid and prostaglandin E synthesis. Mucin deposition has been found in large pulmonary vessels in a patient with PAH, in the kidney, adrenals, cardiac and coronary vessels, eyelids and cornea. The role of mucin in the development of systemic manifestations of disease is still unknown.

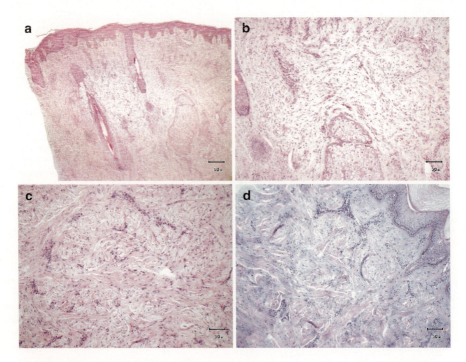

Fig. 32.4 Histological features of scleromyxoedema. (**a**) Low power view of early stage disease showing perivascular inflammatory cell infiltrate and expanded reticular dermis. (**b**) High power view of early stage disease with numerous fibroblasts in the reticular dermis. (**c**) High power view of late stage disease with increased, thickened collagen bundles in the reticular dermis. (**d**) Alcian blue stain showing interstitial mucin deposits in between thickened collagen bundles in the upper dermis

Conclusions

Scleromyxoedema is a potentially fatal skin disease that leads to important complications and for which current treatment strategies are often inadequate. However, there are emerging data that support immunomodulatory therapy and in particular intravenous immunoglobulin as useful therapies. Accurate diagnosis and appropriate patient education and follow-up form an important part of current management.

See Also

Scleroderma, scleroedema, nephrogenic systemic fibrosis, eosinophilic fasciitis, myxoedema

References

1. Boin F, Hummers LK. Scleroderma like fibrosing disorders. Rheum Dis Clin North Am. 2008;34:199.
2. Rongioletti F, Rebora A. Updated classification of papular mucinosis, lichen myxedematosus and scleromyxoedema. J Am Acad Dermatol. 2001;44:273.
3. Dinneen AM, Dicken CH. Scleromyxoedema. J Am Acad Dermatol. 1995;33:37.
4. Dziadzio M, et al. From scleroedema to AL amyloidosis: disease progression or coincidence? Review of the literature. Clin Rheumatol. 2006;25:3.
5. Kucher C, et al. Histopathologic comparison of nephrogenic fibrosing dermopathy and scleromyxoedema. J Cutan Pathol. 2005;32:484.

Chapter 33
Eosinophilic Fasciitis

Yannick Allanore and Camille Frances

Eosinophilic fasciitis (EF) is a rare scleroderma-like disorder, first described by Lawrence Edward Shulman in 1974 [1], in patients with diffuse fasciitis and eosinophilia. Until today, both the aetiology and pathogenesis remain unknown [2–4]. Several potential triggers have been suggested such as extreme physical exercise, ingestion of pharmaceutical agents (statins, L-tryptophan) or toxics, traumas, Lyme borreliosis, haematologic malignant conditions and thyroid disease [2, 5, 6]. Typically, EF affects adults of both sexes in the second to sixth decade of life although paediatric cases have been reported. It is characterised by the sudden onset of painful, tender, oedematous and erythematous extremities. Within weeks to months, patients develop stiffness and sclerodermatous infiltration. The superficial skin may be still superficially wrinkled while there is a deep sclerosis (Fig. 33.1a) leading toward a peau d'orange aspect and the groove sign (Fig. 33.1a, b) which corresponds to an indentation along the course of the superficial veins. Lesions are symmetric with involvement of the upper and lower limbs. The trunk and neck can be affected with typical sparing of the hands and face. Raynaud phenomenon is usually absent. Deep and superficial extension of the fibrosis leads to progressive muscle weakness and morphea-like lesions. Associated morpheas or localised scleroderma lesions are present on other parts of the body in 20–30 % of cases [3, 6]. Synovitis and contractures induce impaired mobility. Some extra-cutaneous manifestations have been reported including arthritis (elbows, wrists, knees or ankles), carpal tunnel syndrome, restrictive lung functions and haematological disturbances [2, 6, 7].

Y. Allanore, M.D., Ph.D. (✉)
Rheumatology A department, Paris Descartes University, Assistance Publique-Hôpitaux de Paris, Cochin Hospital, 27 rue du faubourg, Saint Jacques, 75014 Paris, France
e-mail: yannick.allanore@cch.aphp.fr

C. Frances, M.D.
Department of Dermatology-Allergology, Pierre et Marie Curie University, Assistance Publique-Hôpitaux de Paris, Tenon Hospital, 4 rue de la Chine, 75020 Paris, France
e-mail: camille.frances@tnn.aphp.fr

M. Matucci-Cerinic et al. (eds.), *Skin Manifestations in Rheumatic Disease*,
DOI 10.1007/978-1-4614-7849-2_33, © Springer Science+Business Media New York 2014

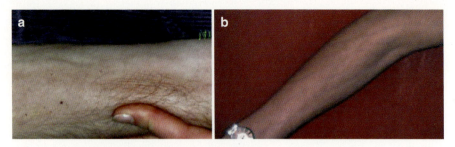

Fig. 33.1 (**a**)"Peau d'orange" feature. The superficial dermis may be wrinkled while the deep dermis and fascias are fibrosed. (**b**) Indentation along the course of the superficial veins (groove sign)

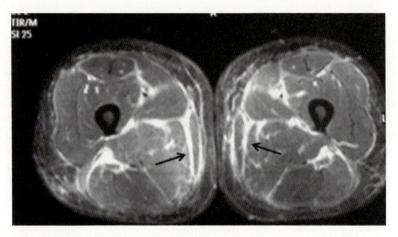

Fig. 33.2 Thigh muscle MRI of a patient with eosinophilic fasciitis. Axial fat-suppressed, T2-weighted fast spin-echo MR image shows markedly increased signal intensity within the superficial and deep fascial layers and mildly increased T2 signal intensity within the superficial muscle fibres adjacent to the fascia (*arrows*)

Biological tests show peripheral eosinophilia and increased inflammatory markers (elevated sedimentation rate and C-reactive protein), at least during the acute phase of the disease. Muscular enzymes may be mildly increased reflecting the underlying muscular involvement. Autoimmune anaemia and hypergammaglobulinemia (sometimes monoclonal gammopathy) are variably present. Immunological markers of autoimmunity such as antinuclear antibodies or rheumatoid factors have not been reported in EF with consistency.

Magnetic resonance imaging of the involved limbs is able to detect fascial thickening and precise the extension of the lesions especially in the muscles (Fig. 33.2). Abnormal signal intensity and contrast enhancement are suggestive of an active inflammation. These findings are useful to make the diagnosis, to guide the location for biopsy and to monitor the response to therapy [8]. High-resolution

Table 33.1 Differential diagnoses of eosinophilic fasciitis

Systemic sclerosis	Presence of Raynaud phenomenon, capillaroscopic abnormalities, antinuclear antibodies, visceral involvements; fibrosis mainly localised in the dermis
Morphea or localised scleroderma	All the areas of the body may be involved. Usually, fibrosis is mainly localised in the dermis; however, in some cases, fibrosis may involve the fascias and the muscles as in EF, especially in the linear forms affecting the limbs. So, EF is frequently considered as a deep variant subset of morphea
Inflammatory myositis and dermatomyositis (DM)	Proximal muscular weakness, general feeling of discomfort, DM skin manifestations, high levels of muscle enzymes, MRI examination and inflammation predominantly localised in the muscles
Hypereosinophilic syndrome	Sustained absolute eosinophil count greater than $>1,500/\mu l$, manifestations of organ involvement (heart, central nervous system, skin, respiratory tract…)
Eosinophilic–myalgia syndrome and toxic oil fibrosis	Epidemic disorders resulting from ingestion of toxic contaminants such as aniline-denaturate rapeseed oil and L-TRYPTOPHAN; sudden onset with more severe manifestations: myalgias, oedema and multi-organ involvement (mainly the lung and central nervous system) leading to a high mortality rate
Sclerodermoid graft versus host disease (GVH)	Onset after allogeneic stem cell transplantation, association with lichen sclerosus and morpheaform lesions mainly on the trunk with sometimes EF-like lesions on the limbs; association with liver abnormalities and gut involvement; initial fibrosis in the superficial dermis [9]

ultrasonography appreciates the extension of the lesions in the dermis. Although these preceding examinations are very useful for managing patients, attempt for confirmation of the diagnosis has to include the examination of a full-thickness skin to muscle biopsy.

Differential Diagnosis

Systemic sclerosis, localised scleroderma, inflammatory myositis, hypereosinophilic syndrome, graft versus host disease, toxic oil syndrome or eosinophilia–myalgia syndrome are considered as differential diagnoses of EF. Lyme disease, vasculitis and cutaneous T-cell lymphoma might also be considered. The most important parameters to be considered for differential diagnosis are listed in Table 33.1.

Biopsy

Histological examination of all tissue layers from the skin to muscle remains the golden standard for the diagnosis. The superficial fascia is markedly thickened and fibrosed. Fibrosis extended to the septa of the hypodermis, to the lower dermis and

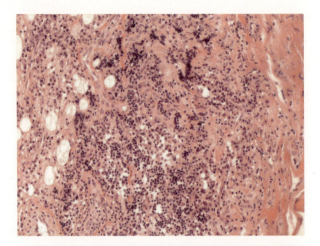

Fig. 33.3 Muscle–fascia–skin biopsy of a patient with eosinophilic fasciitis. Haematoxylin–eosin staining shows a perimysial fascia thickening with an intense inflammatory infiltrate composed of lymphocytes, histiocytes, plasma cells and variable numbers of eosinophils

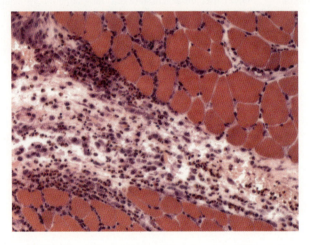

Fig. 33.4 Muscle–fascia–skin biopsy of a patient with eosinophilic fasciitis. Haematoxylin–eosin staining shows adjacent muscles which exhibit mild inflammation but without necrosis

to the underlying perimysium and musculature. The inflammatory infiltrate is mild to heavy and consists of lymphocytes, histiocytes, plasma cells and variable numbers of eosinophils (Fig. 33.3). Eosinophils are not required for diagnosis; the term eosinophilic fasciitis refers to peripheral eosinophilia, not tissue eosinophils.

Adjacent muscles can exhibit mild inflammation but without necrosis (Fig. 33.4). Fibroblast proliferation is associated with an inflammatory infiltrate usually constituted by macrophages and T CD8 lymphocytes.

Treatment

There is substantial agreement among published cases or case series that corticosteroids, initially at high dose (more than 20 mg prednisone/day and often 0.5–1 mg/kg as a starting dose), are the first-line treatment for eosinophilic fasciitis. Corticosteroids are tapered over many months as the disease improves. They are usually effective in more than 70 % of cases. The goal is a complete resolution of fibrotic lesions, but it may take 12–24 months to get a satisfactory response. Other treatments include nonsteroidal anti-inflammatory drugs, hydroxychloroquine, cimetidine, methotrexate, azathioprine, cyclosporin A, mycophenolate mofetil, infliximab, UVA-1 and bath PUVA [3, 5, 10]. These drugs have shown variable results and were more often used in steroid-refractory cases; one may support methotrexate to be the first associated drug to corticosteroids and potential corticosteroid-sparing agent despite no randomised controlled trials. Spontaneous remission rate in patients with eosinophilic fasciitis is 10–20 % at the time of presentation, and this can trouble response to therapy assessment; relapse after discontinuing corticosteroid therapy can also occur. Physical therapy is also needed to try to avoid long-term consequences of contractures.

The lack of response should raise the potential presence of neoplastic disorder. In one study with a systematic review of the literature, the risk factors associated with refractory fibrosis were morphea-like skin lesions, a younger age (under 12 years) at onset and trunk involvement. Histopathologically, the presence of dermal fibrosis was also associated with a higher risk of refractory fibrosis [7].

See Also

Connective tissue disorders
   Scleroderma

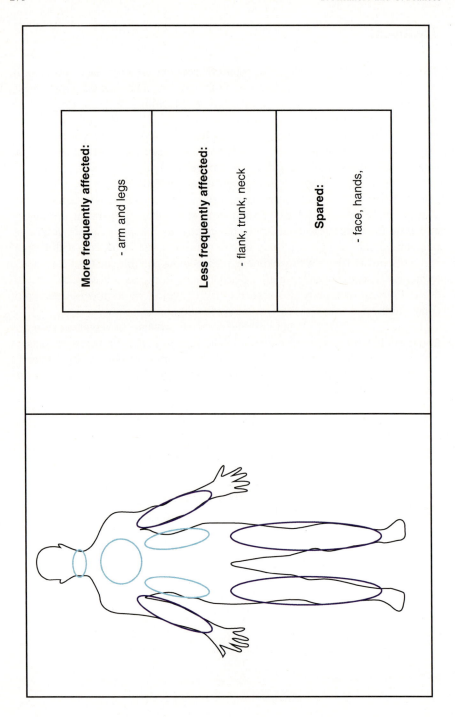

References

1. Shulman LE. Diffuse fasciitis with eosinophilia: a new syndrome? Trans Assoc Am Physicians. 1975;88:70–86.
2. Antic M, Lautenschlager S, Itin PH. Eosinophilic fasciitis 30 years after-what do we really know. Report of 11 patients and review of the literature. Dermatology. 2006;213:93–101.
3. Boin F, Hummers LK. Scleroderma-like fibrosing disorders. Rheum Dis Clin North Am. 2008;34:199–220.
4. Rodnan GP, Di Bartolomeo A, Medsger Jr TA. Proceedings: eosinophilic fasciitis: report of six cases of a newly recognized scleroderma-like syndrome. Arthritis Rheum. 1975;18:525.
5. Bischoff L, Derk CT. Eosinophilic fasciitis: demographics, disease pattern and response to treatment: report of 12 cases and review of the literature. Int J Dermatol. 2008;47:29–35.
6. Lakhanpal S, Ginsburg WW, Michet CJ, Doyle JA, Moore SB. Eosinophilic fasciitis: clinical spectrum and therapeutic response in 52 cases. Semin Arthritis Rheum. 1998;17:221–31.
7. Endo Y, Tamura A, Matsushima Y, Iwasaki T, Hasegawa M, Nagai Y, Ishikawa O. Eosinophilic fasciitis: report of two cases and a systematic review of the literature dealing with clinical variables that predict outcome. Clin Rheumatol. 2007;26:1445–51.
8. Agnew KL, Blunt D, Francis ND, Bunker CB. Magnetic resonance imaging in eosinophilic fasciitis. Clin Exp Dermatol. 2005;30:435–6.
9. Schaffer JV, McNif JM, Seropian S, Cooper DL, Bolognia JL. Lichen sclerosus and eosinophilic fasciitis as manifestations of chronic graft-versus-host disease: expanding the sclerodermoid spectrum. J Am Acad Dermatol. 2005;53:591–601.
10. Khanna D, Agrawal H, Clements PJ. Infliximab may be effective in the treatment of steroid-resistant eosinophilic fasciitis: report of three cases. Rheumatology (Oxford). 2010;49:1184–8.

Part V
Vasculitides

Chapter 34
Kawasaki Disease

Fernanda Falcini

Definition

KD is a febrile systemic vasculitis that generally affects children younger than 5 years. While found worldwide, it is most frequently diagnosed among Asian populations. A probable viral agent entering the respiratory tract causes an oligoclonal IgA response in all tissues and vessel walls and is thought to be pathogenetic. KD is the leading cause of acquired heart disease in children in developed countries. Coronary aneurysms (CAA) develop in about 25 % of untreated children but also in 4 % of those who received IVIG. The mortality rate is 0, 14 %. Along with premature atherosclerosis, KD is regarded as a potential risk factor for adult ischemic heart disease and sudden death in young adults. Male-to-female ratio is 1.8:1. Lacking diagnostic tests, the diagnosis is based on clinical criteria after the exclusion of other febrile diseases with rash. Clinical manifestations include high fever lasting more than 5 days, otherwise explained and unresponsive to antibiotics *plus* (i) bilateral non-exudative conjunctivitis, (ii) rash, (iii) nonsuppurative cervical lymphadenopathy, (iv) mucous membrane changes (fissured lips, redness of pharynx, strawberry-like tongue), and (v) extremity changes (erythema of palms and soles, hands and foot edema, and periungueal digital peeling).

Targetoid cutaneous manifestations are protean. Polymorphous nonspecific rash begins on the face, trunk, and extremities with a confluence on the perineal area.

It may be morbilliform (Fig. 34.1) or scarlet, seldom pruritic, vesicular, or bullous. Strawberry tongue, mucosal redness and cracked lips are typical manifestations helpful in diagnosing Kawasaki disease (Fig. 34.2). Indurate edema of the dorsum of hands (Fig. 34.3) and a diffuse red purple erythema of the palms and soles (Fig. 34.4) may be seen early from fever onset followed by desquamation at fingertips (Fig. 34.5).

F. Falcini, M.D. (✉)
Internal Medicine, Rheumatology Section, University of Florence,
Viale Pieraccini 18, Florence 50139, Italy
e-mail: falcini@unifi.it

M. Matucci-Cerinic et al. (eds.), *Skin Manifestations in Rheumatic Disease*,
DOI 10.1007/978-1-4614-7849-2_34, © Springer Science+Business Media New York 2014

Fig. 34.1 Macular,
morbilliform rash on the
trunk in an 11-month-old boy

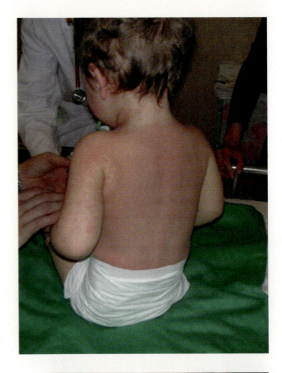

Fig. 34.2 Strawberry tongue,
mucosal redness, and cracked
lips in a 3-year-old boy

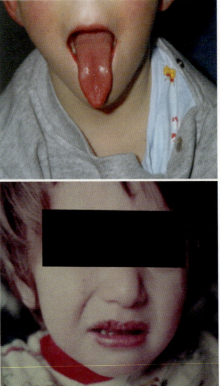

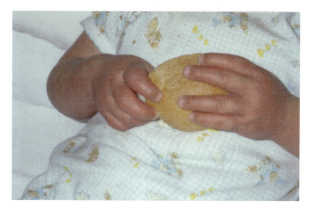

Fig. 34.3 Edema of dorsum of both hands in a 2-year-old girl

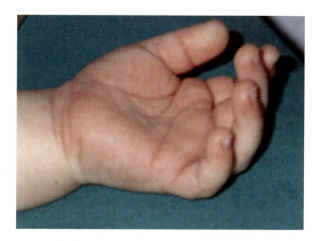

Fig. 34.4 Palmar erythema in a 9-month-old infant with Kawasaki disease

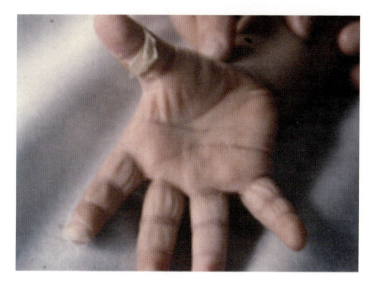

Fig. 34.5 Typical peeling, exfoliation of hands in a 7-month-old baby

Symptoms evolve over the first 10 days and then gradually resolve even in untreated patients. Less common symptoms are urethritis, aseptic meningitis, pneumonia, otitis, and gastroenteritis. Arthritis develops both in the acute and in convalescent phase and usually involves one or more large joints. Fever of 5 days duration plus 4 of the 5 remaining criteria or typical fever and CAA detected on 2D echocardiogram are required to diagnose KD. Patients with fever and two to three of clinical features are defined as "incomplete" KD. In the most recent classification criteria, fever is mandatory, in addition to 4 of the typical clinical findings. Desquamation in the perineal area has been added to changes in peripheral extremities. Digital peeling, a useful diagnostic hint, usually occurs 10–15 days from onset. The therapy includes IVIG (2 g/Kg) within the first 10 days from fever onset and aspirin (50–80 mg/kg). In severe cases, a second IVIG pulse, i.v. methylprednisolone (30 mg/Kg), and anti-TNF drug are required [1–3].

Differential Diagnosis

Among the most common in the differential diagnosis are nonspecific infantile febrile diseases with rash; adenovirus infection (ADV) characterized by prolonged fever, conjunctivitis, lymphadenopathy, mucous membrane changes, high erythrocyte sedimentation rate, and C-reactive protein, and leukocytosis strongly resembles KD.

Scarlet fever at onset mimics KD, but fever promptly responds to penicillin; desquamation usually does not involve periungueal area. Measles may also look like KD; however, dry cough, enanthema, rhinitis, and lower parameters of inflammation differentiate the two conditions.

Biopsy

No biopsy is required to diagnose Kawasaki disease.

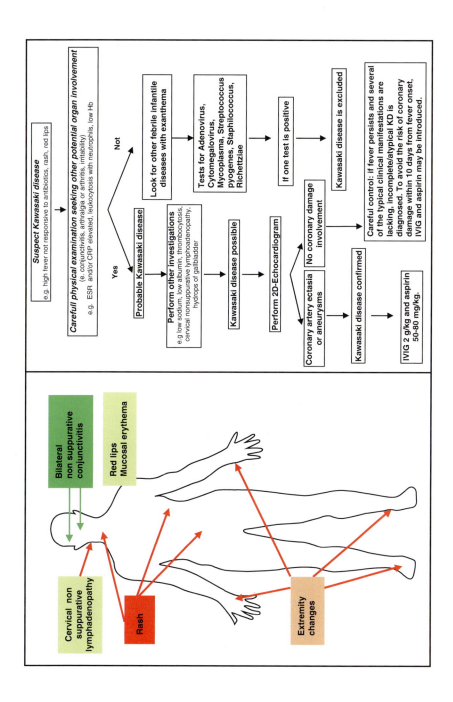

Suspect Kawasaki disease
e.g. high fever not responsive to antibiotics, rash, red lips

Carefull physical examination seeking other potential organ involvement
(e. conjunctivitis, arthralgia or arthritis, irritability)
e.g. ESR and/or CRP elevated, leukocytosis with neutrophils, low Hb

Yes / Not

Probable Kawasaki disease

Perform other investigations
e.g low sodium, low albumin, thrombocytosis, cervical nonsuppurative lymphoadenopathy, hydrops of gallbladder

Kawasaki disease possible

Perform 2D-Echocardiogram

No coronary damage involvement / Coronary artery ectasia or aneurysms

Kawasaki disease confirmed

IVIG 2 g/kg and aspirin 50–80 mg/kg.

Look for other febrile infantile diseases with exanthema

Tests for Adenovirus, Cytomegalovirus, Mycoplasma, Streptococcus pyogenes, Staphilococcus, Richettziae

If one test is positive

Kawasaki disease is excluded

Careful control: if fever persists and several of the typical clinical manifestations are lacking, incomplete/atypical KD is diagnosed. To avoid the risk of coronary damage within 10 days from fever onset, IVIG and aspirin may be introduced.

Bilateral non suppurative conjunctivitis

Red lips Mucosal erythema

Cervical non suppurative lymphadenopathy

Rash

Extremity changes

References

1. McCrindle BW. A childhood disease with important consequences into adulthood. Circulation. 2009;120:6–8.
2. Newburger JW, et al. Diagnosis, treatment, and long-term management of Kawasaki disease: a statement for health professionals from the Committee on Rheumatic Fever, Endocarditis, and Kawasaki Disease, Council on Cardiovascular Disease in the Young, American Heart Association. Pediatrics. 2004;114:1708–33.
3. Rowley AH, Shulman ST. Pathogenesis and management of Kawasaki disease. Expert Rev Anti Infect Ther. 2010;8:197–203.

Chapter 35
Dermatologic Manifestations of Granulomatosis with Polyangiitis (Wegener's Granulomatosis)

Camille Francès, Christian Pagnoux, and Loïc Guillevin

Definition

Dermatologic lesions of granulomatosis with polyangiitis (Wegener's granulomatosis; GPA) are frequently encountered and occasionally may be the initial manifestations (8–13 %). Their frequencies during the course of the disease vary widely, from 12 % to 67 %, depending on the series [1–5]. Specific dermatologic lesions are characterized by leukocytoclastic vasculitis, extravascular palisading granuloma(s), granulomatous vasculitis, or abscess with granulomatous inflammation [6]. Despite being considered specific, they are not observed exclusively in GPA but are also seen in other vasculitides affecting vessels of the same size. Vasculitis and granuloma are not detected in other nonspecific skin lesions that may still be highly suggestive of GPA, such as gingival hyperplasia.

C. Francès, M.D.
Department of Dermatology-Allergology, Pierre et Marie Curie University, Assistance Publique-Hôpitaux de Paris, Tenon Hospital, 4 rue de la Chine, Paris 75020, France
e-mail: camille.frances@tnn.aphp.fr

C. Pagnoux, M.D., MPH
Division of Rheumatology, Mount Sinai Hospital/University Health Network, The Rebecca MacDonald Centre for Arthritis and Autoimmunity, 60 Murray Street, Ste 2-220, Toronto, ON M5T 3L9, Canada
e-mail: cpagnoux@mtsinai.on.ca

L. Guillevin, M.D. (✉)
Department of Internal Medicine, National Referral Center for Rare Systemic and Autoimmune Diseases, Necrotizing Vasculitides and Systemic Sclerosis, Hôpital Cochin, Assistance Publique–Hôpitaux de Paris, Université Paris Descartes, 27, rue du Faubourg Saint-Jacques, Paris Cedex 14 75679, France
e-mail: loic.guillevin@cch.aphp.fr

M. Matucci-Cerinic et al. (eds.), *Skin Manifestations in Rheumatic Disease*,
DOI 10.1007/978-1-4614-7849-2_35, © Springer Science+Business Media New York 2014

Description of GPA Skin Manifestations

Specific Dermatologic Manifestations

The clinical picture is largely dependent on the skin-vessel caliber involved and the presence or absence of granulomatous infiltration, although considerable overlaps exist among vasculitides [6–9].

Palpable purpura, localized mainly on the lower limbs, is the most frequent clinical manifestation. The visible lesion ranges from tiny red macules and pinheads to coin-sized petechiae, but sometimes includes more extensive plaques and ecchymoses. Color range may change from red to purple to brownish yellow as extravasated blood is progressively broken down. Purpura may evolve to necrosis, leading to vesicles, blisters, erosions, ulcerations, and ulcers. Often, different concomitant lesions are observed: erythematous to purpuric macules, papules, and necrotic lesions (Fig. 35.1).

Papulonecrotic lesions are ulcerated papules that are located on the extensor surfaces of the limbs, close to elbows, knees, hands, and feet (Fig. 35.2). They can also develop on the face and scalp. Occasionally, they can resemble erythema elevatum diutinum and may be associated with IgA paraproteinemia. Present in 10 % of GPA patients, these lesions may be mistaken for rheumatoid nodules. However, unlike rheumatoid nodules, they tend to ulcerate and are mobile within the dermis [10].

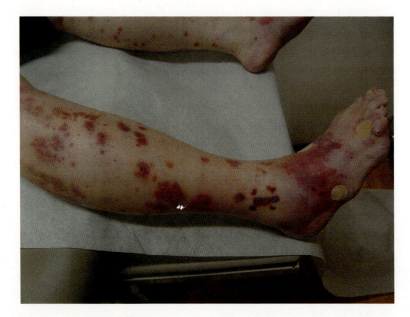

Fig. 35.1 Necrotic purpura on the legs

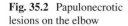

Fig. 35.2 Papulonecrotic lesions on the elbow

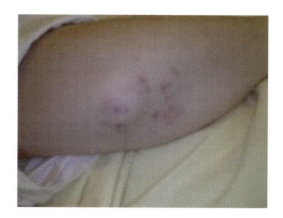

Dermal or hypodermal nodules, the so-called subcutaneous nodules, are always palpable, typically inflammatory, tender, red, and small-sized but can sometimes be barely visible. They should be actively sought overlying lower limb vessel territories, where they can be surrounded by livedo reticularis, but are also seen elsewhere, such as the dorsal face of the upper limbs or, rarely, the trunk.

Livedo reticularis is a reddish-blue mottling of the skin in a "fishnet" reticular pattern, frequently localized on the lower limbs. It may also develop on the lower trunk and the upper limbs. It is rarely isolated in GPA and is usually associated with other cutaneous symptoms, especially nodules and necrosis.

Necrotic lesions are characterized by ulcerations or ulcers. Ulcerations of the mucosae and skin may be observed. They are more frequently nonspecific when present on mucosae [9]. Necrotic skin lesion extension and depth are highly variable, reflecting the extension and depth of histological findings, with massive skin necrosis described in a case report [11]. Extensive and painful cutaneous ulcerations may precede, by weeks to months, other systemic manifestations. Although GPA ulcers are sometimes described as "pyoderma gangrenosum-like lesions," especially when they arise subsequent to localized trauma or the breakdown of painful nodules or pustules [6–8], they usually lack the typical raised, tender, undermined border of pyoderma gangrenosum. Sometimes numerous, they are located on the limbs, trunk, face (preauricular area), breasts (mimicking adenocarcinoma, with possible nipple retraction and galactorrhea), and perineum.

Gangrene resulting from arterial occlusion may be seen in all systemic vasculitides. It is initially characterized by the sharply demarcated blue–black color of the digits. The main differential diagnoses are thrombosis without inflammation of the vessel walls and emboli. Other concomitant cutaneous lesions can be observed in patients with skin-biopsy-proven vasculitis, e.g., nonspecific inflammation, thrombosis, and/or atheromatous embolism [7].

Clinical features that should evoke a diagnosis of cutaneous GPA in patients with pyoderma-like ulcerations include facial involvement (especially preauricular lesions), absence of typical pyoderma gangrenosum features (no undermined violaceous border, erythema, or necrotic centers), and other disease associations.

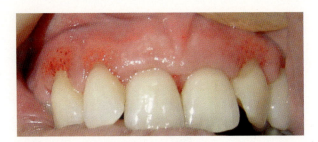

Fig. 35.3 Gingival hyperplasia highly suggestive of granulomatosis with polyangiitis (Wegener's granulomatosis)

Nonspecific Dermatologic Manifestations

Oral ulcers are undoubtedly frequent, present in 10–50 % of GPA patients depending on the series. Unlike aphthae, they are persistent and not recurrent. Their number and localization are highly variable, having been observed on cheeks, tongue, floor of the mouth, lips, palate, gingivae, tonsils, and posterior palate (Fig. 35.3). Genital ulcers are uncommon, although penile necrosis has previously been described. Histologic findings for GPA oral ulcer tend to be nonspecific, showing only acute and chronic inflammation [9]. In a few cases, extravascular granulomas have been found [8].

Gingivitis. Some patients develop an unusual and distinctive gingivitis, which can suggest GPA in its early stages [12]. This gingivitis is characterized by exophytic hyperplasia with petechial flecks and a red, friable, granular appearance that begins focally in the interdental papillae and quickly spreads to produce segmental or pan-oral gingivitis (Fig. 35.4). It may be associated with alveolar bone loss and tooth loosening. Jaw bone pain and gingival bleeding are common. Biopsy specimens generally show nonspecific, chronic inflammation with histiocytes and eosinophils sometimes forming microabscesses. Giant cells are often present. Additional features include pseudoepitheliomatous hyperplasia with focal necrosis without vasculitis. Rarely, extravascular granuloma(s) or granulomatous vasculitis is present [8]. Differential diagnoses include drug-induced hyperplasia, or gingival hyperplasia secondary to leukemia, lymphoma, or Langerhans' histiocytosis.

Skin necrotizing ulcerations may be nonspecific manifestations with histology finding only epitheliomatous hyperplasia, dermal hemorrhages, granulation tissue, and mixed diffuse inflammatory infiltrate(s) [6].

Erythema nodosum-like lesions consist of recurrent erythematous, edematous, and tender subcutaneous nodules. Nodule size is usually around 1 cm or 2 cm but can be much larger. Nodules are primarily located over the extensor surface of the lower limbs. They regress spontaneously without atrophic scarring. Their histomorphology in GPA is characterized by predominantly septal and focal lobular panniculitis, with a mixed inflammatory infiltrate that contains histiocytes, lymphocytes, occasional plasma cells, and singly disposed foreign-body giant cells with neutrophils. Focal lipomembranous and liposclerotic changes have also been seen without vasculitis [13].

Xanthelasmas are yellow cholesterol plaques on the eyelids, predominantly on the nasal side. They do not have any distinctive histological features. When they appear suddenly in a GPA patient, they are usually adjacent to a granulomatous infiltration into the underlying orbit [8]. An orbit X-ray should confirm the infiltration around the eye which may require additional treatment.

Other nonspecific skin manifestations have been described, such as pustules and vesicles [6].

Histopathologic Findings

Palpable purpura is usually secondary to leukocytoclastic vasculitis affecting mainly the small vessels (postcapillary venules) of the upper dermis but also larger vessels, especially when necrosis is associated.

Papulonecrotic lesions correspond to leukocytoclastic or granulomatous vasculitis involving small vessels or extravascular granuloma(s). Cutaneous extravascular necrotizing granulomas are clinically characterized by the presence of rheumatoid-like papules or nodules [14]. Histologically, focal necrobiosis is surrounded by palisading histiocytic granuloma(s). The core consists of degenerated collagen with basophilic necrotizing fibrinoid material and leukocytoclastic polymorphonuclear cells. Numerous epithelioid cells are present in the palisading granuloma(s), which have been described in association with many autoimmune diseases, like GPA, but also in eosinophilic granulomatosis with polyangiitis (Churg–Strauss syndrome), systemic lupus erythematosus, thyroiditis, rheumatoid vasculitis, polyarteritis nodosa, Takayasu's arteritis, infectious hepatitis, inflammatory bowel disease, or lymphoproliferative disease [14–16]. Usually, more eosinophils are present in eosinophilic granulomatosis with polyangiitis (Churg–Strauss syndrome).

Small nodules mainly reflect necrotizing vasculitis involving medium-sized arterioles of the deep dermis or hypodermis that may be suggestive of polyarteritis nodosa for the pathologist. In other cases, these nodules are sites of granulomatous vasculitis of medium-sized arterioles or extravascular granuloma(s).

The skin ulcerations may be secondary to leukocytoclastic or granulomatous vasculitis. The histologic pattern of pyoderma-like ulcerations differs from that observed in pyoderma gangrenosum; it is characterized by foci of palisading neutrophilic and granulomatous dermatitis, prominent granulomatous and neutrophilic necrotizing vasculitis, and basophilic collagen degeneration.

Although GPA is considered a pauci-immune systemic vasculitis based on the absence of immune deposits in renal biopsies of patients with active disease, a substantial number of skin biopsies showed immune deposits (24–71 %). C3 deposition in and around dermal vessels is the most frequent finding. IgM, IgG, and/or IgA deposits may also be detected without similar immune deposits in kidney biopsies [6, 17].

Differential Diagnosis

Serologic antineutrophil cytoplasm antibodies (ANCA) may be positive and support GPA diagnosis, predominantly directed against proteinase 3 or, more rarely, myeloperoxidase [13]. Other vasculitides are to be considered, mainly microscopic polyangiitis, eosinophilic granulomatosis with polyangiitis (Churg–Strauss syndrome), and polyarteritis nodosa. Other differential diagnoses of GPA include sarcoidosis, inflammatory bowel diseases, infection, mainly endocarditis, and toxic or drug-induced vasculitis and vasculopathies (especially related to the use of levamisole-tainted cocaine).

See Also

Chapter 36 – Eosinophilic   Granulomatosis   with   Polyangiitis   (Churg–Strauss Syndrome)

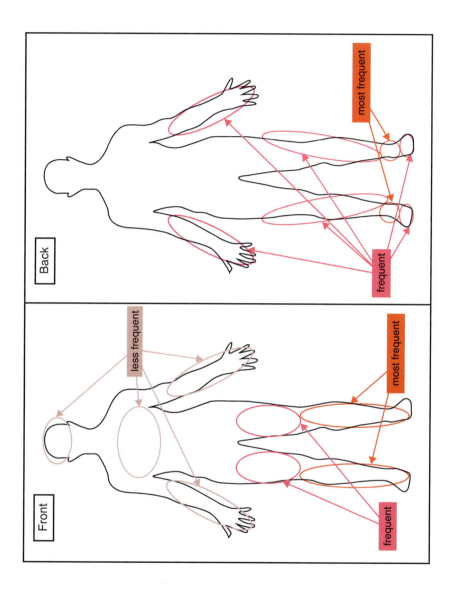

References

1. Guillevin L, Cordier JF, Lhote F, et al. A prospective, multicenter, randomized trial comparing steroids and pulse cyclophosphamide versus steroids and oral cyclophosphamide in the treatment of generalized Wegener's granulomatosis. Arthritis Rheum. 1997;40:2187–98.
2. Pinching AJ, Lockwood CM, Pussell BA, et al. Wegener's granulomatosis: observations on 18 patients with severe renal disease. Q J Med. 1983;52:435–60.
3. Lie JT. Wegener's granulomatosis: histological documentation of common and uncommon manifestations in 216 patients. Vasa. 1997;26:261–70.
4. Fauci AS, Haynes BF, Katz P, Wolff SM. Wegener's granulomatosis: prospective clinical and therapeutic experience with 85 patients for 21 years. Ann Intern Med. 1983;98:76–85.
5. Hoffman GS, Kerr GS, Leavitt RY, et al. Wegener granulomatosis: an analysis of 158 patients. Ann Intern Med. 1992;116:488–98.
6. Daoud MS, Gibson LE, De Remee RA, Specks U, El-Azhary RA, Su WPD. Cutaneous Wegener's granulomatosis: clinical, histopathologic and immunopathologic features of thirty patients. J Am Acad Dermatol. 1994;31:605–12.
7. Kluger N, Francès C. Cutaneous vasculitis and their differential diagnoses. Clin Exp Rheumatol. 2009;27 Suppl 2:S124–38.
8. Francès C, Lê Thi Huong D, Piette JC, et al. Wegener's granulomatosis. Dermatological manifestations in 75 cases with clinicopathologic correlation. Arch Dermatol. 1994;130:861–7.
9. Patten SF, Tomecki KJ. Wegener's granulomatosis: cutaneous and oral mucosal disease. J Am Acad Dermatol. 1993;28:710–8.
10. Fiorentino DF. Cutaneous vasculitis. J Am Acad Dermatol. 2003;48:311–40.
11. Cybulska A, Undas A, Sydor WJ, Flak A, Musial A. Wegener's granulomatosis with massive skin necrosis. J Rheumatol. 2004;31:830–1.
12. Manchanda Y, Tejasvi T, Handa R, Ramam M. Strawberry gingiva: a distinctive sign in Wegener's granulomatosis. J Am Acad Dermatol. 2003;49:335–7.
13. Comfere NI, Macaron NC, Gibson LE. Cutaneous manifestations of Wegener's granulomatosis: a clinicopathologic study of 17 patients and correlation to antineutrophil cytoplasmic antibody status. J Cutan Pathol. 2007;34:739–47.
14. Finan MC, Winkelmann RK. The cutaneous extravascular necrotizing granuloma (Churg–Strauss granuloma) and systemic disease: a review of 27 cases. Medicine (Baltimore). 1983;62:142–58.
15. Wilmoth GJ, Perniciaro C. Cutaneous extravascular necrotizing granuloma (Winkelmann granuloma): confirmation of the association with systemic disease. J Am Acad Dermatol. 1996;34:753–9.
16. Obermoser G, Zelger B, Zangerle R, Sepp N. Extravascular necrotizing palisaded granulomas as the presenting skin sign of systemic lupus erythematosus. Br J Dermatol. 2002;147:371–4.
17. Brons RH, de Jong MC, de Boer NK, Stegeman CA, Kallenberg CG, Tervaert JW. Detection of immune deposits in skin lesions of patients with Wegener's granulomatosis. Ann Rheum Dis. 2001;60:1097–102.

Chapter 36
Eosinophilic Granulomatosis with Polyangiitis (Churg–Strauss Syndrome)

Christian Pagnoux and Loïc Guillevin

Definition

Eosinophilic granulomatosis with polyangiitis (EGPA; formerly and also named Churg–Strauss syndrome) is a rare, systemic, necrotizing vasculitis that predominantly affects small-sized arteries [1–3]. Its annual incidence ranges between 0.6 and 6.8 per million inhabitants, and its prevalence between 10.7 and 14 per million inhabitants [2, 3]. Typically, its onset is characterized, in a middle-aged individual developing late-onset asthma and allergic sinus polyposis, by the onset of vasculitis manifestations, like fever, skin lesions, and/or mononeuritis multiplex, plus blood and tissue eosinophilia. The lung, gastrointestinal tract, and heart are frequently involved, with cardiac manifestations associated with a high mortality rate. The kidney is less frequently involved than in granulomatosis with polyangiitis (Wegener's granulomatosis) [2–6].

EGPA pathophysiological mechanisms are multiple and complex. Inhaled allergens, vaccinations, desensitization, or drugs (like leukotriene-receptor antagonists) have been incriminated as potential triggers and/or precipitating cofactors. Eosinophils may play a role, but several genetic predispositions or immune dysregulations are also being gradually identified [2, 3]. Notably, in nearly 40 % of EGPA patients,

C. Pagnoux, M.D., M.P.H., M.Sc. (✉)
Division of Rheumatology, Mount Sinai Hospital/University Health Network,
The Rebecca MacDonald Centre for Arthritis and Autoimmunity, 60 Murray Street,
Ste 2-220, Toronto, ON M5T 3L9, Canada
e-mail: cpagnoux@mtsinai.on.ca

L. Guillevin, M.D.
Department of Internal Medicine, National Referral Center for Rare Systemic
and Autoimmune Diseases, Necrotizing Vasculitides and Systemic Sclerosis,
Hôpital Cochin, Assistance Publique–Hôpitaux de Paris, Université Paris Descartes,
27, rue du Faubourg Saint-Jacques, Paris Cedex 14 75679, France
e-mail: loic.guillevin@cch.aphp.fr

M. Matucci-Cerinic et al. (eds.), *Skin Manifestations in Rheumatic Disease*,
DOI 10.1007/978-1-4614-7849-2_36, © Springer Science+Business Media New York 2014

antineutrophil cytoplasmic autoantibodies (ANCA) can be detected that usually generate a perinuclear immunofluorescent-labeling pattern, referred to as P-ANCA, most frequently specific to myeloperoxidase (MPO) [2, 5–7].

Description

Skin lesions can be present at diagnosis in 40–75 % of EGPA patients [3, 5, 8]. Palpable purpura, often necrotic, on legs and feet is the most frequent of these manifestations (Fig. 36.1). Cutaneous nodules (one-third of the patients) or papules, sometimes with an urticarial appearance, are also very common, mainly located on the lower limbs or on the elbows and forearms, fingers, scalp, forehead, and/or breasts (Fig. 36.2). Various other cutaneous lesions have been reported, including maculopapules resembling erythema multiforme, ulcerations, livedo reticularis, patchy and migratory urticarial rashes, nail-fold infarctions, deep pannicular vasculitis, and facial edema.

The so-called extravascular granulomas, initially described by Churg and Strauss as a possible manifestation of EGPA, may be seen in other systemic vasculitides and some connective tissue diseases and have, therefore, been given different other names, including Winkelmann's granuloma [1, 8–10]. Clinically, these red-to-violaceous lesions may be linear ("rope sign"), on the trunk or extensor surfaces of the upper arms, but also frequently resemble large, annular, 2-mm to 2-cm-sized papulonodules or plaques.

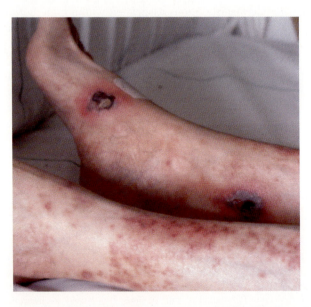

Fig. 36.1 Lower leg and foot purpura with necrotic and superficial ulcerations of a patient with eosinophilic granulomatosis with polyangiitis (Churg–Strauss syndrome)

Fig. 36.2 Diffuse
erythematous plaque with a
palpable subcutaneous nodule
(*circled*) below the calf of a
patient with eosinophilic
granulomatosis with
polyangiitis (Churg–Strauss
syndrome)

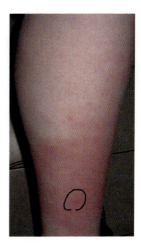

Differential Diagnosis

Because skin lesions are rarely the first and isolated symptoms of EGPA (6 % of the patients), common causes of purpuric lesions, such as thrombocytopenia or Bateman's syndrome, or urticarial rash, e.g., drug or contact allergy, are easily ruled out [3]. Some other diagnoses may be more challenging, because several of these diseases' manifestations may mimic those of EGPA. Other systemic vasculitides like granulomatosis with polyangiitis (Wegener's granulomatosis), parasitic infections, and hypereosinophilic syndromes especially should be evoked and actively looked for. Lymphocyte immunophenotyping, T-cell clonal studies, and molecular analyses to detect Fip1-like 1 (FIP1L1)–platelet-derived growth factor receptor-α (PDGFRA) gene fusion should probably be done in every ANCA-negative patients, to exclude myeloid neoplasms associated with eosinophilia. Other diagnoses to exclude are hypersensitivity vasculitis, Carrington's disease, and malignant hemopathies (especially lymphomas), along with Crohn's disease, sarcoidosis, eosinophilic fasciitis, or Gleich syndrome.

Biopsy

Histologically, vasculitis may be found in two-thirds of the positive skin biopsies of EGPA patients, but the most "typical" and/or eosinophilic granulomas are detected in less than half of them [8–10]. Examination of nodules may show granulomatous vasculitis, necrotizing vasculitis of arterioles in the deep dermis or the subcutis, or extravascular granulomas (Fig. 36.3). Purpuric lesions can reveal vasculitis, usually paired with eosinophil-rich inflammatory infiltrates. Two patterns of extravascular granulomas have been distinguished: the first is classic, with palisading granuloma and eosinophils when

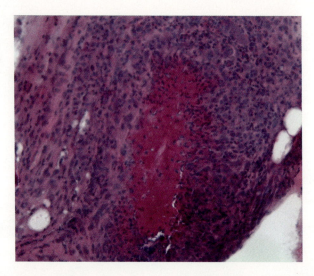

Fig. 36.3 Histological features of necrotizing vasculitis with massive eosinophilic infiltrate, around the vessel and within the necrotic vessel wall, in a patient with eosinophilic granulomatosis with polyangiitis (Churg–Strauss syndrome)

associated with EGPA, or basophilic debris ("blue" granuloma due to neutrophil–mucin degradation) in granulomatosis with polyangiitis (Wegener's) or rheumatoid arthritis, and the second is focal basophilic necrosis, without a palisading organization.

Diagnostic Flow Chart

Diagnosis work-up relies on the combination of suggestive clinical findings, blood eosinophilia (up to >50,000/mm³), exclusion of all the differential diagnoses, and, when feasible, a biopsy of an affected organ, especially the skin or muscle and nerve. Detection of anti-MPO ANCA can further support EGPA diagnosis.

See Also

Urticaria (leukocytoclastic vasculitis)
    Purpura
    Granulomatosis with polyangiitis (Wegener's granulomatosis)
    Skin Manifestations of antiphospholipid syndrome
    Skin Manifestations of Eosinophilic Fasciitis
    Sarcoidosis

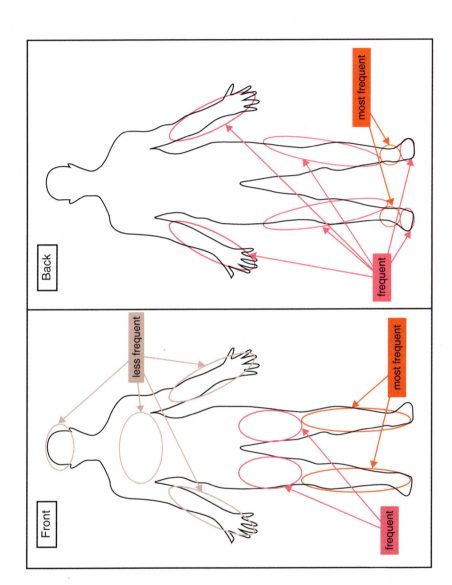

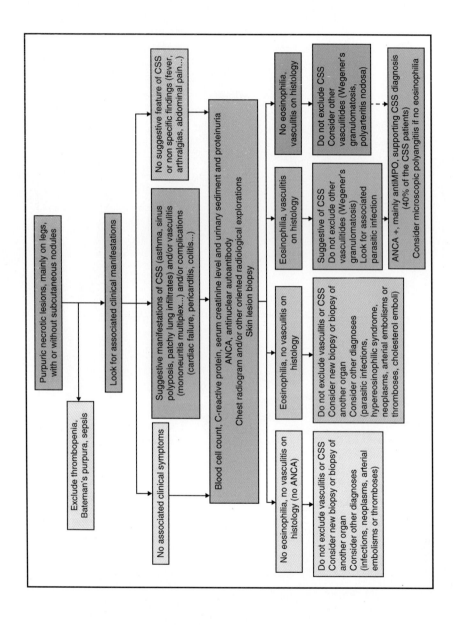

References

1. Churg J, Strauss L. Allergic angiitis and periarteritis nodosa. Am J Pathol. 1951;27:277–301.
2. Pagnoux C, Guillevin L. Churg–Strauss syndrome: evidence for disease subtypes? Curr Opin Rheumatol. 2010;22:21–8.
3. Sinico RA, Bottero P. Churg–Strauss angiitis. Best Pract Res Clin Rheumatol. 2009;23:355–66.
4. Guillevin L, Cohen P, Gayraud M, Lhote F, Jarrousse B, Casassus P. Churg–Strauss syndrome. Clinical study and long-term follow-up of 96 patients. Medicine (Baltimore). 1999;78:26–37.
5. Keogh KA, Specks U. Churg–Strauss syndrome: clinical presentation, antineutrophil cytoplasmic antibodies, and leukotriene receptor antagonists. Am J Med. 2003;115:284–90.
6. Sablé-Fourtassou R, Cohen P, Mahr A, et al. Antineutrophil cytoplasmic antibodies and the Churg–Strauss syndrome. Ann Intern Med. 2005;143:632–8.
7. Sinico RA, Di Toma L, Maggiore U, et al. Prevalence and clinical significance of antineutrophil cytoplasmic antibodies in Churg–Strauss syndrome. Arthritis Rheum. 2005;52:2926–35.
8. Davis MD, Daoud MS, McEvoy MT, Su WP. Cutaneous manifestations of Churg–Strauss syndrome: a clinicopathologic correlation. J Am Acad Dermatol. 1997;37:199–203.
9. Finan MC, Winkelmann RK. The cutaneous extravascular necrotizing granuloma (Churg–Strauss granuloma) and systemic disease: a review of 27 cases. Medicine (Baltimore). 1983;62:142–58.
10. Pagnoux C, Kluger N, Francès C, Guillevin L. Cutaneous granulomatous vasculitis and extravascular granulomas. Expert Rev Dermatol. 2006;1:315–26.

Chapter 37
Polyarteritis Nodosa

Mehmet Tuncay Duruöz

Definition

Polyarteritis nodosa (PAN) is necrotizing inflammation of medium-sized or small arteries without glomerulonephritis or vasculitis in arterioles, capillaries, or venules. This inflammation commonly leads to vessel wall weakening with formation of microaneurysms, stenosis, endothelial dysfunction, and/or thrombotic formation [1].

PAN may present as a systemic disease or may involve a single organ.

PAN may affect any organ except lungs. Skin lesions are present in about 50 % of patients. Livedo reticularis, bullous or vesicular eruptions, infarctions, ulcerations, tender erythematous nodules (subcutaneous), and ischemic changes of the distal digits or a combination may occur. Peripheral nerve (e.g., mononeuritis multiplex), articular (large joints preferentially), renal, hepatic, cerebral, gastrointestinal, and testicular involvements are frequent. Visceral involvement may be present at disease onset [2, 3].

Cases of polyarteritis nodosa limited to skin (cutaneous PAN), gall bladder, pancreas, female and male genital tracts, calf muscles, kidneys, and gastrointestinal tract have also been reported.

Cutaneous PAN causes transmural inflammation of small- and medium-sized arteries of the dermis and subcutaneous tissue, leading to fibrinoid necrosis and formation of cutaneous nodules (4–15 mm) along superficial arteries. Larger inflammatory plaques may be seen. When the plaques heal, they leave patches of postinflammatory pigmentation. Infarcts in the skin present as purple or black patches or blood-filled blisters [1] (Figs. 37.1 and 37.2).

There is no known etiology for PAN, although numerous infectious agents (e.g., hepatitis B and C, cytomegalovirus, parvovirus) have been implicated in the

M.T. Duruöz, M.D. (✉)
Physical Medicine and Rehabilitation Department, Rheumatology Division,
Celal Bayar University Medical School, Uncubozköy, Manisa 45037, Turkey
e-mail: tuncayduruoz@gmail.com

M. Matucci-Cerinic et al. (eds.), *Skin Manifestations in Rheumatic Disease*,
DOI 10.1007/978-1-4614-7849-2_37, © Springer Science+Business Media New York 2014

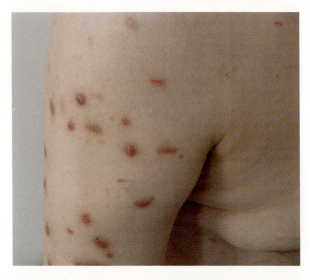

Fig. 37.1 Vesicular eruptions of patient with PAN. The eruptions are more frequent in upper and lower extremities than trunk

Fig. 37.2 Vesicular eruptions of patient with PAN. The eruptions are more frequent in upper and lower extremities than trunk

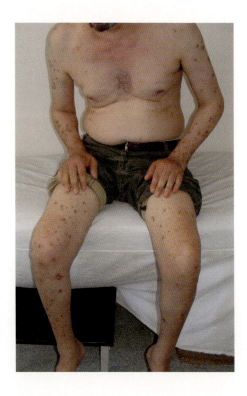

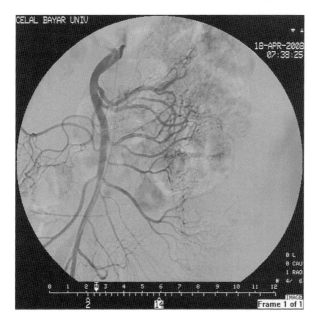

Fig. 37.3 The superior mesenteric artery angiography of the same patient shows the millimetric aneurysms

pathogenesis. The association of PAN with HBV is particularly strong. PAN may develop within the first 6 months of an HBV infection as a result of immune-complex formation [4].

Diagnosis of PAN requires the integration of clinical, angiography, and biopsy findings. The ACR classification criteria of PAN are commonly used with 82.2 % of sensitivity and 86.6 % of specificity. Antineutrophil cytoplasmic antibodies (ANCA) are negative in PAN. The renal, hepatic, and mesenteric vessels are the most frequently involved vessels in PAN. The typical angiographic appearance includes segments of arterial stenosis alternating with normal or dilated artery areas, smooth tapered occlusions, and thrombosis. The dilated segments have saccular and fusiform aneurysms [5, 6] (Figs. 37.3 and 37.4).

Differential Diagnosis

A cutaneous form of polyarteritis, affecting predominantly the lower extremities, is distinguished from systemic PAN by its restriction to the skin and to the neurological and osteo-muscular systems and lack of visceral involvement and benign course. Skin biopsy of a typical lesion is usually performed to make an accurate diagnosis of cutaneous PAN.

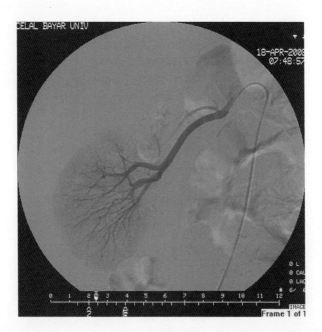

Fig. 37.4 The renal artery angiography of the same patient shows the millimetric aneurysms

The skin involvement in microscopic polyangiitis (MPA) is frequent, typically a purpuric rash, nail bed infarcts, splinter hemorrhages, livedo reticularis, skin infarction, or ulceration may mimic PAN. The frequency of skin lesions in PAN and in MPA is roughly similar. MPA is distinguished by small-vessel vasculitis in the pulmonary and renal vasculature, glomerulonephritis, normal angiography, and the tendency to relapse [2].

Medium-sized vessel vasculitis mimicking PAN may be a manifestation or complication of secondary vasculitis such as systemic lupus erythematosis, rheumatoid arthritis, Sjögren syndrome, hairy cell leukemia, and myelodysplastic syndrome. The visceral angiographic appearance of vasculitis, including bacterial endocarditis, left atrial myxoma, drug abuse, pancreatitis, and abdominal malignancy, can mimic PAN [2, 5].

Biopsy Histopathology

Biopsy of an affected artery can confirm the diagnosis. The demonstration of focal, segmental, panmural, necrotizing inflammation of medium-sized arteries with a predilection for bifurcations is the gold standard for the diagnosis of PAN. Different stages of the inflammatory process may be present simultaneously. PMNs and occasionally eosinophils exist in early lesions; later lesions contain lymphocytes and plasma cells exist in later lesions. Granulomatous inflammation does not exist.

The specimen for biopsy may include the skin, skeletal muscle, sural nerve, liver, and kidney, depending on the clinical features. Muscle biopsy is positive in around 50 % of patients with PAN who have muscle pain or claudication. The sub-dermis should be included into the skin specimen to detect medium-sized vessel involvement [2, 6].

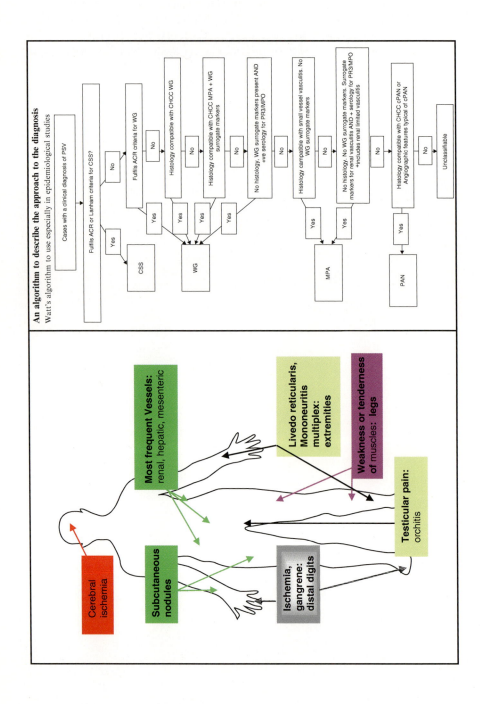

References

1. Jennette JC, Falk RJ, Andrassy K, et al. Nomenclature of systemic vasculitides: proposal of an international consensus conference. Arthritis Rheum. 1994;37:187–92.
2. Guillevin L. Polyarteritis nodosa and microscopic polyangiitis. In: Ball GV, Bridges SL, editors. Vasculitis. New York: Oxford University Press; 2002. p. 300–20.
3. Pagnoux C, Mahr A, Cohen P, Guillevin L. Presentation and outcome of gastrointestinal involvement in systemic necrotizing vasculitides: analysis of 62 patients with polyarteritis nodosa, microscopic polyangiitis, Wegener granulomatosis, Churg-Strauss syndrome or rheumatoid arthritis- associated vasculitis. Medicine (Baltimore). 2005;84:115–28.
4. Guillevin L, Mahr A, Callard P, et al. Hepatitis B virus-associated polyarteritis nodosa. Medicine (Baltimore). 2005;84:313–22.
5. Watts R, Lane S, Hanslick T, et al. Development and validation of a consensus methodology for the classification of the ANCA-associated vasculitides and polyarteritis nodosa for epidemiological studies. Ann Rheum Dis. 2006;66:222–7.
6. Lightfoot RW, Michel BA, Bloch DA, et al. The American College of Rheumatology 1990 criteria for the classification of polyarteritis nodosa. Arthritis Rheum. 1990;33:1088–94.

Chapter 38
Skin Manifestations in Microscopic Polyangiitis

Nicolò Pipitone, Carlo Salvarani, and Gene G. Hunder

Definition

Microscopic polyangiitis (MPA) is a pauci-immune necrotizing small- and medium-vessel vasculitis mainly involving the lung and kidneys but also the peripheral nerves and skin [1]. Anti-neutrophil cytoplasmic antibodies (ANCA) are often positive, mainly with a perinuclear pattern (p-ANCA, ~60 % of cases) and rarely with a cytoplasmic pattern (c-ANCA, ~10 % of cases). Cutaneous manifestations have been described in 20–70 % of MPA patients [2–5], in 13–15 % of cases as the presenting sign [6, 7]. In a large (162 MPA patients) series reported by the French vasculitis study group, the most common skin lesion was palpable purpura (26 % of cases) (Fig. 38.1), followed by livedo racemosa (12 %), nodules (10 %), skin ulcers sometimes evolving into necrosis (6 %), and urticaria (1.2 %) [2]. Other uncommon skin changes described in MPA include diffuse erythema, macules, vesicles, bullae, splinter hemorrhage, annular purpura, erythema elevatum diutinum, facial edema, and pyoderma gangrenosum-like lesions [2, 5, 6, 8].

Differential Diagnosis

MPA has only recently been separated from polyarteritis nodosa on the basis of clinical and laboratory features as well as of the size of the vessels involved [1]. Polyarteritis nodosa involves small- and medium-sized vessels. Both conditions

N. Pipitone, M.D., Ph.D. • C. Salvarani, M.D. (✉)
Department of Rheumatology, Division of Medicine, Arcispedale Santa Maria Nuova,
Viale Risorgimento 80, Reggio Emilia 42100, Italy
e-mail: Pipitone.nicolo@asmn.re.it; Salvarani.carlo@asmn.re.it

G.G. Hunder, M.D.
Emeritus Staff Center, Mayo Clinic, 200 First St SW, Rochester, MN 55905, USA
e-mail: ghunder@mayo.edu

M. Matucci-Cerinic et al. (eds.), *Skin Manifestations in Rheumatic Disease*,
DOI 10.1007/978-1-4614-7849-2_38, © Springer Science+Business Media New York 2014

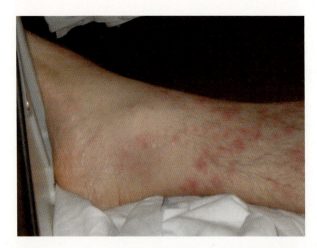

Fig. 38.1 Palpable purpura in a patient with microscopic polyangiitis. Note the relative sparing of the distal limb

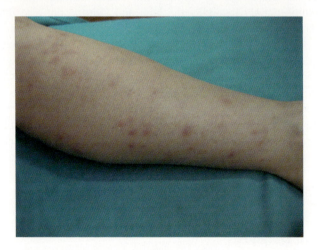

Fig. 38.2 Skin nodules in a patient with polyarteritis nodosa (Image courtesy of Dr. Monica Cattania, Dermatology Department, Arcispedale Santa Maria Nuova, Reggio Emilia, Italy)

may present with similar cutaneous manifestations. Palpable purpura, which reflects vasculitis of the superficial dermis causing damage to the vessels, is more frequent in MPA than in polyarteritis nodosa. Vasculitic purpura must be differentiated from purpura due to trauma, infections, glucocorticoid therapy, systemic amyloidosis, scurvy, and thrombocytopenia [9].

Nodules reflect vasculitis localized in the deep dermis or subcutaneous tissue and tend to occur more frequently in polyarteritis nodosa than in MPA [2] (Fig. 38.2). However, nodules may also be secondary to rheumatoid arthritis, lepromatous leprosy, some skin tumors, secondary deposits, lymphoma, and dermatofibroma [9].

Livedo racemosa is a violaceous mottling of the skin. It can be seen both in MPA and in polyarteritis nodosa but also in the antiphospholipid antibody syndrome, the cholesterol emboli syndrome, cryofibrinogenemia, calciphylaxis, and cryoglobulinemic vasculitis [9, 10]. Livedo racemosa should be differentiated from livedo reticularis, which is a functional disorder due to impaired blood flow of the cutaneous vessels leading to a netlike cyanotic pattern in the legs, especially in cold weather [10]. Clues to the diagnosis of livedo racemosa over that of livedo reticularis are a more widespread localization and a shape characterized by irregular, broken circular segments [10].

Skin ulcers can be vasculitic in origin but can also be due to noninflammatory vasculopathy, infections, pyoderma gangrenosum, and malignancies, particularly squamous cell carcinoma [9]. The most common causes of leg ulcers are venous hypertension and atherosclerosis. Venous hypertension typically underlies leg ulcers over the medial malleolus, while atherosclerotic ulcers most commonly occur over the toes and dorsum of the feet [9].

Despite some differences between MPA and polyarteritis nodosa, a distinction between these two conditions cannot reliably be made in the individual patient on the basis of the cutaneous manifestations alone because of a substantial overlap of the different types of skin lesions in these vasculitides [2]. In order to reliably distinguish MPA from polyarteritis nodosa, other features beyond clinical picture and histological alterations need to be taken into account. Both conditions can present with constitutional symptoms, arthralgia, and peripheral nerve disease. However, while MPA mainly causes capillaritis of the lungs and glomerulonephritis, polyarteritis nodosa rarely affects the lungs and kidneys, and when renal involvement occurs, the typical manifestation is of renal infarction instead of glomerulonephritis. In terms of serology, ANCA (usually with a perinuclear pattern) are often positive in MPA, but only occasionally seen in polyarteritis nodosa, whereas polyarteritis nodosa, but not MPA, may be associated with hepatitis B virus. Finally, angiography may show characteristic aneurysms of visceral arteries in polyarteritis nodosa, which are not a feature of MPA.

The vasculitis seen in MPA is often undistinguishable from that observed in Wegener granulomatosis and Churg-Strauss syndrome. All these conditions are associated with circulating ANCA, although ANCA are absent in 60 % of cases of Churg-Strauss syndrome and have mostly a cytoplasmic pattern (c-ANCA) in granulomatosis with polyangiitis (Wegener) [8]. The presence of granulomata and of upper respiratory tract involvement would point to Wegener granulomatosis, while asthma, eosinophilia, and extravascular granulomata would rather suggest Churg-Strauss syndrome.

Finally, the absence or scarcity of immunoglobulin and complement deposits in the vessel walls can help distinguish MPA from immune complex-mediated small-vessel vasculitides such as cryoglobulinemic vasculitis, urticarial vasculitis, and Henoch-Schönlein purpura [11]. A detailed clinical history and physical examination complemented by the appropriate investigations can further help discriminate between MPA and immune complex-mediated small-vessel vasculitides. The differential diagnosis between MPA and vasculitis mimickers such as scurvy and the cholesterol emboli syndrome is usually straightforward since histology in these latter cases will not show evidence of vasculitis proper.

Biopsy

Histology of skin lesions shows a leukocytoclastic picture with fibrinoid degeneration, neutrophil infiltration, nuclear dust, and sometimes erythrocyte extravasation in and around the affected capillaries and small vessels in the dermis, while direct immunofluorescence studies show absence of immunoglobulin deposits [3, 12] (Fig. 38.3). In later stages the cellular infiltration becomes predominantly lymphocytic. In contrast, polyarteritis nodosa vasculitis is localized in the deep dermis or subcutaneous tissue/hypodermis (Fig. 38.4).

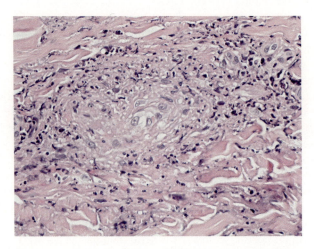

Fig. 38.3 Histology of a skin biopsy from a patient with microscopic polyangiitis showing a typical leukocytoclastic vasculitis (H&E, 400x) (Image courtesy of Dr. Simonetta Piana, Pathology Department, Arcispedale Santa Maria Nuova, Reggio Emilia, Italy)

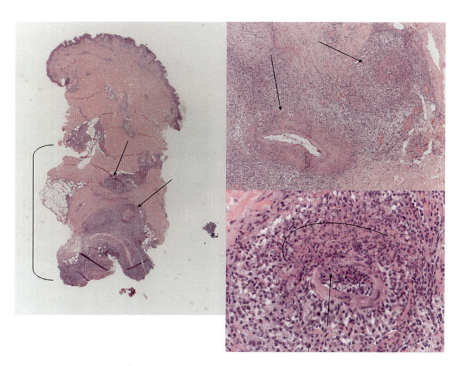

Fig. 38.4 Polyarteritis nodosa, histology. Vasculitis of the hypodermis with sparing of the epidermis and dermis. *Left* (H&E, 20x): the epidermis and dermis appear unremarkable, while in the hypodermis two vessels show an extensive inflammatory infiltrate. *Top right* (H&E, 100x): two vessels show an extensive inflammatory infiltrate and fibrinoid necrosis (*pink*). *Bottom right* (H&E, 400x), marked, predominantly mononuclear, vessel wall inflammatory infiltrate spreading beyond the vessel wall, fibrinoid necrosis (*pink*), and leukocytoclastia (cell fragmentation and nuclear dust) (Images courtesy of Dr. Alberto Cavazza, Pathology Department, Arcispedale Santa Maria Nuova, Reggio Emilia, Italy)

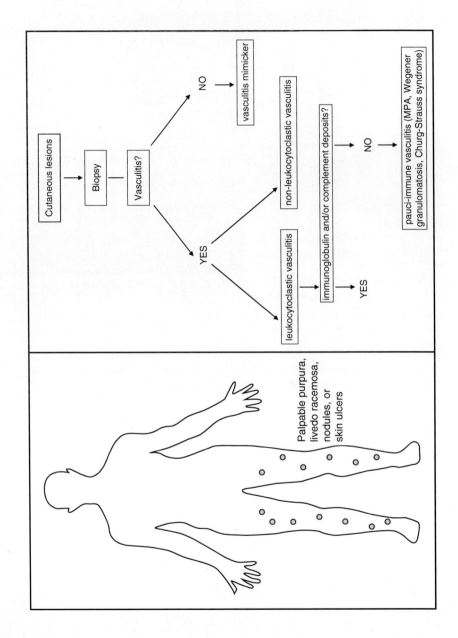

References

1. Jennette JC, Falk RJ, Andrassy K, et al. Nomenclature of systemic vasculitides. Proposal of an international consensus conference. Arthritis Rheum. 1994;37:187–92.
2. Kluger N, Pagnoux C, Guillevin L, Frances C. Comparison of cutaneous manifestations in systemic polyarteritis nodosa and microscopic polyangiitis. Br J Dermatol. 2008;159:615–20.
3. Nagai Y, Hasegawa M, Igarashi N, Tanaka S, Yamanaka M, Ishikawa O. Cutaneous manifestations and histological features of microscopic polyangiitis. Eur J Dermatol. 2009;19:57–60.
4. Kawakami T, Kawanabe T, Saito C, et al. Clinical and histopathologic features of 8 patients with microscopic polyangiitis including two with a slowly progressive clinical course. J Am Acad Dermatol. 2007;57:840–8.
5. Seishima M, Oyama Z, Oda M. Skin eruptions associated with microscopic polyangiitis. Eur J Dermatol. 2004;14:255–8.
6. Lane SE, Watts RA, Shepstone L, Scott DG. Primary systemic vasculitis: clinical features and mortality. QJM. 2005;98:97–111.
7. Agard C, Mouthon L, Mahr A, Guillevin L. Microscopic polyangiitis and polyarteritis nodosa: how and when do they start? Arthritis Rheum. 2003;49:709–15.
8. Wiik A. Clinical and pathophysiological significance of anti-neutrophil cytoplasmic autoantibodies in vasculitis syndromes. Mod Rheumatol. 2009;19:590–9.
9. Savin JA, Hunter JA. Hepburn NC Skin signs in clinical medicine. London: Mosby-Wolfe; 1997.
10. Kramer M, Linden D, Berlit P. The spectrum of differential diagnosis in neurological patients with livedo reticularis and livedo racemosa. J Neurol. 2005;252:1155–66.
11. Kluger N, Frances C. Cutaneous vasculitis and their differential diagnoses. Clin Exp Rheumatol. 2009;27:S124–38.
12. Niiyama S, Amoh Y, Tomita M, Katsuoka K. Dermatological manifestations associated with microscopic polyangiitis. Rheumatol Int. 2008;28:593–5.

Chapter 39
Henoch-Schönlein Purpura

Fernanda Falcini

Definition

Henoch-Schönlein purpura (HSP) is the most common systemic vasculitis in childhood of small-sized blood vessels, resulting from an IgA-mediated inflammation. It is typically seen in school-aged children, with an estimated incidence of 13.5–18 per 100.000 children per year. HSP is more common in autumn and winter and often preceded by an upper respiratory tract infection. It mainly affects the skin, gastrointestinal tract, joints and kidney. Petechiae and palpable purpura, the typical skin lesions, involve the lower extremities and buttocks and rarely the upper extremities, face and trunk (Figs. 39.1, 39.2, 39.3, 39.4, and 39.5). The purpuric rash is a mandatory criterion to the diagnosis although may not be the presenting feature of the disease. Subcutaneous oedema over the dorsum of hands, feet, forehead and around the eyes may be also observed. Skin lesions appear on crops and may often recur. Arthralgia or arthritis may precede the purpura by 1–3 days with the ankles, knees and wrists mainly affected. Abdominal pain, gastrointestinal bleeding, haematemesis and melena develop in two-third of children and often precede the purpuric lesions. Vasculitis of the bowel may provoke intussusceptions and gut perforation. One-third of children will have glomerulonephritis but only 10 % nephritic or nephrotic syndrome, hypertension or renal failure. Isolated microhaematuria and/or proteinuria is common within the first 4–6 weeks and can continue for months though urinalysis generally normalizes in a few weeks. HSP is a benign self-limiting condition that lasts 2–4 weeks; only one-third of patients may have a recurrent disease which usually subsides within 3–6 months. Longer course has been reported in patients with renal involvement. Only 1–3 % of cases reach end-stage renal

F. Falcini, M.D. (✉)
Internal Medicine, Rheumatology Section, University of Florence, Viale Pieraccini 18,
Florence 50139, Italy
e-mail: falcini@unifi.it

M. Matucci-Cerinic et al. (eds.), *Skin Manifestations in Rheumatic Disease*,   321
DOI 10.1007/978-1-4614-7849-2_39, © Springer Science+Business Media New York 2014

Fig. 39.1 Palpable purpura lesions involve the leg; there is also the sock's sign

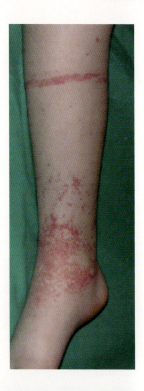

Fig. 39.2 A boy with petechiae, ecchymoses and palpable purpura involving the upper and lower extremities, arms and hands

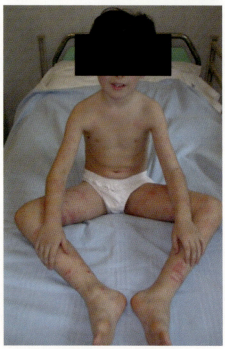

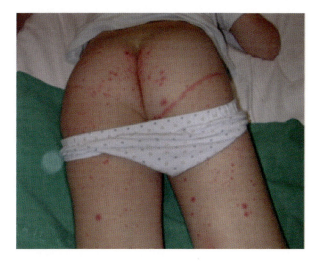

Fig. 39.3 Typical palpable purpura on the buttocks

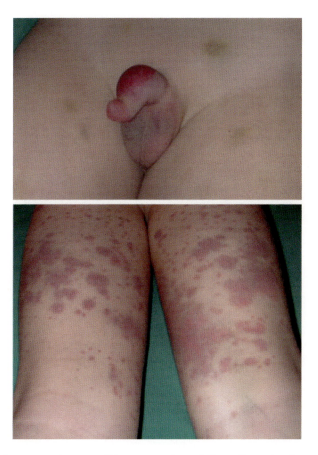

Fig. 39.4 Ecchymoses and purpura of the scrotum; the penis is swollen and ecchymotic. Different skin lesions, ranging from palpable purpura and petechiae to ecchymoses, on the legs

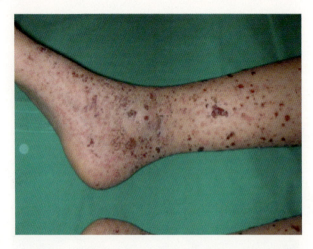

Fig. 39.5 Bullous evolution of purpuric lesions; a rare awful evolution of palpable purpura in an 8-year-old girl with HSP

disease. There is no specific treatment of HSP. No significant benefit of short-course prednisone given at HSP onset has proved to be helpful in preventing persistent renal disease. According to PRES/EULAR criteria, at least one of the following four may be present in addition to palpable purpura: (i) diffuse abdominal pain, (ii) any biopsy showing predominant IgA deposition, (iii) arthritis or arthralgia and (iv) renal involvement (any haematuria and/or proteinuria) [1–3].

Differential Diagnosis

HSP may be differentiated from other systemic vasculitis in which purpura is the skin manifestation. They include panarteritis nodosa, hypersensitivity angiitis, hypocomplementemic urticarial vasculitis and vasculitis associated with connective tissue diseases. As purpura is the first symptom of other vasculitis, the diagnosis may be missed when the accompanying features have not yet developed. A careful evaluation of blood tests and visceral involvement may help in the correct definition of the underlying disease.

Biopsy

Skin biopsy usually shows a leukocytoclastic vasculitis in the dermal capillary and postcapillary venules with the presence of perivascular infiltrates of IgA. Immunofluorescence confirms the presence of IgA, and in addition of IgG, fibrin, and complement around the small vessels of involved and uninvolved areas. Renal biopsy shows proliferative glomerulonephritis with features of focal and segmental lesions up to severe multiple crescents. Renal biopsy may be indistinguishable from IgA nephropathy.

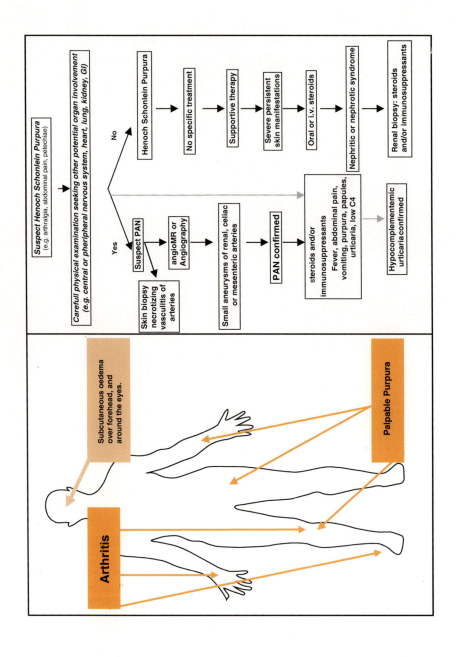

References

1. Chartapisak W, et al. Prevention and treatment of renal disease in Henoch-Schönlein purpura: a systematic review. Arch Dis Child. 2009;94:132–7.
2. Eleftheriou D, Brogan PA. Vasculitis in children. Best Pract Res Clin Rheumatol. 2009;23: 309–23.
3. Gardner-Medwin JM, et al. Incidence of Henoch-Schönlein purpura, Kawasaki disease, and rare vasculitides in children of different ethnic origins. Lancet. 2002;360:1197–202.

Chapter 40
Skin Manifestations and Cryoglobulinemia

**Chiara Baldini, Elisabetta Bernacchi, Rosaria Talarico,
Alessandra Della Rossa, and Stefano Bombardieri**

Definition

The term cryoglobulinemia (C) refers to the presence in the serum of single or
mixed immunoglobulins (Ig), which precipitates at a temperature below 37 °C and
redissolves on rewarming [1]. Cryoglobulinemia is an in vitro phenomenon which
can be associated with various infections, malignancies, and immune-mediated diseases. According to the cryoglobulins' composition, cryoglobulinemia is classified
as type I, type II, and type III. *Type I* cryoglobulinemia (10–15 %) is composed of a
single monoclonal Ig (IgG, IgM, or IgA) with self-aggregating activity, invariably
associated with lymphoproliferative-hematological disorders, and is frequently
asymptomatic. *Type II and III* cryoglobulinemia are immune complexes composed
of polyclonal IgG autoantigens and mono- or polyclonal IgM with RF activity autoantibodies, respectively; they are mainly detected in mixed cryoglobulinemia (MC)
[1]. MC is a systemic vasculitis first described by Meltzer and Franklin in 1961.
Orthostatic skin purpura, weakness, arthralgias, low C4 levels, and circulating
mixed cryoglobulins are the hallmarks of the disease; the kidney, the gastrointestinal
system, and the peripheral nervous system are sometimes involved in the vasculitic
process [1]. MC is quite frequent (1:100,000) in Southern Europe; since 1990 it has
been strongly associated with hepatitis C virus (HCV) infection [2, 3]. MC represents a crossroads among infections, autoimmunity, and lymphoproliferative disorders,
involving humoral and cellular immunity.

C. Baldini, M.D. • R. Talarico, M.D., Ph.D. • S. Bombardieri, M.D. (✉)
Department of Internal Medicine, Rheumatology Unit, University of Pisa,
Via Roma 67, Pisa 56126, Italy
e-mail: chiara.baldini74@gmail.com; sara.talarico76@gmail.com;
s.bombardieri@int.med.unipi.it

E. Bernacchi, M.D. • A.D. Rossa, M.D.
Malattie Muscolo Scheletriche e Cutanee, Ospedale S. Chiara, Unità Operativa di
Reumatologia, AOUP, Via Roma 67, Pisa 56126, Italy
e-mail: bettibernacchi@libero.it; a.dellarossa@ao-pisa.toscana.it

M. Matucci-Cerinic et al. (eds.), *Skin Manifestations in Rheumatic Disease*,
DOI 10.1007/978-1-4614-7849-2_40, © Springer Science+Business Media New York 2014

Description

Cryoglobulinemia type I is mainly found in patients with lymphoproliferative disorders (immunocytoma, Waldenstrom macroglobulinemia, multiple myeloma). Clinical manifestations derive from hemorheological disturbances and include cold-induced circulatory symptoms, from moderate acrocyanosis to severe Raynaud's phenomenon and gangrene. Rarely, cerebrovascular accidents occur during the course of MC type I. Acrocyanosis and gangrene can occur associated with cryoglobulinemia type I. The differential diagnosis is outlined in Table 40.1 [1].

   Cryoglobulinemia types II and III with RF activity affect small and medium vessels and are immune complexes-mediated (DIF+) systemic leukocytoclastic vasculitis, with various organs involvement including the skin, liver, and kidney; peripheral neuropathy; and, less frequently, lung and endocrine gland disorders. Purpura and ulcers are the most frequent symptoms and can be present in up to 90 % of the MC patients. Purpura and skin ulcerations, especially of the lower extremities, can be intermittent, and their severity can vary from mild purpura to severe vasculitic ulceration. Ulcers appear torpid and deep and are associated with high levels of pain, inflammation, and tissue necrosis [1–4].

   In particular, purpura is currently one of the major proposed classification criteria for this disease. Moreover, a possible MC complication is the appearance of a B-cell lymphoma [1–4]. Serological, pathological, and clinical criteria for the diagnosis of MC patients are reported in Table 40.2 [3, 4]. A careful patient evaluation is necessary for a correct classification of MC syndromes, with regard to a wide range of infectious, neoplastic, and other RF-positive, systemic rheumatic disorders (Table 40.1)

Table 40.1 Cryoglobulinemic skin lesions and their differential diagnosis

Cryoglobulinemia skin lesions	Differential diagnosis
Type I monoclonal	Other pseudovasculitis: *hemorrhage, embolism, thrombosis, vasospasm*
Type II–III mixed	HBV-HCV-related vasculitis and cutaneous manifestation, autoimmune hepatitis, systemic autoimmune disorders RF positive (AR, SS, UCTD), B lymphoproliferative diseases
Orthostatic purpura	**Cutaneous leukocytoclastic vasculitis (hypersensitivity vasculitis, allergic vasculitis) –** *Idiopathic exercise-induced* **drugs:** *almost every class, chemicals, food, vitamins, nutritional supplements, tumor necrosis factor alpha.* **Infections:** *all virus, bacteria, fungi, and parasites.* **Malignancy:** *homeopatie, myelodysplastic syndrome, lymphoma, carcinomas.* **Systemic leukocytoclastic vasculitis:** *autoimmune disorders, CTD, CM, hypocomplementemic vasculitis, SH purpura, Kaposi sarcoma, malignancy, hepatitis B and C infections, endocarditis, ANCA-associated vasculitis, Becket's disease.* **Hemorrhagic disorders:** senile purpura (Bateman), thrombotic thrombocytopenic purpura, CID
	Lymphocytic vasculitis: *rickettsial-viral infections, drugs, CTD, Behcet's disease, Degos'disease*
Skin ulcers	Necrotizing cutaneous and systemic vasculitis, APL antibodies syndrome, pyoderma gangrenosum, IVC ulcer

Table 40.2 Serological, pathological, and clinical criteria for the diagnosis of MC patients

Criteria	Serologic	Pathologic	Clinical
Major	Mixed cryoglobulins low C4	Leukocytoclastic vasculitis	Purpura
Minor	Rheumatoid factor HCV+, HBV+	Clonal B-cell infiltrates (liver and/or bone marrow)	Chronic hepatitis, MPGN, peripheral neuropathy, skin ulcers

Definite MC:

1. Serum MC ± low C4 + purpura + leukocytoclastic vasculitis

2. Serum MC ± low C4+ 2 minor clinical symptoms + 2 minor serological/pathological findings

Essential or secondary MC

Absence or presence of well-known disorders (infectious, immunologic, or neoplastic)

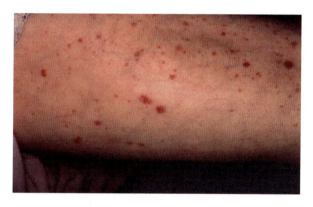

Fig. 40.1 Orthostatic purpura: active sporadic palpable purpura lesions, associated lesions (i.e., telangiectasies, livedo reticularis), and residual brown-ochraceous hyperpigmentation consequently to the repeated purpuric pousses

[3, 4]. In particular, pSS and MC can share various overlap symptoms [5]. Histopathological alterations of salivary glands and specific pSS autoantibody patterns (anti-SSA/SSB) are rarely found in MC patients. On the contrary, HCV infection, orthostatic purpura, ulcers, and peripheral neuropathy are rare in pSS. Patients with MC/pSS overlap syndrome are often characterized by a more severe evolution. With regard to skin manifestations, the association of MC with FAN positivity, generalized morphea, Raynaud's phenomenon, and sclerodattilia can be found. Finally, the coexistence of HCV-related skin diseases (i.e., lichen planus, porphyria cutanea tarda, pruritus, erythema nodosum, urticaria and urticarial vasculitis, erythema multiform, necrolytic acral erythema) and MC can be taken into account. Generally, the association of MC with other HCV-related cutaneous skin manifestations is low [3–5].

MC purpura appeared isolated in 54 % of the cases, and in 46 %, it is associated with asthenia and arthralgia (i.e., Melzer and Franklin triad) [4–6]. Purpura is usually on the lower extremities and usually intermittent (days, months) and symmetrically distributed (Fig. 40.1). Lesions might be formed by prolonged standing (orthostatic),

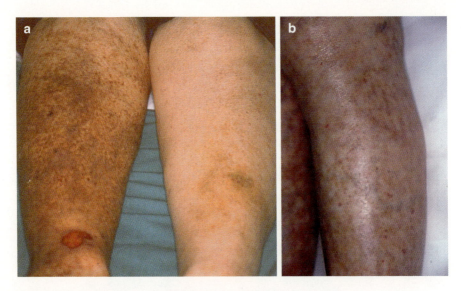

Fig. 40.2 (**a** and **b**) Orthostatic palpable purpura: florid lesions

trauma, and/or physical exercise [4–6]. Chronic venous insufficiency (VCI) may be an additional aggravating factor. The dimension and diffusion of skin lesions largely vary, from sporadic, isolated elements to severe vasculitic lesions (Figs. 40.1 and 40.2) [5]. After repeated episodes of purpura, two-thirds (40 %) of patients developed confluent areas of post-inflammatory hyperpigmentation. This ocherous coloration of the skin with a socklike distribution is caused by chronic erythrocytes extravasations and hemosiderin tissue deposition (Fig. 40.1) [4–6]. Purpuric (not palpable), telangiectasic, and livedo reticularis lesions may occur. The presence of more than ten purpuric lesions and/or the spreading on the upper part of the legs must be considered as a more severe prognostic index of the disease. Moreover, palpable purpura is a nonspecific and common skin symptom of other diseases, such as systemic vasculitis, purpura senilis, SHA, and VCI [4–6] (Table 40.1).

MC ulcers of the legs and malleolar areas often complicate purpura (Fig. 40.3) [6]. Ulcers appear torpid and deep and are associated with high levels of pain, inflammation, and tissue necrosis [6]. The ulcers are usually late complications of MC and are often slow-healing [1, 2]. Skin vasculitic ulcers are considered to be severe manifestations of MC and might require aggressive therapies [1, 2]. The differential diagnosis may be made with VCI malleolar ulcer, other necrotizing leukocytoclastic vasculitic lesions, and antiphospholipid antibodies syndrome [4].

In a small number (3 %) of MC cases, atypical cryoglobulinemic lesions such as "annular" purpura and urticarial vasculitis may be present, while in 30 % of the cases, edema of lower extremities may be found. It is often a poor prognostic factor potentially reflecting both the kidney and liver involvement and cardiovascular age-related complications of the patients. Finally, in 35 % of MC, Raynaud's phenomenon can be detected [1, 2, 4].

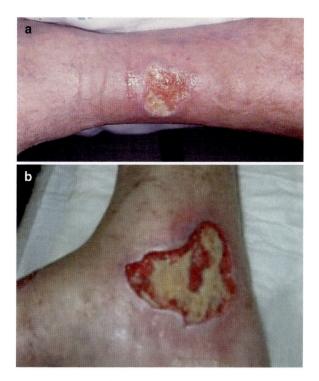

Fig. 40.3 (**a** and **b**) Typical CM ulceration of the lower extremities

Differential Diagnosis

Biopsy

Purpura: Purpura has been histopathologically referred to as the leukocytoclastic vasculitis of the small superficial venules characterized by an inflammatory infiltrate composed predominantly by neutrophils, many of which are fragmented. Moreover, the lesions typically display fibrinoid necrosis, lumen occlusion, and extravasations of red blood cells in the dermis with large hemosiderin deposits. Leukocytoclastic vasculitis features disappeared after 24–48 h. Then a perivascular lymphocytic-neutrophilic infiltrate can be detected [4, 6].

See Also

Raynaud's phenomenon, Sjogren's syndrome, Systemic leukocytoclastic vasculitis, HCV cutaneous lesions

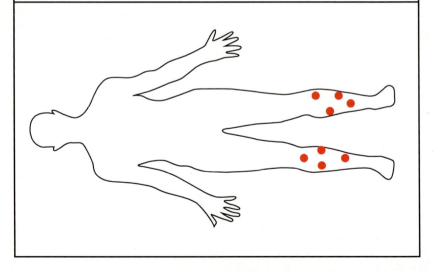

Skin lesions	Treatment
Purpura	Low-medium corticosteroids + LAC-diet
Skin ulcers	Corticosteroids, Plasmapheresis, Cyclophosphamide, Rituximab

Acknowledgment We thank Laura Maria Fatuzzo for her valuable contribution in reviewing the text.

References

1. Atzeni F, Carrabba M, Davin JC, Francès C, Ferri C, Guillevin L, Jorizzo JL, Mascia MT, Patel MJ, Pagnoux C, Vulpio L, Sarzi-Puttini P. Skin manifestations in vasculitis and erythema nodosum. Clin Exp Rheumatol. 2006;24(1 Suppl 40):S60–6.
2. La Civita L, Zignego AL, Bernacchi E, Monti M, Fabbri P, Ferri C. Hepatitis C virus infection and cutaneous vasculitis in mixed cryoglobulinemia. Mayo Clin Proc. 1996 Jan;71(1):109–10.
3. Antonelli A, Ferri C, Galeazzi M, Giannitti C, Manno D, Mieli-Vergani G, Menegatti E, Olivieri I, Puoti M, Palazzi C, Roccatello D, Vergani D, Sarzi-Puttini P, Atzeni F. HCV infection: pathogenesis, clinical manifestations and therapy. Clin Exp Rheumatol. 2008;26(1 Suppl 48):S39–47.
4. Kluger N, Francès C. Cutaneous vasculitis and their differential diagnoses. Clin Exp Rheumatol. 2009;27(52):SI24–38.
5. Bernacchi E, Civita LL, Caproni M, Zignego AL, Bianchi B, Monti M, Fabbri P, Pasero G, Ferri C. Hepatitis C virus (HCV) in cryoglobulinaemic leukocytoclastic vasculitis (LCV): could the presence of HCV in skin lesions be related to T CD8+ lymphocytes, HLA-DR and ICAM-1 expression? Exp Dermatol. 1999;8(6):480–6.
6. Carlson JA. The histological assessment of cutaneous vasculitis. Histopathology. 2010;56:3–23.

Chapter 41
Skin Manifestations in Giant Cell Arteritis

Nicolò Pipitone, Carlo Salvarani, and Gene G. Hunder

Definition

Giant cell arteritis (GCA) is a primary systemic vasculitis involving large- and medium-sized vessels which affects almost exclusively patients aged 50 years or older [1]. GCA rarely presents with cutaneous manifestations because it spares the small vessels which are typically associated with skin lesions [1]. The most common visible "skin involvement" in GCA is related to the inflammation of the cranial arteries, especially the temporal arteries, i.e., visible temporal artery thickening or nodularity and erythema over the superficial temporal arteries (Fig. 41.1). The temporal arteries are often tender, while their pulses may be decreased or absent [1].

Much less frequently severe vascular inflammation in GCA can be associated with ischemic skin lesions such as necrosis of the scalp or tongue (Figs. 41.2, 41.3, and 41.4) [2]. Scalp necrosis usually occurs in active GCA before the initiation of glucocorticoid treatment and is often associated with other ischemic manifestations. In a review of the literature which identified 24 patients with GCA who presented with scalp necrosis, 16 patients suffered visual loss, 4 had tongue gangrene, and 1 had necrosis of the nasal septum [3]. Nineteen patients developed scalp necrosis before receiving glucocorticoids, while in 21 cases out of 24, scalp necrosis occurred before temporal artery biopsy was performed [3]. Temporal artery biopsy was positive in 14/16 cases in which it was performed [3]. Therefore, scalp necrosis appears to be due to active GCA and is not an ischemic complication of temporal artery biopsy.

N. Pipitone, M.D., Ph.D. • C. Salvarani, M.D. (✉)
Department of Rheumatology, Division of Medicine, Arcispedale Santa Maria Nuova,
Viale Risorgimento 80, 42100 Reggio Emilia, Italy
e-mail: Pipitone.nicolo@asmn.re.it; Salvarani.carlo@asmn.re.it

G.G. Hunder, M.D.
Emeritus Staff Center, Mayo Clinic, 200 First St SW, 55905 Rochester, MN, USA
e-mail: ghunder@mayo.edu

M. Matucci-Cerinic et al. (eds.), *Skin Manifestations in Rheumatic Disease*,
DOI 10.1007/978-1-4614-7849-2_41, © Springer Science+Business Media New York 2014

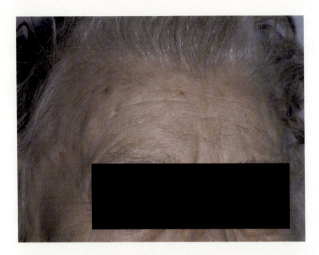

Fig. 41.1 GCA in an 80-year-old woman. Frontal view

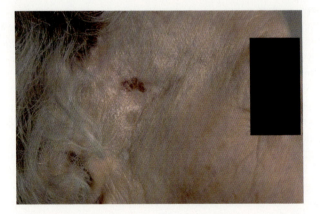

Fig. 41.2 GCA in a 75-year-old woman. GCA of 2 months' duration. On glucocorticoid treatment for 3 weeks. Two areas of scalp necrosis with loss of surrounding hair can be seen

Other mucocutaneous changes occasionally seen in GCA are necrosis of the tongue or lips, glossitis, and facial swelling [2, 4, 5]. Necrosis of the tongue and lips is due to ischemia secondary to inflammation, while facial swelling might be related to the underlying inflammation.

Differential Diagnosis

Rarely, the temporal arteries can be involved in ANCA (anti-neutrophil cytoplasmic antibodies)-associated vasculitis [6] and in amyloidosis [7]. Biopsy is diagnostic.

Fig. 41.3 GCA in an 80-year-old woman. Ischemic necrosis of tongue due to GCA

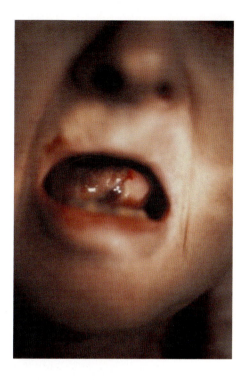

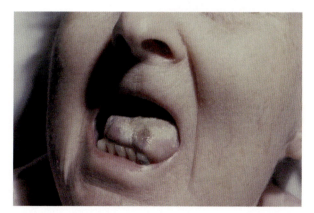

Fig. 41.4 GCA in an 80-year-old woman. Two months after treatment. There has been sloughing of skin of tip of tongue and healing

Skin changes due to small vessel involvement such as purpura or nodules are not part of the clinical manifestations of GCA. If such lesions are present, one should suspect a small-vessel vasculitis mimicking GCA [6]. However, skin lesions of several types may occasionally be seen in Takayasu arteritis, a disease similar to GCA [8, 9]. These lesions commonly appear as erythematous nodules over the legs. Biopsy generally reveals vasculitis [8, 9].

Biopsy

Histology of the temporal arteries typically shows a transmural lymphomononuclear infiltrate and a disrupted internal elastic lamina with or without giant cells and occasionally an adventitial/*vasa vasorum* vasculitis surrounding a spared artery [1, 10] (Fig. 41.5).

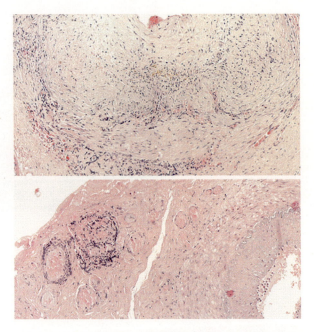

Fig. 41.5 Temporal artery biopsy in patients with giant cell arteritis (H&E, 100x). *Top picture*: transmural inflammatory cell infiltrate. *Bottom picture*: adventitial cell infiltrate (Image courtesy of Dr. Alberto Cavazza, Pathology Department, Arcispedale Santa Maria Nuova, Reggio Emilia, Italy)

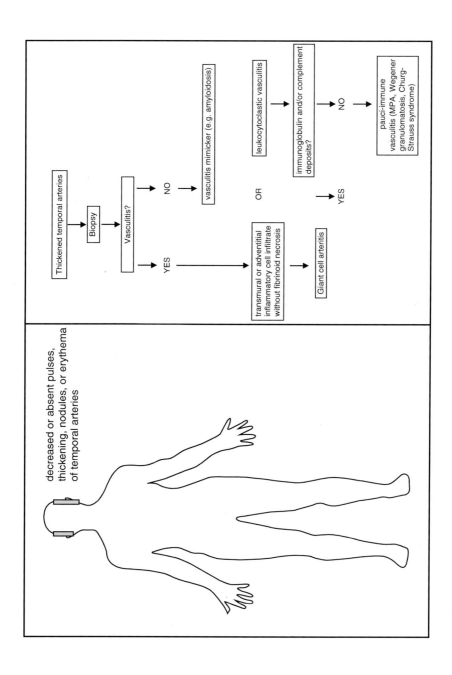

References

1. Salvarani C, Cantini F, Hunder GG. Polymyalgia rheumatica and giant-cell arteritis. Lancet. 2008;372:234–45.
2. Kinmont PD, McCallum DI. Skin manifestations of giant cell arteritis. Br J Dermatol. 1964;76:299–308.
3. Currey J. Scalp necrosis in giant cell arteritis and review of the literature. Br J Rheumatol. 1997;36:814–6.
4. Friedman G, Friedman B. The sensation of facial swelling in temporal arteritis: a predictor for the development of visual disturbance. Postgrad Med J. 1986;62:1019–20.
5. Liozon E, Ouattara B, Portal MF, Soria P, Loustaud-Ratti V, Vidal E. Head-and-neck swelling: an under-recognized feature of giant cell arteritis. A report of 37 patients. Clin Exp Rheumatol. 2006;24:S20–5.
6. Nishino H, DeRemee RA, Rubino FA, Parisi JE. Wegener's granulomatosis associated with vasculitis of the temporal artery: report of five cases. Mayo Clin Proc. 1993;68:115–21.
7. Salvarani C, Gabriel SE, Gertz MA, Bjornsson J, Li CY, Hunder GG. Primary systemic amyloidosis presenting as giant cell arteritis and polymyalgia rheumatica. Arthritis Rheum. 1994;37:1621–6.
8. Perniciaro CV, Winkelmann RK, Hunder GG. Cutaneous manifestations of Takayasu's arteritis. A clinicopathologic correlation. J Am Acad Dermatol. 1987;17:998–1005.
9. Frances C, Boisnic S, Bletry O, et al. Cutaneous manifestations of Takayasu arteritis. A retrospective study of 80 cases. Dermatologica. 1990;181:266–72.
10. Esteban MJ, Font C, Hernandez-Rodriguez J, et al. Small-vessel vasculitis surrounding a spared temporal artery: clinical and pathological findings in a series of 28 patients. Arthritis Rheum. 2001;44:1387–95.

Chapter 42
Skin Manifestations of Behçet's Disease

Ayhan Dinç and İsmail Şimşek

Introduction

Behçet's disease (BD) is a multisystem, inflammatory disorder of unknown etiology with vasculitis as its main underlying pathological process. BD is characterized by recurrent oral and genital ulcers, skin lesions, and uveitis. Other features are arthritis, thrombophlebitis, a positive pathergy test, and central nervous system and gastrointestinal lesions. The usual course is of exacerbations and remissions, and in most patients, the disease is nearly silent between the events. The disease usually occurs in adults between 20 and 40 years of age. The prevalence was between 20 and 421 per 100,000 adults in five field surveys carried out in Turkey. It is less frequent in the rest of the world; the estimated prevalence ranges from 0.64 per 100,000 in the UK and 6.4 per 100,000 in Spain to 8.6 per 100,000 in the USA [1].

The disease has a quite heterogeneous presentation in which patients with the disorder may manifest all or only some of these clinical features [2]. Due to the lack of a generally accepted diagnostic test, diagnosis of BD usually relied on recognition of several of its more distinctive clinical features [3]. It is important to note that none of these features is specific for BD. Furthermore, each and every one of these features might be associated with diseases other than BD, and some might also be seen as an isolated finding. Given the heterogeneity of organ system involvement, the International Study Group for Behçet's Disease (ISGBD) established a classification criteria in 1990 which require the presence of recurrent oral ulceration plus any two of the following: recurrent genital ulceration, eye lesions, skin lesions

A. Dinç, M.D. (✉)
Rheumatology, Patio Clinic, Kıbrıs Sok. 1/3, Çankaya, Ankara 06540, Turkey
e-mail: ayhandincmd@gmail.com

İ. Şimşek, M.D.
Rheumatology, Gulhane School of Medicine, GATA Romatoloji Bilim Dali,
Etlik, 06018 Ankara, Turkey
e-mail: drisimsek@gmail.com

M. Matucci-Cerinic et al. (eds.), *Skin Manifestations in Rheumatic Disease*,
DOI 10.1007/978-1-4614-7849-2_42, © Springer Science+Business Media New York 2014

Table 42.1 International Study Group diagnostic (classification) criteria for Behçet's disease (1990)[a]

Recurrent oral ulceration	Minor aphthous, major aphthous, or herpetiform ulceration observed by physician or patient recurring at least three times in one 12-month period
Plus two of:	
Recurrent genital ulceration	Aphthous ulceration or scarring, observed by physician or patient
Eye lesions	Anterior uveitis, posterior uveitis, cells in the vitreous on slit-lamp examination, or retinal vasculitis observed by ophthalmologist
Skin lesions	Erythema nodosum observed by the physician or patient, pseudofolliculitis, papulopustular lesions, or acneiform nodules observed by physician in post adolescent patients not on corticosteroids treatment
Pathergy test	Read by physician at 24–48 h

[a]Findings applicable only in the absence of other clinical explanations

(erythema nodosum, folliculitis, pustules), or positive finding on pathergy test (Table 42.1). The findings are not valid if any other clinical explanation is present. Although it is not proposed to serve for diagnosis, the criteria permit diagnosis in the absence of concomitant happening of individual findings.

Mucocutaneous features are the most common presenting symptoms of the disease. In the absence of ophthalmologic, neurological, or vascular involvement, the disease generally runs a benign course with a rather good prognosis [4]. Other less frequent cutaneous features of BD, which are not discussed in this chapter, are extragenital ulcers, Sweet's syndrome, pyoderma gangrenosum, and palpable purpura.

Oral Ulcer/Oral Aphthae

Definition

The most common (97–100 %) and characteristic lesion of Behçet's disease, and often the initial sign, is oral aphthosis. The term *aphthae* means ulcer and is used to describe areas of ulceration on mucous membranes. An aphthous ulcer is a painful mouth ulcer, resulting from a break in the mucous membrane. The severity may be such that the patient is unable to eat, swallow, and even speak during the acute period.

The most common sites of the lesions are the mucous membranes of the lips, the buccal mucosa, the floor of the mouth, the soft palate, and the tongue. Although rare, hard palate, gums, tonsillar fauces, and pharynx can also be involved. The lesions mostly start as an erythematous, circular, slightly raised area evolving into an oval or round ulcer within 48 h.

There are three well-differentiated clinical forms: minor aphthae, major aphthae, and herpetiform aphthae. Minor aphthae have a diameter <10 mm, are superficial, covered by a gray membranous slough, surrounded by an erythematous rim, and heal without scarring in 1–2 weeks. Major ulcers are morphologically similar but larger

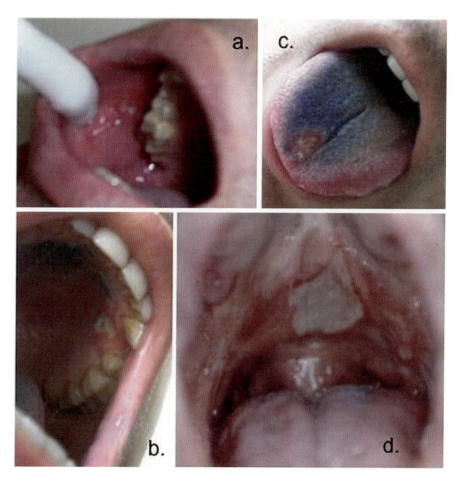

Fig. 42.1 Oral ulcers: (**a**) a minor ulcer on the buccal mucosa; (**b**) a minor ulcer on the gingiva; (**c**) a minor ulcer on the tongue; (**d**) a single major ulcer and minor ones on the hard palate

(>10 mm), deeper, more painful, and heal in 10–30 days or more often with scarring and tissue loss. In herpetiform ulceration, numerous (up to 100), small pinpoint (1–2 mm), yellowish, papular lesions become confluent and form larger plaques and can heal with scarring. Minor aphthae are seen in most patients, with major aphthae in approximately half, and herpetiform ulcers rarely. More than one type of aphthous ulcer may be present in an individual patient simultaneously (Fig. 42.1).

Differential Diagnosis

There are no specific tests available for BD, and the diagnosis is largely based on history and clinical features. Therefore, in a patient with recurrent oral aphthae, it is essential to reveal the existence of other clinical features of BD (genital ulcer, uveitis, acne, etc.) to establish a diagnosis [5].

Oral aphthosis is a very common complaint and can be related to various conditions developing within the oral cavity other than BD. One of the most striking feature of oral aphthosis associated with BD is its recurrent nature which may help to eliminate some sporadic causes of aphthosis in the differential diagnosis.

Recurrent multiple ulcers, especially in the absence of concomitant genital ulcers, are most typical (but not limited) of the following conditions: recurrent aphthous stomatitis (RAS), systemic lupus erythematosus (SLE), inflammatory bowel disease, celiac disease, HIV infection, and iron, B12, and folate deficiency. PFAPA syndrome (periodic fever, aphthous stomatitis, pharyngitis, and cervical adenitis) should also be included in the differential diagnosis, especially in pediatric patients with recurrent oral ulcers. Among the entities listed above, RAS is the most common affecting up to 25 % of the general population. Since RAS describes aphthous ulcers in the absence of systemic disease, its diagnosis is one of exclusion.

The pattern of aphthous ulceration is not a reliable guide to underlying causes, and it can be difficult to differentiate oral aphthae of BD from RAS on the basis of severity, duration, and frequency. Nevertheless, some reports suggested that patients with BD tend to have more ulcers (>6 simultaneously) and more frequent involvement of the soft palate and oropharynx than in RAS.

It should also be kept in mind that diagnostic clinical features may not be present at the onset of disease, and therefore, BD should be considered in patients diagnosed previously with RAS on development of potentially related clinical problems.

Biopsy

Histopathologic and immunofluorescent findings may exclude certain entities in the differential diagnosis and may lend support to the diagnosis of BD, but histopathologic findings are not diagnostic. The biopsies of oral lesions from BD show a mononuclear cell infiltrate in all sections. Although the ulcer itself is contained and surrounded by polymorphonuclear cells and contained cell debris, outside this zone and extending diffusely throughout the lamina propria, large numbers of infiltrating lymphocytes and macrophage-like cells can be seen. It is also important to note that histologically, there is no difference between the lesions in BD and those with RAS.

See Also

Aphthae.

Genital Ulcer/Genital Aphthae

Definition

Genital ulcers are the second most common manifestation of BD, present in 60–80 % of patients, and rarely are the first manifestation of the disease. They can be painful, leading to problems both sitting down and walking, pain on intercourse, as well as dysuria. Ulcers may be preceded by papules or pustules, and morphologically their appearance is similar to oral aphthae with round and sharp erythematous border (punched-out), covered with grayish-white pseudomembrane or central yellowish fibrinous base; they tend to occur less often than oral ulcers. They usually occur on the scrotum in the male while they are uncommon on the shaft or on the glans penis (Fig. 42.2). In the female, both major and minor labia are affected most

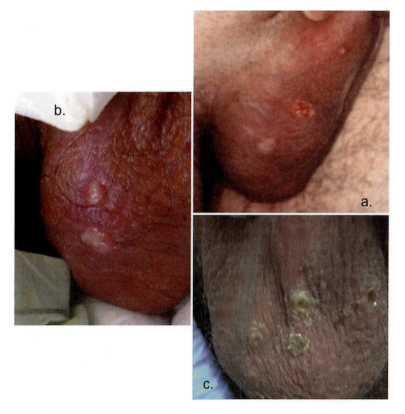

Fig. 42.2 Genital ulcers. (**a**) Three scrotal genital ulcer on different stages: upper while as a papule, middle while as a punch out ulcer, bottom while as a healed cicatrix; (**b**) two scrotal ulcer covered by a pseudomembrane; (**c**) several scrotal ulcer covered by a crust during healing

commonly, but vaginal and cervical ulcers occur and may be associated with vaginal discharge. They usually heal in 2–4 weeks. Since they are usually deeper than oral aphthae, scarring may eventuate from intensely inflamed, deep lesions. It is therefore important to search for scars even if there are no signs of active ulcer at the time of examination. The ulcers located at the labia minor, however, may heal without scar formation. Furthermore, vaginal and cervical ulcers may be asymptomatic making speculum examination of the female patient essential.

Differential Diagnosis

Clinically identical genital ulcers may be seen in a variety of disorders, either alone or together with oral ulcers. Differential diagnosis of patients presenting with recurrent genital ulceration accompanied by oral aphthae (orogenital ulceration) should include Reiter's syndrome, mouth and genital ulcers with inflamed cartilage (MAGIC), inflammatory bowel disease, cyclical neutropenia, and Sweet's syndrome. Recurrent orogenital ulceration may also be associated with bullous skin disorders, fixed drug reaction, and erythema multiforme.

Genital ulcers can sometimes be the initial manifestation of BD. When a patient is referred for assessment of genital ulcer without accompanying symptom suggestive of BD, sexually transmitted diseases figure more prominently in the possibilities. The three major diseases characterized by genital ulcers – genital herpes, syphilis, and chancroid – are common, with genital herpes being most common in industrialized countries and chancroid being most common in developing countries. In the differential diagnosis, conditions presenting with recurrent GU should be considered in the first place. In this regard, the recurrent nature of the genital lesions might mislead the unwary into assuming that herpes could be the diagnosis. In herpes simplex infection, lesions arise as multiple, painful, small, grouped vesicles on an erythematous base and recur at the same location each time.

There is considerable overlap in the clinical signs and symptoms of both infectious and noninfectious genital ulcers. Therefore, diagnosis of genital ulceration based solely upon morphologic examination is fraught with difficulty and subject to a high degree of inaccuracy and should be investigated aggressively with laboratory tests.

Biopsy

The histopathology is similar to that seen in oral aphthous lesions. Early lesions are characterized by neutrophil-predominating infiltrate, while in older lesions, the inflammatory cells are mostly lymphocytes. Presence of lymphocytic vasculitis has been reported in almost half of the cases, while leukocytoclastic vasculitis was rare.

See Also

Ulcers.

Papulopustular Lesions

Definition

Papulopustular lesions are commonly seen in patients with BD, while their frequency shows wide diversity (56–96 %) in different studies. They are heterogenous, folliculitis-like (when the lesion is around a hair follicle) or acne-like (acneiform) lesions on an erythematous base which appear as a papule and in the course of a 24–48 h become pustule. Although long considered to be sterile, the pustular lesions of BD were shown to be infected in a recent study [6]. They usually appear as multiple small papules and pustules most commonly located on the trunk, followed by extremities, but they can be seen everywhere. They usually heal within 2–3 days. Although pseudofolliculitis, papulopustular lesions, and acneiform nodules are listed as separate entities consisting one diagnostic criterion of BD, the use of papulopustular lesions might be a more appropriate term which covers both pseudofolliculitis and acneiform nodules. It is important to note that the pustular lesions are more common in BD patients with arthritis, which supports the view that pustular lesions and arthritis are associated.

Differential Diagnosis

The clinical appearance of papulopustular lesions seen in BD is not enough to determine whether any given specific lesion is due to BD or not. Thus, the differential diagnosis for papulopustular skin disorders is widespread and includes Reiter's disease, acneiform drug eruptions, acne vulgaris, SAPHO syndrome, perioral dermatitis, and suppurative folliculitis. However, the distribution of the lesions and the age of the patient are characteristics that may provide strong clues to the cause of cutaneous papulopustular eruptions. It is challenging even for an experienced dermatologist to differentiate acneiform lesions of BD from the acne vulgaris (ordinary acne) morphologically. The only feature that may help to differentiate is the presence, in BD, of these lesions at sites (limbs and buttocks) atypical for ordinary acne.

Biopsy

The histopathology of papulopustular lesions seen in BD is an area where much of the research as well as controversy exists [7]. Some studies suggest that the pustular lesions of BD lack the histopathologic findings of vasculitis and only show perivascular mononuclear or neutrophilic infiltration, or features of folliculitis and/or perifolliculitis. Such histopathological features cannot distinguish papulopustular lesion of BD from acne vulgaris. Others, on the other hand, suggest that both leukocytoclastic vasculitis and lymphocytic vasculitis can be observed in pustular lesions of BD, and specificity of the papulopustular lesions in BD can be improved by histopathological examination. Indeed, findings of the recent study support both of the followers, as showing four types of lesions (leukocytoclastic vasculitis 16.7 %, lymphocytic vasculitis 7.1 %, superficial and/or deep perivascular infiltration 64.3 %, and folliculitis and/or perifolliculitis 11.9 %) can be observed in papulopustular lesions of BD with varying frequencies.

See Also

Papules.

Erythema Nodosum-like Lesions

Definition

Erythema nodosum-like lesions are acute inflammatory nodules of the subcutaneous adipose tissue and presenting feature in about half of the patients with BD, especially in females. The typical eruption consists of a sudden onset of tender, erythematous, warm nodules (few or many) and raised plaques usually located on the shins (Fig. 42.3). Although lower extremities are the most commonly affected site, they can also appear in the face, neck, and buttocks. The nodules, which range from 2 to 6 cm in diameter with poorly defined borders may become confluent resulting in erythematous plaques. As the nodules age, they become bluish purple, brownish, yellowish, and finally green, similar to the color changes that occur in a resolving bruise. They usually subside over a period of 2–6 weeks without scarring, while some degree of post-inflammatory hyperpigmentation can be seen.

Differential Diagnosis

As similar to the other mucocutaneous manifestations of BD, differentiation of erythema nodosum-like lesions of BD from other causes of erythema nodosum is not possible clinically. Therefore, a search for an associated disease should always accompany the diagnosis of EN. The list of etiologic factors which can lead to

Fig. 42.3 Erythema nodosum-like lesions. Tender, erythematous nodules on the leg

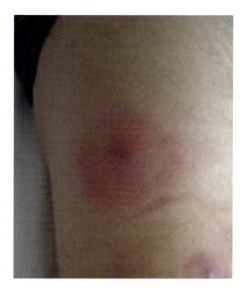

erythema nodosum is long and varied, including infections (e.g., tuberculosis, streptococcal, Mycoplasma pneumoniae, Yersinia, and Epstein-Barr virus), drugs (sulfonamides, oral contraceptives, bromides), malignant diseases (lymphoma), and a wide group of miscellaneous conditions (e.g., pregnancy, connective tissue diseases). There are also some diseases which have more than one feature resembling BD (e.g., EN plus aphthae) and present a diagnostic dilemma. Both erythema nodosum and oral ulcers are well-known features of inflammatory bowel disease. In fact, there is a considerable clinical overlap between inflammatory bowel disease with extragastrointestinal involvement and Behcet's disease with predominantly gastrointestinal involvement. Sarcoidosis can also present with erythema nodosum, uveitis and arthralgia, but genital ulcers are not a feature. While being a totally different clinical entity, superficial thrombophlebitis looks like erythema nodosum and might be difficult to differentiate them by naked eye. Ultrasonography may differentiate the two.

Biopsy

Histopathological features of the erythema nodosum-like lesions include a neutrophilic (rarely lymphocytic) infiltrate both in lobules and septum of subcutaneous tissue and vasculitis. Vasculitis in EN-like lesions of BD is leukocytoclastic or lymphocytic, and sometimes both can be observed in different vessels in the same specimen. Since classical EN lesions typically lack features suggestive of vasculitis, detection of vasculitis may help distinguish EN-like lesions of BD from EN associated with other diseases [8].

See Also

Erythema nodosum, panniculitis.

Superficial Thrombophlebitis

Definition

Thrombosis of the superficial veins has been termed superficial vein thrombosis (SVT) or superficial thrombophlebitis. It is a common manifestation of BD and seen in about 25 % of the patients. A diagnosis is established primarily on the basis of clinical signs: SVT appears as a red, hot, palpable tender cord in the course of a superficial vein (Fig. 42.4). Although most often detected in the veins of the lower extremities (most commonly affected site is great saphenous vein), it has also been reported in many other locations. Inflammation may extend further to some distance into surrounding tissue, making the distinction from infection or erythema nodosum sometimes difficult. There is no peripheral limb edema unless accompanied by a deep vein thrombosis.

Differential Diagnosis

Superficial thrombophlebitis is frequently confused with erythema nodosum. It is difficult clinically to differentiate the two entities, while nodular lesions seen in EN

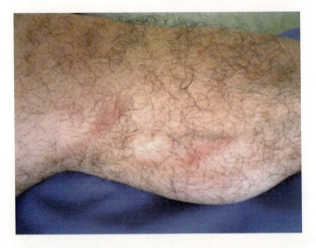

Fig. 42.4 Superficial thrombophlebitis. Two palpable tender cord-like erythema over the leg

may be differentiated from superficial thrombophlebitis because of the absence of a well-circumscribed cord-like structure. Ultrasonography may be useful in this setting, and it may also be a decisive factor in the presence of clinically difficult differential diagnosis with cellulitis, panniculitis, insect bites, and lymphangitis. Patients who present with spontaneous thrombophlebitis without a previous indwelling intravenous catheter or other precipitating cause (without obvious risk factors) should be considered for evaluation for a hypercoagulable state. Likewise, migratory thrombophlebitis, especially without good explanation, may be an indication for a more detailed evaluation of the patient in search of a malignant lesion.

Biopsy

Microscopically, superficial thrombophlebitis is an acute vasculitis usually accompanied by thrombosis involving veins of the upper subcutis and lower dermis. In early lesions, there is a moderate inflammatory cell infiltrate mainly composed of neutrophils within the vessel wall. A very constant feature is the presence of thrombi occluding the lumina of the affected veins that eventually undergo recanalization.

See Also

Erythema nodosum.

Pathergy Reaction

Definition

Defined as a state of altered (*path*-ological) tissue reactivity (−*ergy*), it is the non-specific hyperreactivity of the skin following minor trauma. The reaction is a unique feature of BD and, according to the International Study Group, is among the major criteria required for the diagnosis/classification. The formal pathergy test involves the intradermal puncture of the skin with a 20-gauge needle under sterile conditions with positive reactions manifesting as a papule or pustule surrounded by an erythematous halo developing by 48 h (Fig. 42.5). Despite being highly specific for BD, its sensitivity is moderate in Mediterranean, Near and Far Eastern countries (50 %), and even poor in Continental Europe or the Americas due to its lower rate of positivity. The reaction has been noted to be more strongly positive among male patients with Behçet's although the prevalence of positivity is similar in males and females [9].

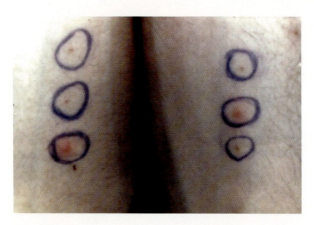

Fig. 42.5 Pathergy test. There are six puncture sites on the forearms. At the two of them, presence of a red papule is regarded as positive reaction

Differential Diagnosis

Although the reaction was found to be highly specific for BD, there are some diseases which can show positive results upon testing. Pyoderma gangrenosum is an ulcerative skin disorder that can exhibit clinical pathergy. The provocation of new lesions by trauma such as needle sticks or incisions was reported in 20–30 % of these cases. Likewise, a positive pathergy reaction was reported in 24 % of interferon-treated CML patients while none of those patients tested positive prior to interferon therapy. Although quite rare, pathergy can also occur in rheumatoid arthritis, Crohn's disease, and genital herpes.

Biopsy

A mononuclear cell infiltration composed of lymphocytes, neutrophils, and eosinophils around dermal blood vessels is a characteristic histopathological finding. A neutrophilic vasculitis (leukocytoclastic or Sweet-like vasculitis) can also be seen in some cases while, some reports suggest that the histopathology of pathergy lesions demonstrate mixed inflammatory infiltrate without vasculitis. It has been suggested that the variability of the reported histopathologic features of the pathergy may be related to individual differences in immune responses to inciting agents or different stages of the skin response.

See Also

Pyoderma gangrenosum.

References

1. Yurdakul S, et al. Behçet's syndrome. Best Pract Res Clin Rheumatol. 2008;22(5):793.
2. Dinc A, et al. The proportional Venn diagram of Behçet's disease-related manifestations among young adult men in Turkey. Clin Exp Rheumatol. 2005;23(4 Suppl 38):S86–90.
3. Simsek I, et al. Accuracy of recall of the items included in disease activity forms of Behçet's disease: comparison of retrospective questionnaires with a daily telephone interview. Clin Rheumatol. 2008;27(10):1255–60.
4. Alpsoy E, et al. Mucocutaneous lesions of Behçet's disease. Yonsei Med J. 2007;48(4):573.
5. Keogan MT. Clinical immunology review series: an approach to the patient with recurrent orogenital ulceration, including Behçet's syndrome. Clin Exp Immunol. 2009;156(1):1.
6. Hatemi G, et al. The pustular skin lesions in Behçet's syndrome are not sterile. Ann Rheum Dis. 2004;63(11):1450.
7. Ilknur T, et al. Histopathologic and direct immunofluorescence findings of the papulopustular lesions in Behçet's disease. Eur J Dermatol. 2006;16(2):146.
8. Demirkesen C, et al. Clinicopathologic evaluation of nodular cutaneous lesions of Behçet syndrome. Am J Clin Pathol. 2001;116:341.
9. Varol A, et al. The skin pathergy test: innately useful? Arch Dermatol Res. 2010;302(3):155.

Chapter 43
Familial Mediterranean Fever

Murat İnanç and Can Baykal

Definition

Familial Mediterranean fever (FMF) is the most common hereditary recurrent fever syndrome that may cause serositis, synovitis, and/or cutaneous inflammation [1]. Pathogenetically FMF belongs to the group of autoinflammatory diseases, and inflammasome activation has been proposed as the main mechanism [2]. FMF is an autosomal recessive disease with mutations in MEFV gene that encodes pyrin, which usually affects people from Mediterranean origin like Sephardic Jews, Turks, Arabs, and Armenians [1]. The clinical picture of FMF consists of attacks with rapid development of high-grade fever and constitutional symptoms accompanied by acute-phase response (leukocytosis, elevated erythrocyte sedimentation rate, fibrinogen, C reactive protein). Duration of attacks is generally short (6–96 h) with irregular occurrences. The main clinical features during attacks are peritonitis (95 %), arthritis (>50 %) (mono-oligoarticular), pleuritis (40 %), and less frequently pericarditis, scrotal swelling (inflammation of the tunica vaginalis testis), myalgia, and erysipeloid skin rash [3]. The first attack appears before the age of 20 in more than 85 % of the patients. The most important chronic manifestation of FMF is secondary AA amyloidosis which generally presents with proteinuria and may cause chronic renal insufficiency. The prevalence of amyloidosis in FMF was reported 12.9 % in a recent large survey from Turkey [4]. Erysipeloid erythema (ELE) is the typical skin rash of FMF [3]. The reported frequency of ELE is variable

M. İnanç, M.D. (✉)
Department of Internal Medicine, Division of Rheumatology, Istanbul Faculty
of Medicine, Istanbul University, Capa, Topkapi, Istanbul 34390, Turkey
e-mail: drinanc@istanbul.edu.tr

C. Baykal, M.D.
Department of Dermatology, Istanbul University, Istanbul Medical Faculty,
Capa, Topkapi, Istanbul 34390, Turkey
e-mail: baykalc@istanbul.edu.tr

M. Matucci-Cerinic et al. (eds.), *Skin Manifestations in Rheumatic Disease*, 357
DOI 10.1007/978-1-4614-7849-2_43, © Springer Science+Business Media New York 2014

Fig. 43.1 Sharply
demarcated erythematous
patch on the calf (Courtesy
of Orhan Aral, Istanbul
University, Division of
Rheumatology)

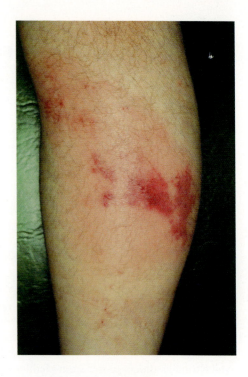

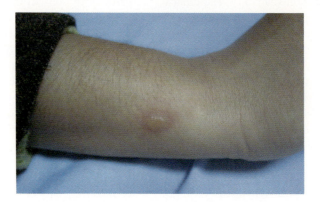

Fig. 43.2 Bullae on an erythematous base on the forearm (Courtesy of Ayşe Akman-Karakas, Akdeniz University, Department of Dermatology)

(3–46 %) and it is prevalent in childhood-onset patients [5]. ELE may be an early sign and sometimes precedes systemic symptoms. The erythematous patches with well-defined borders mostly involve the lower legs (Fig. 43.1), especially the area around the ankle joint, the dorsum of the foot and calf unilaterally, and occasionally bilaterally [6]. The lesions may be warm and tender in the acute stage and frequently disappear within 24–72 h with rest. Bullous lesions (Fig. 43.2), urticaria, and pyoderma have been reported as additional skin manifestations in patients with

FMF [7]. Other diseases with skin manifestations may accompany FMF (or patients with MEVF mutations) like polyarteritis nodosa, Henoch-Schonlein purpura, Behçet's disease, and relapsing polychondritis [8, 9].

Differential Diagnosis

Erythematous patches resembling FMF lesions may be caused by other dermatoses. Erysipelas and cellulitis are common streptococcal infections of skin causing erythematous warm patches and plaques accompanied with fever and chills [6]. In contrast to ELE these lesions do not subside in a few days spontaneously but respond to systemic antibiotic treatment. Sweet's syndrome presents with fever, systemic symptoms, and long-lasting well-demarcated erythematous nodules and plaques with some common histopathological features with ELE. Lesions of Sweet's syndrome are often multiple and elevated, and histopathologically the dermal edema is prominent. These lesions are not confined to lower extremities, and treatment with systemic corticosteroids is preferred [10]. Other hereditary recurrent fever syndromes, for example, HIDS (hyperimmunoglobulinemia D syndrome) and TRAPS, with various skin manifestations are included in the differential diagnosis of FMF [11]. HIDS begins usually under 1 year of age and the presence of high serum level of IgD is diagnostic. Various types of skin manifestations including maculopapular and papular eruptions are seen nearly in all of the patients [1]. Histopathologically a mild vasculitis may be observed. Skin manifestations are common in TRAPS and may be generalized in contrast to FMF. Large erythematous migratory patches and swollen plaques with indistinct borders are accompanied by painful myalgia. The rash shows perivascular infiltration of lymphocytes and monocytes [1, 11].

Biopsy

The histopathological features of ELE and nonspecific skin lesions are not diagnostic for FMF [11]. Histopathological examination of ELE shows slight edema of the superficial dermis, a sparse mixed perivascular infiltration composed of lymphocytes, neutrophils, histiocytes, and nuclear dust. Vasculitis is not seen. Direct immunofluorescence examination of these patches reveals deposits of C3 in the wall of superficial vessels. IgM and fibrinogen can be detected in some patients. The nonspecific bullous lesions show a subepidermal cleavage without any specific immunoglobulin deposition in the direct immunofluorescence examination [6].

See Also

Henoch-Schonlein purpura, neonatal onset autoinflammatory diseases (TRAPS), Behçet's disease.

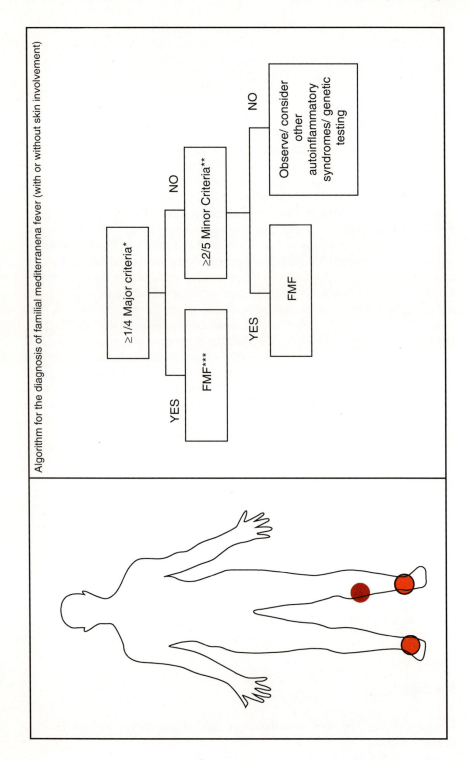

Algorithm for the diagnosis of familial mediterranena fever (with or without skin involvement)

Explanation of Algorithm

*Major Criteria**

1. Peritonitis (generalized)
2. Pleuritis or pericarditis
3. Monoarthritis (hip, knee, ankle)
4. Fever

*Minor Criteria***

1. Incomplete attacks (chest/joint)
2. Exertional leg pain
3. Favorable response to colchicine

*FMF****

Consider that diagnostic criteria set does not include skin involvement because of low sensitivity and specificity [12]. On the other hand, rarely skin manifestations can be the only clinical manifestation in a patient with MEFV mutations [9].

It has been proposed that these criteria is more appropriate for use in patients from Mediterranean origin and in patients with atypical features or different origin, a search for MEVF mutations and other autoinflammatory syndromes is warranted [13].

Family history of FMF considered as a major criterion by other investigators [14].

References

1. Grateu G. Clinical and genetic aspects of the hereditary periodic fever syndromes. Rheumatology. 2004;43:410–5.
2. Kastner D, Aksentijevich I, Goldbach-Mansky R. Autoinflammatory disease reloaded: a clinical perspective. Cell. 2010;140:784–90.
3. Livneh A, Langevitz P. Diagnostic and treatment concerns in familial Mediterranean fever. Baillieres Clin Rheumatol. 2000;14:477–98.
4. Turkish FMF Sudy Group. Familial mediterranean fever in Turkey: results of a nationwide multicenter study. Medicine. 2005;84:1–11.
5. Sayarlıoğlu M, Çefle A, İnanç M, et al. Characteristics of patients with adult onset familial Mediterranean fever in Turkey: analysis of 401 cases. Int J Clin Pract. 2005;59:202–5.
6. Barzilai A, et al. Erysipelas-like erythema of familial Mediterranean fever: clinicopathologic correlation. J Am Acad Dermatol. 2000;42:791–5.

7. Akman A, et al. Recurrent bullous lesions associated with familial Mediterranean fever: a case report. Clin Exp Dermatol. 2008;34:216–8.
8. Salihoğlu A, Seyahi E, Çelik S, Yurdakul S. Relapsing polychondritis in a patient with familial Mediterranean fever and amyloidosis. Clin Exp Rheumatol. 2008;26 Suppl 50:S-125.
9. Ben-Chetrit E, Peleg H, Aamar S, Heyman SN. The spectrum of MEVF clinical presentations – is it familial mediterranean fever only? Rheumatology. 2009;48:1455–9.
10. Cohen PR, Kurzrock R. Sweet's syndrome revisited: a review of disease concepts. Int J Dermatol. 2003;42:761–78.
11. Kanazawa N, Furukawa F. Autoinflammatory syndromes with a dermatological perspective. J Dermatol. 2007;34:601–18.
12. Livneh A, et al. Criteria for the diagnosis of familial Mediterranean fever. Arthritis Rheum. 1997;40:1879–85.
13. Federici L, et al. A decision tree for genetic diagnosis of hereditary periodic fever in unselected patients. Ann Rheum Dis. 2006;65:1427–32.
14. Yalçınkaya F, et al. A new criteria for the diagnosis of familial mediterranean fever in childhood. Rheumatology. 2009;48:395–8.

Chapter 44
Cryopyrin-Associated Periodic Syndromes

Marco Gattorno

Definition

An "urticaria-like eruption" is the hallmark of the three clinical entities grouped under the term of cryopyrin-associated periodic syndromes (CAPS). It consists in a migratory eruption characterized by edematous papules and plaques involving all part of the body (arms, trunk, face) without a particular distribution.

In the most severe form, named CINCA (chronic infantile neurologic cutaneous articular) syndrome or NOMID (neonatal-onset multi-systemic inflammatory disease), the rash usually develops at birth or during the first weeks of life (Fig. 44.1). Wheals of 0.2–3 cm in size with associated redness appear daily with migration into different parts of the body throughout the day (Fig. 44.2) [1]. Confluence of the skin manifestations can be observed. Other associated clinical features are (i) a typical "facies" characterized by frontal bossing, saddle back nose, and midface hypoplasia, causing a sibling-like resemblance; (ii) bone involvement characterized by bony overgrowth that predominantly involve the knees (including the patella) and the distal extremities of hands and feet; (iii) chronic inflammatory polyarthritis; and (iv) central nervous system manifestations, such as chronic aseptic meningitis, increased intracranial pressure, cerebral atrophy, ventriculomegaly, sensorineural hearing loss, and chronic papilledema, with associated optic-nerve atrophy and loss of vision [2].

In the Muckle-Wells syndrome, the cutaneous rash may be present at birth, but a late onset is also described, even in the second or third decade of life. The skin manifestations may appear daily but also once or twice weekly or even less frequently. The rash is usually non-pruritic, even if some patients may define it as itchy. Conjunctivitis (Fig. 44.3), limb pain and acute arthritis (Fig. 44.4), and

M. Gattorno, M.D. (✉)
Genoa and Department of Pediatrics, UO Pediatria, Istituto G. Gaslini, University of Genoa,
UO Pediatria II, Largo G. Gaslini 5, 16147 Genoa, Italy
e-mail: marcogattorno@ospedale-gaslini.ge.it

M. Matucci-Cerinic et al. (eds.), *Skin Manifestations in Rheumatic Disease*,
DOI 10.1007/978-1-4614-7849-2_44, © Springer Science+Business Media New York 2014

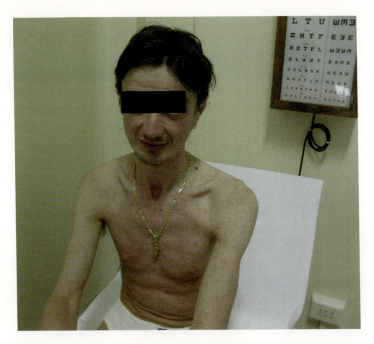

Fig. 44.1 Urticarial rash at trunk and face in a 32-year-old man with NOMID

Fig. 44.2 Early phase of skin
eruption in a 43-year-old
woman with Muckle-Wells
syndrome with E255K
mutation

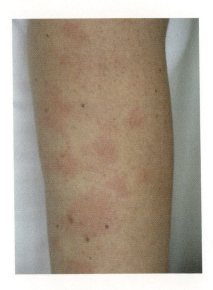

late-onset hearing loss are other associated features. Renal amyloidosis is the classical long-term complication [3].

In familial cold urticarial autoinflammatory (FCAS) syndrome, the skin rash is typically associated to the exposure of the whole body to cold [4]. Typically, also the parts not directly exposed to the cold present the skin rash after a mean of

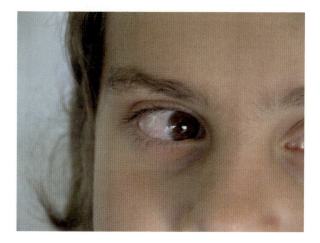

Fig. 44.3 Conjunctivitis in an 8-year-old girl with Muckle-Wells syndrome

Fig. 44.4 Swollen joint associated to urticarial rash in a 12-year-old girl with NOMID

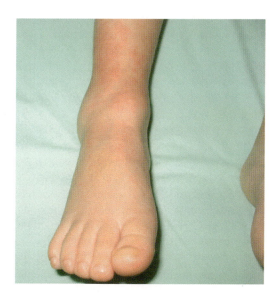

2 h after cold exposure for a duration of approximately 12 h. Fever, limb pain, conjunctivitis, and elevation of acute phase reactants are usually associated with skin eruption.

FCAS, Muckle-Wells syndrome, and chronic CINCA represent the clinical spectrum of a syndrome associated with mutations of *NLRP3* gene, coding for cryopyrin [5], and gathered under the term of cryopyrin-associated periodic syndromes (CAPS). Cryopyrin is a member of NOD-like receptor protein family. In the presence of a number of stimuli, cryopyrin oligomerizes and binds the adaptor protein ASC. This association activates directly two molecules of Caspase-1 which, in turn converts pro-IL-1β to the mature, active 17 kDa form. Mutations in the cryopyrin gene in humans are associated with its gain of function that lead to an excessive and faster production of IL-1β. Treatment with IL-1 blockers dramatically controls disease activity.

Differential Diagnosis

Other autoinflammatory diseases are characterized by a wide range of skin manifestations. An urticarial rash can be present during fever attacks observed in **hyper IgD syndrome** (or mevalonate kinase deficiency) or **TNF receptor-associated periodic syndrome** (TRAPS). As for FCAS, in these two diseases, the skin rash is observed only during the fever attacks, but is not induced by cold exposure. Moreover, while urticarial rash represents a constant manifestation in CAPS, its appearance in other autoinflammatory diseases is much more sporadic [6].

Mutations of **NLRP12** gene are associated to a clinical phenotype similar to FCAS, with episodes of urticarial rash and arthralgia after cold exposure [7].

In **Schnitzler syndrome** an urticarial rash is combined with a monoclonal IgM gammopathy. The first symptoms usually start at the age of 50, and it seems to be an acquired disorder. Apart from intermittent attacks of fever, the clinical manifestations are bone and muscle pain, arthralgia or arthritis, and lymphadenopathy [8]. A lymphoproliferative disease cannot be detected. The pathogenesis and the part played by IgM are unknown.

Due to the presence of a skin rash, fever, arthritis, and persistent elevation of acute phase reactants, **systemic-onset juvenile idiopathic arthritis** and **adult Still's disease** may enter into differential diagnosis with CAPS. The skin rash of these two latter conditions is characterized by a salmon-like evanescent eruption to the arms and trunk that characteristically coincides with fever peaks [8].

Chronic urticaria represents an important differential diagnosis for CAPS. Chronic urticaria has no obvious cause, although some factors (e.g., drugs, infections, emotional stress, and food) can serve as eliciting stimuli. An autoimmune origin caused by the presence of autoantibodies to FceRIa or to IgE itself can be identified in some patients. The primary lesion is a wheal characterized by a transient edema of the papillary dermis and which appears as a circumscribed cutaneous elevation with elastic consistency, pink or pale in color, and a variable erythematous surrounding flare. Usually the distribution on the body surface is usually random and asymmetric. Individual wheals last no longer than 24–36 h, and the lesions disappear without leaving skin marks. Wheals are typically pruritic or, in rare instances, are associated with a burning sensation. In about 40 % of patients, urticaria is associated with angioedema, which is determined by transient swelling of the reticular dermis and/or subcutaneous tissue. No other symptoms (e.g., fever, arthralgia, or muscular pain) are present.

At histologic examination, some dermal edema and mild dilatation of dermal blood vessels, without signs of wall damage or leukocytoclasia are seen. A sparse

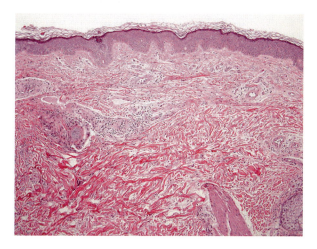

Fig. 44.5 Skin biopsy of an urticarial lesion in a CAPS patient shows a mild perivascular inflammatory infiltrate in the superficial dermis. The epidermal changes are minimal (H&E, 100x) (Courtesy of Dr. R. Goldbach-Mansky and Dr. C. Richard Lee)

perivascular infiltrate is composed of macrophages, lymphocytes, eosinophils, and neutrophils [9].

Urticarial vasculitis is a discrete disease entity, distinct from urticaria, in which the urticarial lesions persist for more than 24 h and heal leaving brownish residues. Because leukocytoclastic vasculitis involves leakage of erythrocytes from blood vessels, hyperpigmentation remains after resolution of the urticarial lesion. In contrast, the exanthema seen in acute or chronic urticaria resolves completely within 24 h. If the vasculitis also involves deeper vessels, angioedema may be found. Urticarial vasculitis can be also observed in the context of **systemic lupus erythematosus**.

The hallmark of UV diagnosis is demonstration of leukocytoclastic vasculitis in dermal biopsy samples (Fig. 44.5). This involves a leukocytoclastic reaction, vessel wall destruction, and deposits of fibrinogen. Immune complexes and complement should be visible in the blood vessels on immunohistochemical analysis [10].

Hypocomplementemic urticarial vasculitis syndrome (HUVS) is a severe systemic form of urticarial vasculitis. All HUVS patients exhibit extremely low levels of C1q. Through activation of the classical complement pathway, complement factors C3 and C4 are also nearly always markedly reduced. A C1q antibody can regularly be detected but is not specific for HUVS [10].

HUVS is a specific autoimmune disease with involvement of the skin, joints, kidneys, and gastrointestinal tract manifested by vasculitis and polyserositis. Arthralgia and arthritis of various joints are the most frequent systemic manifestations of HUVS. Renal involvement is often only mild, but dialysis may be required. The frequently found proteinuria and hematuria is seen histologically as membranous, membranoproliferative, or intra- and extracapillary glomerulonephritis. Lung involvement goes along with shortness of breath, coughing, hemoptysis, pleural effusion, and chronic obstructive pulmonary disease (COPD) and is the most frequent cause of death among HUVS patients.

Cogan syndrome preferentially affects young adults in the third decade of life. Following a reovirus III infection, antibodies to the virus core protein can cross-react with the inner ear and eye. The clinical presentation is characterized by fainting attacks, hearing loss, and interstitial keratitis with reddened, painful eyes and visual impairment [11].

Several other conditions that may present with urticaria-like skin lesions have been recently reviewed [11]. Among them are urticarial dermatitis, contact dermatitis (irritant or allergic), arthropod bite reactions, exanthematous drug eruption, mastocytosis (children), and autoimmune bullous diseases (subepidermal – bullous pemphigoid, gestational pemphigoid, linear IgA dermatosis, epidermolysis bullosa acquisita, and dermatitis herpetiformis of Duhring).

Biopsy

Histologic examination of the papules and plaques shows a normal epidermidis but a superficial and deep perivascular infiltrate predominantly composed by neutrophils, few lymphocytes and occasional eosinophils. Unlike classical urticaria, mast cells are absent. Neutrophilic eccrine hidradenitis has been also reported (Fig. 44.6) [12].

In FCAS patients, 15 min after cold exposure, a moderate dermal edema with dilatation of lymphatics and small vessels can be observed. Neutrophils and few

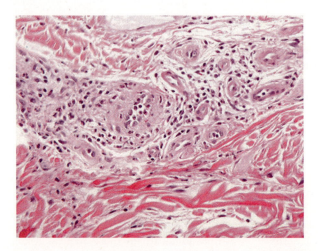

Fig. 44.6 Perivascular inflammatory infiltrate composed of predominantly neutrophils. There is no histologic evidence of vasculitis (H&E, 400x) (Courtesy of Dr. R. Goldbach-Mansky and Dr. C. Richard Lee)

eosinophils are present in the upper dermis. After 1 h a more marked neutrophilic infiltration, with some sparse mononuclear cells and eosinophils is detected in the upper and mid-dermis. Fibrinoid deposits may be observed around some blood vessels. After 3 h the number of neutrophils had decreased in the upper dermis with a more pronounced involvement in the lower dermis [13].

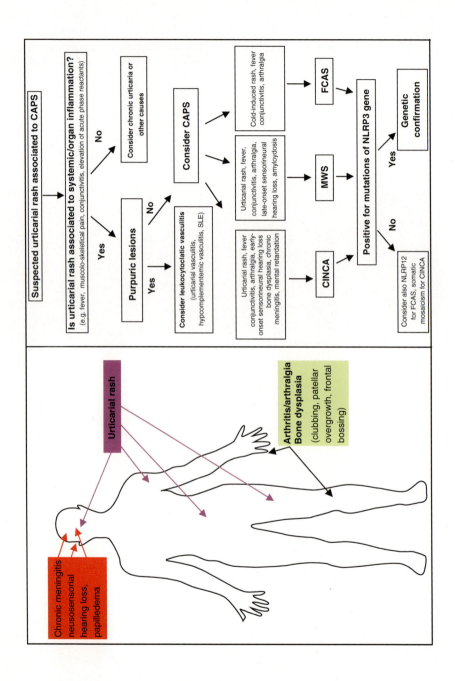

References

1. Neven B, et al. Molecular basis of the spectral expression of CIAS1 mutations associated with phagocytic cell-mediated autoinflammatory disorders CINCA/NOMID, MWS, and FCU. Blood. 2004;103:2809.
2. Prieur AM, et al. A chronic, infantile, neurological, cutaneous and articular (CINCA) syndrome. A specific entity analysed in 30 patients. Scand J Rheumatol. 1987;Suppl 66:57.
3. Muckle TJ, et al. Urticaria, deafness, and amyloidosis: a new heredo-familial syndrome. Q J Med. 1962;31:235.
4. Kile RL, et al. A case of cold urticaria with an unusual family history. JAMA. 1940;114:1067.
5. Hoffman HM, et al. Mutation of a new gene encoding a putative pyrin-like protein causes familial cold autoinflammatory syndrome and Muckle-Wells syndrome. Nat Genet. 2001;29:301.
6. Gattorno M, et al. Diagnosis and management of autoinflammatory diseases in childhood. J Clin Immunol. 2008;28:S73.
7. Borghini S, et al. Clinical presentation and pathogenesis of cold-induced autoinflammatory disease in a family with recurrence of an NLRP12 mutation. Arthritis Rheum. 2011;63:830–9.
8. Krause K, et al. How not to miss autoinflammatory diseases masquerading as urticaria. Allergy. 2012;67:1465–74.
9. Greaves MW, et al. Chronic urticaria: recent advances. Clin Rev Allergy Immunol. 2007;33:134.
10. Marzano AV, et al. Skin involvement in cutaneous and systemic vasculitis. Autoimmune Rev. 2013;12:467.
11. Peroni A, et al. Urticarial lesions: if not urticaria, what else? The differential diagnosis of urticaria: part I. Cutaneous diseases. J Am Acad Dermatol. 2010;62:541.
12. Shinkai K, et al. Cryopyrin-associated periodic syndromes and autoinflammation. Clin Exp Dermatol. 2008;33:1.
13. Haas N, et al. Muckle-Wells syndrome: clinical and histological skin findings compatible with cold air urticaria in a large kindred. Br J Dermatol. 2004;151:99.

Part VI
Other Rheumatic Conditions

Chapter 45
Sarcoidosis

**Diletta Bonciani, Federico Perfetto, Costanza Marchiani,
and Alberto Moggi Pignone**

Definition

Sarcoidosis is a multisystemic disorder of unknown origin characterized by the accumulation of lymphocytes and mononuclear phagocytes that induce the formation of noncaseating epithelioid granulomas with secondary derangement of normal tissue or organ anatomy and function. It occurs throughout the world, at any age, in person of either gender, and in all races. The incidence peaks between the second and third decades, with a second upsurge occurring in women between the fourth and sixth decades.

Virtually any organ can be affected; however, granulomas most often appear in the lungs or the lymph nodes. The disease also often affects the eyes and the liver. Although less common, sarcoidosis can affect the heart and brain. Symptoms usually appear gradually but can occasionally appear suddenly. The clinical course generally varies and ranges from asymptomatic disease to a debilitating chronic condition that may lead to death [1].

Cutaneous disease occurs in up to 20 % of cases; lesions often appear at the onset of systemic illness, providing a valuable opportunity for early diagnosis. The cutaneous manifestations are variable, sometimes being very obvious and at other time perplexing. They mimic a wide array of dermatological conditions posing a diagnostic challenge to dermatologists worldwide.

D. Bonciani, M.D.
Area Critica Medico-Chirurgica, Dermatologia, Casa Di Cura Santa Chiara, Florence, Italy

F. Perfetto, M.D. • C. Marchiani, M.D.
Department of Internal Medicine, Azienda Ospedaliera Universitaria Careggi, Florence, Italy

A.M. Pignone, M.D., Ph.D. (⊠)
Department of Internal Medicine, University of Florence, Largo Brambilla No. 3,
50134 Florence, Italy
e-mail: alberto.moggipignone@unifi.it

M. Matucci-Cerinic et al. (eds.), *Skin Manifestations in Rheumatic Disease*,
DOI 10.1007/978-1-4614-7849-2_45, © Springer Science+Business Media New York 2014

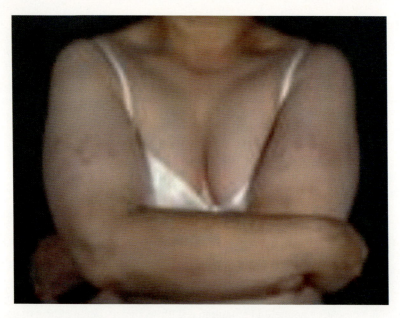

Fig. 45.1 Specific lesions of sarcoidosis: Erythematous maculopapules, in a patient with cutaneous sarcoidosis, involving in a symmetrical way the upper extremities

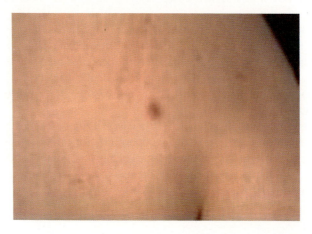

Fig. 45.2 The same patient of Fig. 45.1. Erythematous-isolated nodule on the back, this is the first lesion appeared

Based on the histological findings, skin lesions of sarcoidosis have been classified as "specific" (when a typical granulomatous infiltrate is present in the sample tissue) and "nonspecific" (not contain granulomas and represent a reactive process).

Specific lesions include lupus pernio, maculopapular eruptions, subcutaneous nodules, infiltrative scars, and plaques. Of these, maculopapular and nodular eruptions are the most common (Figs. 45.1 and 45.2). Nonspecific manifestations, except for erythema nodosum, are uncommon, such us calcifications, erythema multiforme, prurigo, nail clubbing, and Sweet syndrome (an acute febrile neutrophilic dermatosis).

If the diagnosis of sarcoidosis is strongly suspected on clinical and pathological grounds, then further investigation should be tailored to identify systemic disease and establish a baseline of disease activity. Mandatory baseline investigations should include chest X-ray, pulmonary function tests (including measurement of transfer factor), electrocardiogram, full blood count, biochemistry, serum immunoglobulins, and a 24-h urinary calcium assay. Measurement of serum angiotensin-converting enzyme (ACE), which is produced by sarcoidal granulomas, may be helpful in monitoring disease activity. It is not a particularly useful diagnostic test as levels may be raised in other conditions such as diabetes and alcoholic liver disease.

Differential Diagnosis

There is a large group of skin diseases that can enter in the differential diagnosis with cutaneous sarcoidosis manifestations, either clinically or/and pathologically. In fact cutaneous sarcoidosis is known as the "great imitator" because of its widely variable morphologies. A high index of clinical suspicion is needed to consider sarcoidosis.

Papules and maculopapules, the most common types of specific lesion, may resemble xanthelasma, acne, rosacea, syphilis, polymorphous light eruption, lupus erythematosus, adenoma sebaceum, lichen planus, syringoma, and granuloma annulare. Micropapular sarcoidosis is an unusual variant; it should be included in the differential diagnosis of lichen nitidus and lichen scrofulosorum.

Sarcoidal plaques (angiolupoid and annular plaques) may mimic lupus vulgaris, necrobiosis lipoidica, morphea, leprosy, leishmaniasis, lichen planus, nummular eczema, cutaneous T-cell lymphoma, B-cell lymphoma, Kaposi sarcoma, secondary syphilis, and gyrate erythema. Moreover, sarcoidosis may manifest as psoriasiform plaques.

Subcutaneous nodules are an unusual manifestation that should be clinically distinguished from tuberculosis, deep mycosis, cutaneous metastases of visceral neoplasm and melanoma, epidermoid cysts, lipomas, rheumatoid nodules, and erythema induratum.

Lupus pernio is the most characteristic skin lesion of sarcoidosis; the differential diagnosis includes lupus erythematosus, benign or malignant lymphocytic infiltrate, and rhinophyma.

In the differential diagnosis of scar sarcoidosis, keloid should be considered.

Scalp sarcoidosis is a rare manifestation, but insidious progressive alopecia caused by sarcoidosis should also be differentiated from lupus erythematosus, lichen planopilaris, pseudopelade, and alopecia neoplastica.

The clinical differential diagnosis of hypopigmented lesions includes postinflammatory hypopigmentation, pityriasis alba, pityriasis lichenoides chronica, mycosis fungoides, pityriasis versicolor, leprosy, vitiligo, idiopathic guttate hypomelanosis, and chemical-induced hypopigmentation.

Nail involvement is rare, and usually it is a marker of chronic disease, the differential diagnosis including fungal infection, psoriasis, lichen planus, trauma, drug eruption, and subungual warts [2].

Histology

Punch or incisional wedge biopsy is typically used to obtain a sample of skin that includes the dermis. If noncaseating granulomas are found, tissue culture may be necessary to exclude infectious causes.

The characteristic histological features of sarcoidosis are noncaseating epithelioid granulomas, with minimal or absent associated lymphocytes or plasma cells (naked granuloma), and within the giant cells, Schaumann bodies and asteroid bodies may be found but are not specific for sarcoidosis. Schaumann bodies are rounded, laminated basophilic inclusions that represent degenerating lysosomes, whereas asteroid bodies represent engulfed collagen seen as eosinophilic stellate inclusions (Figs. 45.3 and 45.4).

See Also

Identify in the book where the lesion or the disease is also mentioned and described

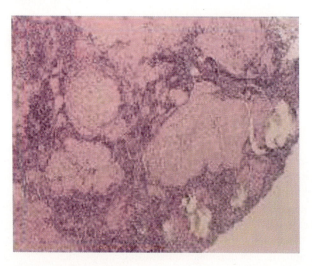

Fig. 45.3 The dermis is replaced by uniform circumscribed nests of noncaseating granuloma

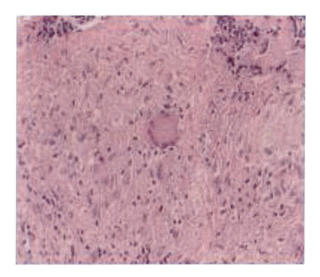

Fig. 45.4 The dermis is replaced by uniform circumscribed nests of noncaseating granuloma

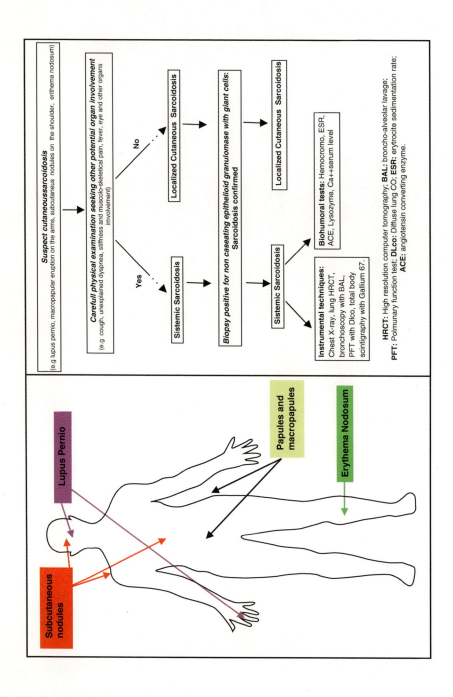

References

1. Ali MM, Atwan AA, Gonzalez ML. Cutaneous sarcoidosis: updates in the pathogenesis. J Eur Acad Dermatol Venereol. 2010;24(7):747–55.
2. Fernandez-Faith E, McDonnell J. Cutaneous sarcoidosis: differential diagnosis. Clin Dermatol. 2007;25:276–87.

Chapter 46
Amyloidoses

Federico Perfetto, Costanza Marchiani, and Alberto Moggi Pignone

Definition and Description

The amyloidoses are a group of diseases characterised by extracellular proteinaceous tissue deposit, which shows green polarisation birefringence after Congo red staining. Deposition of amyloid can be localised (restricted to one organ of the body) or systemic. Three types of systemic amyloidoses are important for the clinician: AL (related to a monoclonal light chain production), AA (associated with chronic inflammation) and heredo-familial amyloidosis (due to underlying hereditary mutations of several proteins) [1]. Cutaneous amyloidosis could be restricted to the skin (i.e. cutaneous localised amyloidosis) or can be one of the systemic manifestations of the disease. In AL amyloidosis, skin involvement is characterised by petechiae and ecchymoses occurring spontaneously or after a minor trauma in eyelids and flexural regions. Bilateral periorbital lesions and macroglossia are the presenting manifestations of the disease in 15 % of cases and provide a clue to early diagnosis (Figs. 46.1 and 46.2). Papules, nodules or non-pruritic waxy plaques in retroauricular, umbilical, inguinal and anogenital regions are also possible during the course of the disease. Acral cutaneous infiltrative lesion with scleroderma-like findings is also reported [2]. There are three types of cutaneous localised amyloidoses (CLA): lichen, macular and nodular amyloidosis. Lichen amyloidosis is the most frequent type of CLA characterised by multiple pruritic brownish or red-lichenoid papules distributed on the shins, thighs, feet and legs. Macular amyloidosis presents as brownish patches with reticular or rippled pattern usually distributed symmetrically over the upper back, the forearms and legs. Nodular amyloidosis is the rarest form.

F. Perfetto, M.D. • C. Marchiani, M.D.
Department of Internal Medicine, Azienda Ospedaliera Universitaria Careggi, Florence, Italy

A.M. Pignone, M.D., Ph.D. (✉)
Department of Internal Medicine, University of Florence, Largo Brambilla No. 3,
50134 Florence, Italy
e-mail: alberto.moggipignone@unifi.it

M. Matucci-Cerinic et al. (eds.), *Skin Manifestations in Rheumatic Disease*,
DOI 10.1007/978-1-4614-7849-2_46, © Springer Science+Business Media New York 2014

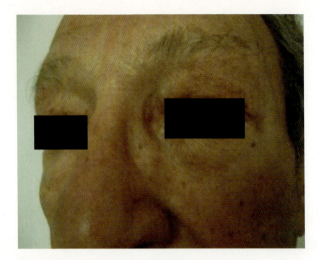

Fig. 46.1 Macroglossia in a patient with AL amyloidosis. The tongue is firm to palpation. Note the non-reducible impression in the tongue caused by the teeth

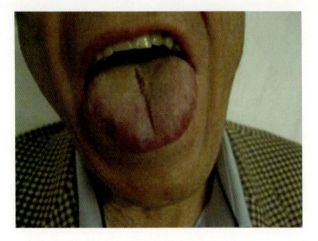

Fig. 46.2 The same patient of Fig. 46.1. Periorbital purpura. Frequently the purpura is bilateral, and the patient gives no history of trauma to the area of ecchymoses

Nodules may occur on the trunk, limbs, extremities and genitals and may be a few millimetres to several centimetres in size and are brownish or red in colour. There is little or no itching.

Differential Diagnosis

Petechiae and ecchymoses in systemic amyloidosis may resemble many causes of purpura or coagulopathy. Lesions around eyes may resemble simple bruising. Amyloidosis waxy plaques of eyelids may resemble syringomas in its early stages;

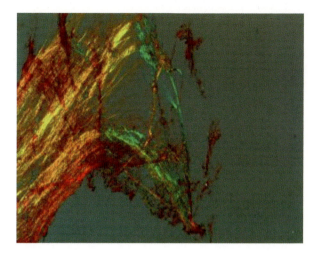

Fig. 46.3 Subcutaneous fat aspirate stained with Congo red and viewed under polarised light amyloid shows apple-green birefringence

the differential, later, might include histiocytoses, mucinoses, xanthomatoses, necrobiotic xanthogranuloma and cutaneous metastases. Lichen amyloidosis requires differential diagnoses with lichen simplex chronicus and hypertrophic lichen planus. Lichen amyloidosis could be misdiagnosed almost be confused with prurigo nodularis, papular mucinosis, pemphigoid nodularis, epidermolysis bullosa pruriginosa and underlying scleroderma. The differential diagnosis for macular amyloidosis includes lichenification, the so-called atopic dirty neck and notalgia paresthetica. The so-called atopic dirty neck shares with amyloidosis the same rippled pigmented appearance. Differential diagnoses to consider with nodular amyloidosis include cutaneous sarcoidosis, lupus vulgaris and granuloma annulare and primary skin tumours such as basal cell carcinoma, xanthomas, granuloma faciale and skin lymphoma.

Biopsy

The diagnosis of amyloidosis requires the histological demonstration of amyloid deposits. This is a positive Congo red-stained tissue specimen with the characteristic apple-green birefringence in polarised light. In systemic amyloidosis, abdominal subcutaneous fat aspiration (Fig. 46.3) or biopsy of minor salivary glands is convenient and a non-invasive method that demonstrates amyloid deposits in 70–85 % of patients (Figs. 46.4 and 46.5). The diagnosis of cutaneous localised amyloidosis is based on the presence of amyloid fibrils in skin biopsy. In macular and lichenoid forms, the amyloid deposits are confined to the papillary dermis. Immunohistochemistry stains are negative for cytokeratin, and electron microscopy shows characteristic fibrillar and linear amyloid. In nodular cutaneous amyloidosis,

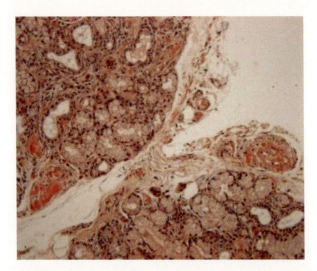

Fig. 46.4 The biopsied specimen of the minor (labial) salivary gland shows amyloid deposits (*arrows*) mainly in the interstitium (Congo red staining)

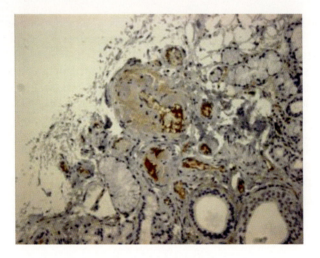

Fig. 46.5 The same biopsy of Fig. 46.2. On immunohistochemistry these amyloid deposits (*arrows*) are positively stained with anti-λ light chain antibody

the amyloid deposits are located in the papillary, subpapillary and reticular dermis, with infiltration of the blood vessel wall. Immunohistochemistry stains are negative for cytokeratin and positive for kappa and/or lambda immunoglobulin light chains.

See Also

Identify in the book where the lesion or the disease is also mentioned and described.

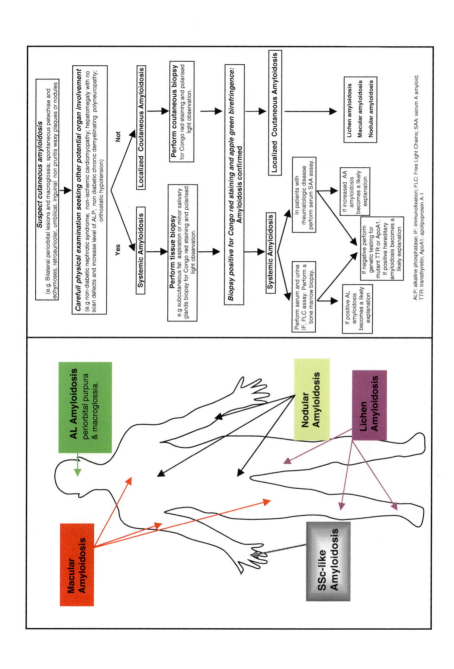

Suspect cutaneous amyloidosis
(e.g. Bilateral periorbital lesions and macroglossia; spontaneous petechiae and ecchymoses; retroauricolar, umbilical, inguinal non pruritis waxy plaques or nodules)

Carefull physical examination seeking other potential organ involvement
(e.g non-diabetic nephrotic syndrome; non-ischemic cardiomyopathy; hepatomegaly with no scan defects and increase level of ALP; non diabetic chronic demyelinating polyneuropathy; orthostatic hypotension)

Yes → Systemic Amyloidosis

Not → Localized Coutaneous Amyloidosis

Perform tissue biopsy
e.g subcutaneous fat aspiration or minor salivary glands biopsy for Congo red staining and polarised light observation.

Perform coutaneous biopsy
for Congo red staining and polarised light observation.

Biopsy positive for Congo red staining and apple green birefringence:
Amyloidosis confirmed

Systemic Amyloidosis

Localized Coutaneous Amyloidosis

Lichen amyloidosis
Macular amyloidosis
Nodular amyloidosis

Perform serum and urine IF, FLC assay. Perform a bone marrow biopsy.

In patients with rheumatologic disease perform serum SAA assay.

If positive AL amyloidosis becomes a likely explanation

If negative perform genetic testing for mutant TTR or ApoA1. If positive hereditary amyloidosis becomes a likely explanation.

If increased AA amyloidosis becomes a likely explanation

ALP: alkaline phosphatase; IF: immunofixation; FLC: Free Light Chains; SAA: serum A amyloid; TTR: transthyretin; ApoA1: apolipoprotein A-1

AL Amyloidosis
periorbital purpura & macroglossia.

Nodular Amyloidosis

Lichen Amyloidosis

Macular Amyloidosis

SSc-like Amyloidosis

References

1. Obici L, Perfetti V, Palladini G, Moratti R, Merlini G. Clinical aspects of systemic amyloid diseases. Biochim Biophys Acta. 2005;1753:11–22.
2. Steciuk A, Dompmartin A, Troussard X, Verneuil L, Macro M, Comoz F, Leroy D. Cutaneous amyloidosis and possible association with systemic amyloidosis. Int J Dermatol. 2002;41:127–32.

Chapter 47
Hypertrophic Osteoarthropathy

Manuel Martínez-Lavín

Definition

Hypertrophic osteoarthropathy (HOA) is a syndrome characterized by abnormal proliferation of the skin and osseous tissues at the distal parts of the extremities. Three clinical features are typically present: a peculiar bulbous deformity of the tips of the digits conventionally described as "clubbing" (Fig. 47.1), periostosis of the tubular bones (Fig. 47.2), and synovial effusions [1].

HOA may be secondary to a severe internal illness such as cyanotic heart disease, lung cancer, chronic liver failure, or Graves' disease, among many others. HOA can also be present as idiopathic or "primary" form that is also known as pachydermoperiostosis [2].

Physical examination is of foremost importance in diagnosis, because the bulbous deformity of the fingertips is unique (Fig. 47.1). Effusions into the large joints are frequently observed and are more easily detected in the knees and wrists.

Primary HOA is characterized by a clear-cut hereditary predisposition, with 33 % of cases having a close relative with the same illness. The male–female ratio is 9:1. Primary cases are prone to display a more disseminated skin hypertrophy, hence the term "pachydermoperiostosis." This overgrowth roughens the facial features, and it can reach the extreme of cutis verticis gyrata, the most advanced stage of cutaneous hypertrophy. In such cases, the scalp takes on a cerebroid appearance. Another cutaneous alteration more frequently seen in idiopathic cases is glandular dysfunction manifested as hyperhidrosis, seborrhea, or acne [3].

Plain radiographs of the extremities may detect abnormalities in an asymptomatic patient; long-standing clubbing is characterized by a bone remodeling process

M. Martínez-Lavín, M.D. (✉)
Rheumatology Department, National Institute of Cardiology, Juan Badiano 1,
14080 Mexico City, Mexico
e-mail: drmartinezlavin@gmail.com

M. Matucci-Cerinic et al. (eds.), *Skin Manifestations in Rheumatic Disease*,
DOI 10.1007/978-1-4614-7849-2_47, © Springer Science+Business Media New York 2014

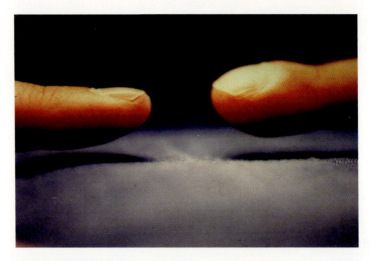

Fig. 47.1 Digital clubbing: the bulbous deformity of the finger on the *right* is compared to the normal finger shape on the *left*

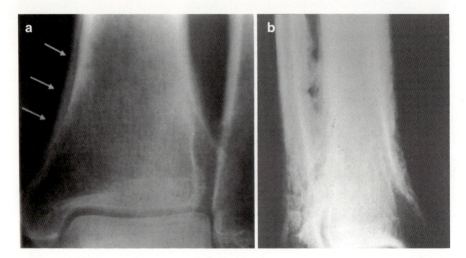

Fig. 47.2 (**a**) Early hypertrophic osteoarthropathy. Anterior-posterior view of the ankle, showing monolayer periosteal apposition on the tibial cortex (*arrows*). (**b**) Advanced periostosis. Anterior-posterior view of the ankle. Chunky irregular periosteal proliferation that generates bone thickening

that usually takes the form of acroosteolysis or more rarely tuftal overgrowth. Periosteal apposition has a symmetric distribution and evolves in a centripetal fashion (Fig. 47.2) [4].

Differential Diagnosis

Drumstick fingers are so unique that its recognition usually poses no dilemma. Diagnostic criteria for HOA are the combined presence of clubbing and radiographic evidence of periostosis of the tubular bones. Synovial effusion is not essential for the diagnosis. Nevertheless, it should be emphasized that in some patients – particularly those with malignant lung tumors – painful arthropathy may be the presenting manifestation of the syndrome in advance of clubbing. Such cases could be misdiagnosed as suffering from an inflammatory type of arthritis. Here, important clinical features in the differential diagnosis are the location of pain – in HOA not only the joint is involved but also the adjacent bone – plus the fact that rheumatoid factor is usually absent and synovial fluid is "noninflammatory" in nature.

Some patients with HOA have an exuberant skin hypertrophy that may resemble acromegaly. The presence of clubbing and periostosis plus the absence of prognathism, enlarged sella turcica, or abnormal circulating concentrations of growth hormone should lead to the correct diagnosis. A patient should be classified as having the primary form of the syndrome only after a careful scrutiny fails to reveal an underlying illness [5].

Biopsy

The bulbous deformity of the digits is secondary to excessive laying down of collagen fibers and interstitial edema. There is also vascular hyperplasia and thickening of the vessels walls, with a perivascular infiltrate of lymphocytes.

Electron microscopic studies have confirmed the structural vessel damage demonstrated by the presence of Weibel-Palade bodies and the prominence of Golgi complexes [6]. Similar changes have been observed in the bones. At this level, excessive connective tissue elevates the periosteum and new osteoid matrix is deposited beneath.

Histologic studies of the joints have found minimal synovial cell proliferation but a prominent artery wall thickening, with intravascular deposition of electron dense material

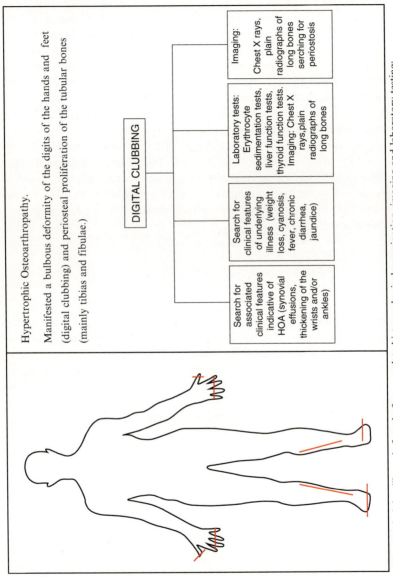

Hypertrophic Osteoarthropathy.

Manifested a bulbous deformity of the digits of the hands and feet (digital clubbing) and periosteal proliferation of the tubular bones (mainly tibias and fibulae.)

DIGITAL CLUBBING

Search for associated clinical features indicative of HOA (synovial effusions, thickening of the wrists and/or ankles)

Search for clinical features of underlying illness (weight loss, cyanosis, fever, chronic diarrhea, jaundice)

Laboratory tests: Erythrocyte sedimentation tests, liver function tests, thyroid function tests. Imaging: Chest X rays, plain radiographs of long bones

Imaging: Chest X rays, plain radiographs of long bones serching for periostosis

If no underlying illness is found after complete history physical examination, imaging and laboratory testing; Primary HOA is a likely diagnosis

References

1. Martinez-Lavin M, Matucci-Cerinic M, Jajic I, Pineda C. Hypertrophic osteoarthropathy: consensus on its definition, classification, assessment and diagnostic criteria. J Rheumatol. 1993;20:1386–7.
2. Martinez-Lavin M. Exploring the cause of the most ancient clinical sign of medicine: finger clubbing. Semin Arthritis Rheum. 2007;36:380–5.
3. Martínez-Lavín M, Pineda C, Valdez T, et al. Primary hypertrophic osteoarthropathy. Semin Arthritis Rheum. 1988;17:156–62.
4. Pineda C, Fonseca C, Martínez-Lavín M. The spectrum of soft tissue and skeletal abnormalities of hypertrophic osteoarthropathy. J Rheumatol. 1990;17:626–32.
5. Martinez-Lavin M, Pineda C. Hypertrophic osteoarthropathy. In: Hochberg MC, Silman AJ, Smolen JS, Weinblatt ME, Weisman MH, editors. Rheumatology. 5th ed. Philadelphia: Elsevier; 2011. p. 1701–5.
6. Matucci-Cerinic M, Lotti T, Calvieri S, Ghersetich I, Sacerdoti L, Teofoli P, Jajic I, Cagnoni M. The spectrum of dermatological symptoms of pachydermoperiostosis (primary hypertrophic osteoarthropathy): a genetic, cytogenetic and ultrastructural study. Clin Exp Rheumatol. 1992;10 Suppl 7:45–8.

Index